# CHOLELITHIASIS
## Causes and Treatment

**Fumio Nakayama, M.D.**
Professor Emeritus
Kyushu University Faculty of Medicine
Department of Surgery I
Fukuoka, Japan

IGAKU-SHOIN, LTD. TOKYO NEW YORK

Published and distributed by

IGAKU-SHOIN Ltd.
5-24-3 Hongo, Bunkyo-ku, Tokyo

IGAKU-SHOIN Medical Publishers, Inc.
One Madison Avenue, New York, N.Y. 10010

**Library of Congress Cataloging-in-Publication Data**

Nakayama, Fumio, 1928–
Cholelithiasis: causes and treatment / Fumio Nakayama.
p. cm.
Includes bibliographical references and index.
ISBN 4-260-14334-4. —ISBN 0-89640-334-3
1. Gallstones. I. Title.
[DNLM: 1. Cholelithiasis. WI 76 N163c 1997]
RC850.N35 1997
616.3′65—dc20
DNLM / DLC 96-42979
for Library of Congress CIP

ISBN 4-260-14334-4 (Tokyo)
ISBN 0-89640-334-3 (New York)



Printed and bound in Japan

Dedicated to

The late Professor Hiroshi Miyake, my lifelong mentor

The late Professor Charles G. Johnston
with whom I ventured into the unknown sea
of oral cholelitholysis

The late Professor Haruo Saikachi
who introduced me to the field of chemistry

Last, if not least, my wife Hanna
who never failed to support me
during all these years of gallstone research
culminating in the publication of this book

"The road we plodded together was indeed long and stretched far beyond."

Translated from the inscription written by his own hand in his great classic Cholelithiasis (Miyake Jr, 1970), given to the author by the late Professor Hiroshi Miyake.

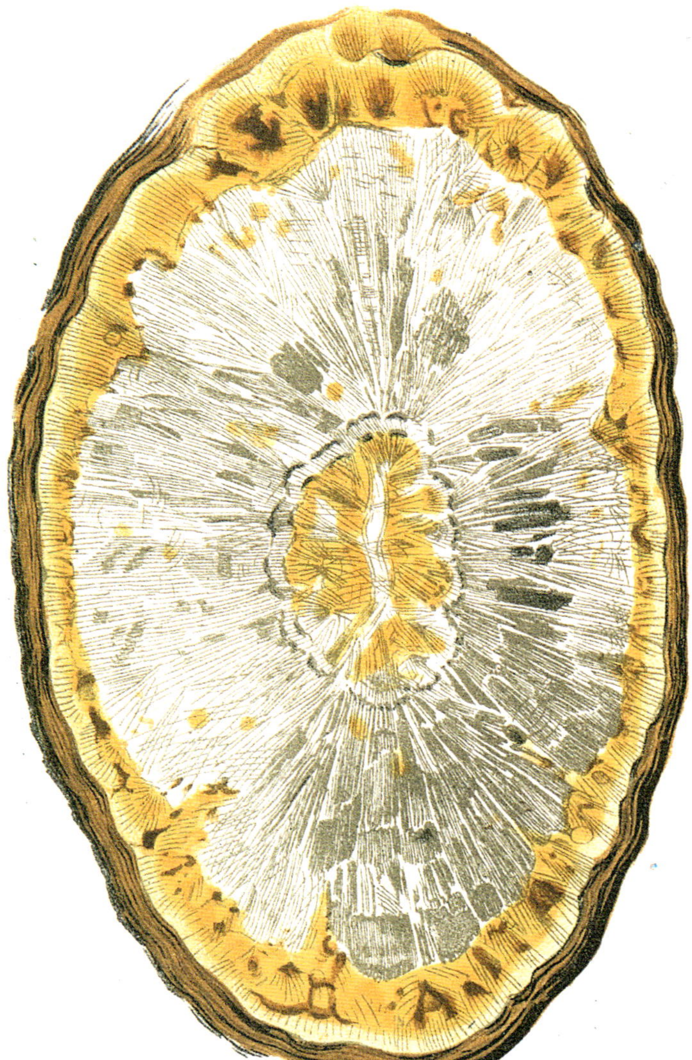

Legend to figure: Combination stone (Kombinationsstein). A lithograph from Aschoff L and Bacmeister A (1909) Die Cholelithiasis. Jena, Verlag von Gustav Fischer, Tafel XIV, Fig. 57.

# Preface

It all happened one day in 1952 when I was just beginning my graduate study Professor Hiroshi Miyake, Chairman of the Department of Surgery I, Kyushu University Faculty of Medicine, asked if I would like to do research on gallstones—the main subject of study at the department since the time of his father, Professor Hayari Miyake. I said "Yes," because I had not much idea either what research meant or any particular field which might be exciting. Taking my lead, he said that gallstones are formed from bile, and hence, that it is mandatory to understand what bile is. In order to pursue this question, one has to have a sound understanding of chemistry before embarking on the project. He thought it was best to go to the Pharmaceutical Department of the university, where much chemical research was being carried out. So he took me to meet his good friend, Professor Haruo Saikachi, who introduced me to organic chemistry. Subsequently, I was sent to the laboratory of his dear friend, Professor Charles G. Johnston, Chairman of the Department of Surgery, Wayne State University College of Medicine, Detroit, Michigan. There I helped to develop oral cholelitholytic agents and began to do research on gallstones.

During the 16 years of my professorship at the Department of Surgery I, Kyushu University Faculty of Medicine, Fukuoka, I attempted several times to write a book on cholelithiasis. I never succeeded, chiefly because of the lack of time, but enthusiasm for this endeavour persisted. Finally, I began this task after my retirement in 1991 as Professor Emeritus.

I have tried to put together all the material accumulated during my research career of over 30 years. The result is the present book, Cholelithiasis: Causes and Treatment. This book is designed to meet the needs of investigators in the field of gallstone research by providing details of the various topics, together with comprehensive references which, I hope, will help to update the view of the subject and plan the development of future research. Hopefully, this book will assist clinicians who are primarily interested in the treatment of gallstones to plan their treatment of particular cases on a rational basis by providing the detailed mechanisms underlying the formation of gallstones.

The first chapter explains the classification of gallstones, a matter of great controversy for over a century. The following chapters deal with the pathology and epidemiology of gallstones, whose variety has aroused much interest worldwide for centuries. The pathogenesis of gallstones is dealt with separately for each kind of gallstones, as the causes of each type seem to be quite different. The chapter on the pathogenesis of gallstones starts with the composition of bile and the physiology of the gallbladder. It then moves on to the pathogenesis of cholesterol gallstones; the formation of supersaturated bile, nucleation and growth of cholesterol crystals, role of the gallbladder, and, finally, various risk factors are discussed. The pathogenesis of black pigment stones and brown pigment stones (calcium bilirubinate stones) is considered in separate chapters. Other kinds of gallstones are also treated, including fatty acid calcium stones, inorganic stones, porphyrin-containing gallstones, parasite stones, and combination stones. The following section is devoted to gallstone formation in animals, which may give important clues to the pathogenesis of gallstones in man.

Clinical aspects of gallstone disease form the latter part of this book beginning with a presentation of symptoms and signs and then moving to diagnosis. The main emphasis is placed on the treatment of cholelithiasis, since the field is at present in a state of flux due to the introduction of many new modalties in recent years. First, nonsurgical treatments are considered such as oral cholelitholysis, contact dissolution agents, extracorporeal shock wave lithotripsy (ESWL), and contact lithotripsy. Next, in addition to standard cholecystectomy, new operative modalties such as percutaneous cholecystolithotomy and laparoscopic cholecystectomy are presented, with their advantages and disadvantages.

Intrahepatic calculi, or hepatolithiasis, are dealt with in a separate chapter as their epidemiology, pathology and pathogenesis are quite different from those of ordinary cholelithiasis. Furthermore, their treatment seems to be difficult, if not impossible, and poses a serious threat to the patient.

Sincere gratitude is due to the late Professors Hiroshi Miyake, Charles G. Johnston, and Haruo Saikachi, as well as my colleagues in several institutions. My wife, Hanna, has spared no effort to help me throughout the years, starting with my young assistant days in Professor Miyake's department, compiling references, deciphering my difficult handwritings, and typing my manuscripts. Thus, this book is a product of the concerted efforts of those who came into contact with me and helped me to concentrate on gallstone research throughout my professional career.

# Contents

# Introduction

The oldest known gallstone specimens are those discovered in an Egyptian mummy of the 21st dynasty of 1500 B.C. from Thebes dissected at the Royal College of Surgeons of England (Rains, 1964). The gallbladder was found to be filled with numerous calculi – probably stones consisting mainly of cholesterol. The second oldest gallstones are from the cadaver of a Western Han Dynasty (25–220 A.D.) tomb near Changsha, Hunan province, China (Wei, 1973). At dissection, Chinese scientists discovered stones in the common bile duct—probably brown pigment or calcium bilirubinate stones. Therefore, it seems that cholesterol stones predominating in the West and calcium bilirubinate or brown pigment stones predominating in the East have not changed for centuries. Apparently, gallstones have been occurring since ancient times. However, an understanding of the disease and its treatment came only in the nineteenth century.

Around 500 B.C., Alexander of Tralle, Lydia described gallstones as dried-up humor in the liver, while in 1000 A.D. the great Avicenna (Ali ibn Sina) of Armenia recommended the use of ox gallstones as a remedy for gallstones. In the fifteenth century, Beniverius of Florence discovered gallstones in the lowest part of the membrane of the liver. In the sixteenth century, Vesalius, at the University of Padua, also described gallstones found at autopsy. Gabriel Fallopius, of Fallopian tube fame, found gallstones in the gallbladder as well as in the common bile duct. In the seventeenth century, Glisson, of Anatomica hepatis fame, described gallstones found in feces. Fabricius and Lieberger removed gallstones by opening an abdominal abscess. In 1667, Stalpat von der Weil and Thilesius opened an abdominal abscess. Gallstones and bile were expelled but left a permanent biliary fistula. Rains gives a good review of the early history of our knowledge on gallstones (Rains 1964).

During this period, there was no specific treatment for gallstone disease and cholelithiasis followed its natural course. When the gallbladder adheres to the alimentary tract following the cholecystitis accompanying cholelithiasis and forms a bilioenteric fistula, gallstones are expelled into the gastrointestinal tract and inflammation of the biliary tract subsides. If the gallbladder adheres to the abdominal wall, an abscess into the abdominal wall is formed. Subsequent disruption of the abscess expells gallstones, but a persistent biliary fistula remains. When gallstones present in the gallbladder move to the bile duct via the cystic duct, they may cause cholangitis and/or obstructive jaundice, which may lead to hepatic insufficiency and death.

An understanding of the pathology of cholelithiasis and the development of rational treatment had to wait until the mid-ninteenth century. In 1878, Tait of Birmingham, England, performed the first cholecystolithotomy and external cholecystostomy (Tait, 1879, 1885). In 1882, a young surgeon at Lazarus Hospital in Berlin—Langenbuch, a student of

Esmarch—performed the first cholecystectomy in man on July 15, 1882 (Langenbuch, 1882). The common bile duct was entered for the first time by Kümmell (1890), followed by Kehr (1897). A good review of biliary surgery for the past 100 years was given by Praderi (1982). With the introduction of operative cholangiography by Mirizzi (1937), gallstone surgery became the mainstay in the treatment of cholelithiasis. With the recent introduction of oral cholelitholysis, extracorporeal shock wave lithotripsy, and laparoscopic cholecystectomy, the treatment of cholelithiasis is at present in a state of flux. However, the choice of treatment depends on how to effect permanent cure with minimal risk to the patient and should be individualized to suit the particular situation. Standard open cholecystectomy is still considered a gold standard (McSherry, 1989) in the treatment of cholelithiasis.

Hepatolithiasis, or intrahepatic calculi, has attracted much attention recently because of the difficulty of management and its intractable course, sometimes requiring multiple operations. Since the epidemiology, pathology, and etiology are quite different from those of ordinary cholelithiasis, requiring particular attention to treatment (Nakayama, 1994), this condition will be dealt with separately later in the book.

# CHAPTER ONE

# Classification of Gallstones

## Historical perspective

A gallstone is defined as a concrement present in the biliary tract. Gallstones vary greatly in composition. One of the main components of human gallstones is cholesterol, a term coined from the Greek words chole for "bile," and stereos, for "solid," by Chevreul (1815). In fact, cholesterol was first isolated from gallstones by Poulletier de la Salle in 1770 (quoted by Rains, 1964). A good historical review of the study of cholesterol is given by Dam (1958). Numerous attempts have been made to classify gallstones. In 1863, Thudichum proposed the first scientific classification of gallstones based on their chemical analysis (Thudichum, 1863) (Table 1). Because of the inadequacy of the analytical method available at that time, his classification has certain limitations when judged by the standards of present knowledge. In his treatise on gallstones, Naunyn, of the University of Strassburg, proposed that all gallstones are formed as a result of inflammation of the biliary tract (Naunyn, 1892). He stated that bile is rendered stagnant by obstruction or that the gallbladder wall becomes infected. The decomposition products of the bile irritate the wall and cause excessive secretion of mucus and cholesterol. Cholesterol saturates the bile and separates out together with pigment on particulate matter, forming the nucleus of a gallstone. However, Aschoff and Bacmeister, at the University of Freiburg, thought that certain gallstones are formed without the presence of inflammation, and divided gallstones into noninflammatory and inflammatory stones (Aschoff and Bacmeister, 1909) (Table 2). They were the first to postulate clearly that the transient increase in hepatic secretion of

**Table 1**

| Classification of Gallstones |
|---|
| First class—pellucid or pure cholesterine calculi |
| Second class—mixed calculi with prevalence of cholesterine |
| Third class—calculi with prevalence of cholochrome (bile pigment) |
| Fourth class—calculi with modified cholochrome |
| Fifth class—calculi with bile acid |
| Six class—calculi with fatty acid |
| Seventh class—calculi with carbonate of lime |

Source: Thudichum (1863).

Table 2

Classification of Gallstones

**Nichtentzündliche Gallensteine** (noninflammatory gallstones)
  **Radiäre Cholesterinsteine** (radial cholesterol stones)

**Entzündliche Gallensteine** (inflammatory gallstones)
  **Kombinationssteine (manteltragende, radiäre Cholesterinsteine)** (combination stones)

  **Kalksteine** (calcium stones)
    **Geschichtete Cholesterinkalksteine** (layered cholesterol-calcium stones)
    **Cholesterinpigmentkalksteine** (cholesterol-pigment calcium stones)
    **Bilirubinkalksteine** (bilirubin calcium stones)
    **Choledochussteine** (common bile duct stones)
  **Seltene Steine** (rare stones)
    **Parasitensteine** (parasite stones)
    **Reine Bilirubinsteine** (pure pigment stones)
    **Karbonat-kalk Steine** (calcium carbonate stones)

Source: Aschoff and Bacmeister (1909).

cholesterol in bile due to the metabolic defect far exceeding its solubilizer (i.e. bile salts) is responsible for the formation of so-called radiäre Cholesterinsteine (radial cholesterol stones). The ratio between the two is fundamental to cholesterol stone formation. Even today their so-called pure or radial cholestrerol gallstones (Figure 1a) consisting almost completely of cholesterol with a very small admixture of other constituents such as bile pigment and calcium, are thought to be formed without inflammation. Today their "layered cholesterol calcium stones" (geschichtete Cholesterinkalksteine) and "cholesterol pigment calcium stones" (Cholesterinpigmentkalksteine)" (Figure 1b) are also thought to be formed without the presence of inflammation, although they were grouped together with the inflammatory gallstones in the original classification of Aschoff and Bacmeister. Combination stones (Kombinationssteine) (Figure 1c) are those in which cholesterol is present in the center, coated with a clearly demarcated crust of a pigmented layer. Bilirubin calcium stones (Bilirubinkalksteine) in their classification are thought to be black pigment stones (Figure 1d) or black stones, as judged from their original drawings in the classic Die Cholelithiasis published in 1909 (Aschoff and Bacmeister 1909), and not brown pigment stones (Figure 1e).

# Newer classification of gallstones and controversies

In 1986 a new classification of gallstones was proposed by the Japan Gastroenterological Society (Table 3) (Japanese Society of Gastroenterology, Committee for the Study of Cholelithiasis, 1986). This classification, with some improvement, subdivides cholesterol stones into pure cholesterol stones, combination stones, and mixed stones. However, the

Table 3

**Classification of Gallstones**

Cholesterol gallstones
- Pure cholesterol stone
- Combination stone
- Mixed stone

Pigment gallstone
- Black stone
- Calcium bilirubinate stone

Rare gallstone
- Calcium carbonate stone
- Fatty acid calcium stone
- Other combination stone
- Miscellaneous stone

Source: Japanese Society of Gastroenterology, Committee for the Study of Cholelithiasis (1986).

question of subdividing cholesterol stones is far from settled. The subdivision proposed above seems to have little meaning, as these stones are composed mainly of cholesterol with a more or less similar mechanism of formation, with or without multiple centers of growth. Mixed stones are essentially the same as the so-called cholesterol pigment calcium stones (Cholesterinpigmentkalksteine). They are composed of cholesterol, calcium bilirubinate, and fatty acid calcium, are multiple and are often faceted. The classification of gallstones in our department is shown in Table 4 (Nakayama, 1981); in it, no subdivision is made among cholesterol stones. The cardinal point to be considered in the formation of gallstones is the precipitation of the major constituents of gallstones such as cholesterol, bilirubin, fatty acid, and calcium for each class of gallstones commonly encountered. Whether or not the classifications currently available survive the test of time remains to be seen and depends on how frequently they are used in the scientific community and how convincing they turn out to be.

Table 4

**Classification of Gallstones**

Cholesterol stones

Pigment stones
- Black pigment stones (black stones)
- Brown pigment stones (calcium bilirubinate stones)

Fatty acid calcium stones

Inorganic stones

Porphyrin-containing stones

Parasite stones

Combination stones

Source: Nakayama (1981).

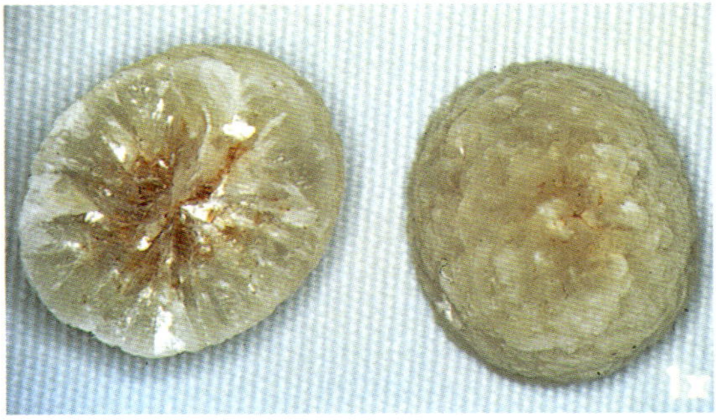

**Figure 1a** Cholesterol stones (radial cholesterol stones)

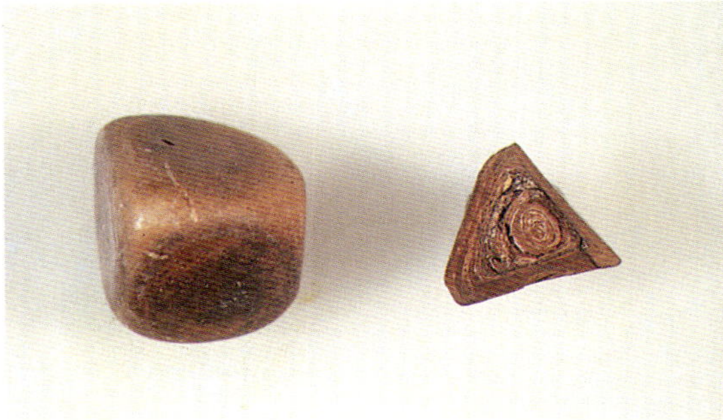

**Figure 1b** Cholesterol stones (cholesterol pigment calcium stones)

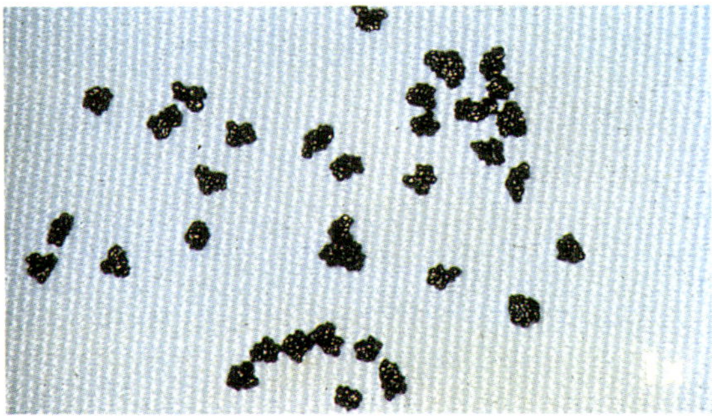

**Figure 1c** Black pigment stones

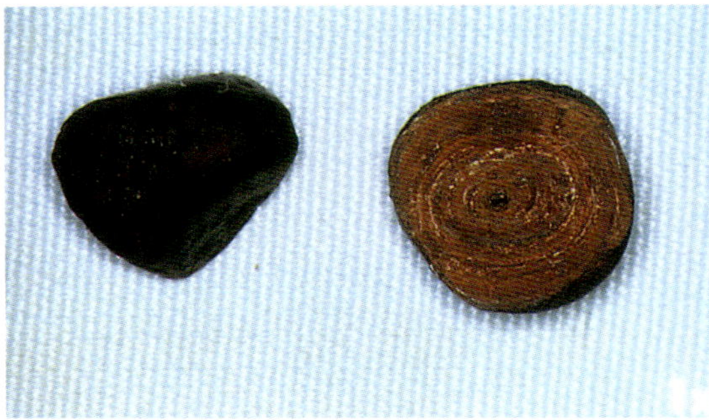

**Figure 1d** Brown pigment sotnes (calcium bilirubinate stones)

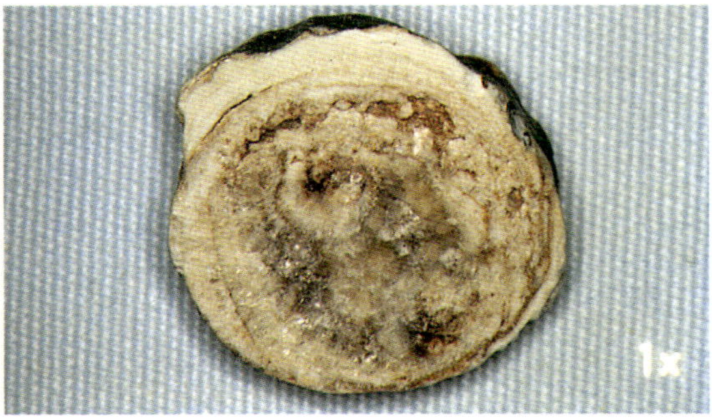

**Figure 1e** Fatty acid calcium stones

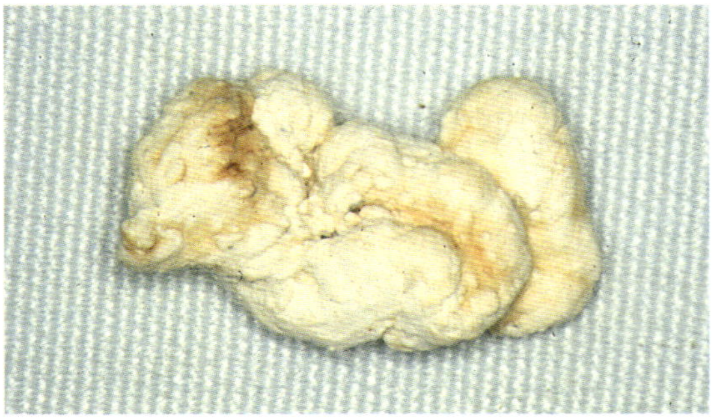

**Figure 1f** Inorganic stones

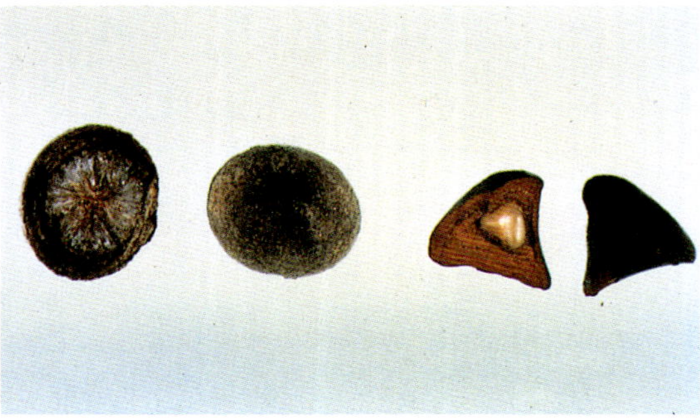

**Figure 1g** Combination stones

# Cholesterol stones

Since the main event in the formation of cholesterol gallstones is the precipitation or nucleation and growth of cholesterol crystals, no distinction is made between so-called radial cholesterol stones and multiple, often faceted, cholesterol pigment calcium stones or mixed stones, since both are composed mainly (over 70 %) of cholesterol. In addition, there seems to be no clear-cut demarcation between the two types of stones either morphologically or in composition. Hence, they are treated, as a whole, as cholesterol stones when considering their etiology. Scanning electron microscopy with windowless energy-dispersive X-ray microanalysis in a core of cholesterol stones shows the presence of calcium salts in 88 % of the cases, calcium bilirubinate in 54 % and calcium palmitate in 39 % (Kaufmann et al., 1994). Cholesterol stones often show pigmented concentric rings (so-called Liesegang rings) which may reflect the changes in bile composition during their growth with the concomitant change in the composition of gallstones in layers (Nakayama, 1971). Microdistribution of three polymorphs of calcium carbonate, namely aragonite, calcite, and vaterite, shows they are mutually exclusive (Taylor et al., 1993). The distribution of calcium carbonate polymorphs in pigmented areas of cholesterol stones reflects periodic changes over time in bile composition. Organic matrix of cholesterol stones is sometimes colorless but more usually is an orange, yellow, or brown, amorphous, organic gel-like substance (Sutor et al., 1974a). The matrix contains a macromolecular complex of mucin and bilirubin (Smith and LaMont, 1985), which constitutes 12.5 % of solitary radial cholesterol stones and 3.5 % of multiple cholesterol-pigment calcium stones or mixed stones. It is present in the central nidus and also in radial or lamellar bands in the periphery of stones (Womack et al, 1963). Bile pigment is eluted together with glycoprotein at the void volume of exclusion gel chromatography, suggesting the presence of a high molecular weight complex (Mr $2 \times 10^6$). Major bile pigments present in the matrix are said to be bilirubin (84 %) and bilirubin monoglucuronide (15 %) which are trapped in mucous gel (Smith and LaMont, 1985). Cholesterol stones sometimes show radiate radiolucencies on plain abdominal X-rays due to the presence of gas which is composed of $CO_2$ (6–7 %), $O_2$ (0.5 %) and noninflammable gas probably $N_2$ (Vakil and Everbach, 1991). Combination stones (Figure 1c) or Kombinnationssteine (Aschoff and Bacmeister, 1909), i.e., "Mit scharfer Grenze setzt sich auf dem radiären Stein ein kalkreicher geschichteter Mantel auf (Kombinationsstein)" – radial cholesterol stones coated with clearly demarcated, calcium-rich, layered shell (combination stone) – are listed separately from cholesterol stones, although the center is often of cholesterol stone coated with a pigment (brown pigment stone) layer, indicating growth in two stages, starting with cholesterol stone formation followed by the formation of brown pigment stone shell. In rare instances, there are stones with a pigmented center surrounded by a cholesterol-rich shell. The use of the term "mixed stones" is somewhat confusing in regard to combination stones and best avoided.

# Pigment stones

Pigment stones are composed mainly of bilirubin and its derivatives. However, there are two kinds of pigment stones (Table 4)—black and brown—distinguished by their color, surface characteristics, consistency, cross-sectional appearance, and finally, chemical composition (Maki et al, 1982; Trotman and Soloway 1982; Malet et al, 1984; Soloway et al, 1986).

## Black pigment stones (black stones)

Black pigment stones, or black stones, are dark brown to black in color, brittle, extremely hard, and with numerous projections or spikes on their surface (Figure 1c) resembling those of Kompeitoh, a Japanese confection, a word originally derived from Portugese word "confeitos". Mathematical simulation of the growth process of these spikes of Kompeitoh has been presented elsewhere (Murai and Nakata 1988). They occur multiple and are located mainly in the gallbladder, accompanied by a very low bacterial infection rate (Tabata and Nakayama 1981). They are composed of bilirubin (5–15 %) and its polymer (5–25 %) and all almost devoid of cholesterol (Yamashita et al, 1988). Their cross-sectional appearance seems to be devoid of any particular structures, with very fine spherical particles 30 nm in diameter (Koga and Todo 1977). Black pigment stones are sometimes associated with hemolysis, cirrhosis or old age (Kaufman et al, 1989).

## Brown pigment stones (calcium bilirubinate stones)

The other group of pigment stones are brown pigment stones, or calcium bilirubinate stones (Figure 1d), composed of bilirubin (20–40 %), cholesterol (1–10 %), fatty acid (5–15 %), and calcium (1.5–2.5 %). They are brown to dark brown color, soft, and pliable. Their cross-sectional appearance shows concentric pigmented layers. They occur commonly in the extrahepatic bile duct but are also found in the gallbladder and the intrahepatic bile ducts. They are either solitary or multiple. In the latter case, the stones become faceted. They occur primarily or secondarily as recurrent stones.

# Fatty acid calcium stones, inorganic stones, porphyrin-containing stones, parasite stones, and combination stones

Fatty acid calcium stones (Fig. 1e) are dark brown to black on the surface but yellow to yellowish-white and lustrous inside consisting mainly of calcium palmitate (Nishimura,

1938; Nakayama, 1968 Cowie et al 1973). They are usually found in the common bile duct. Inorganic stones (Fig. 1f) are composed mainly of calcium carbonate, with a small proportion of calcium phosphate. They are solitary or multiple. Gallstones with a high porphyrin content may occur. Parasite stones are classified separately from brown pigment stones or calcium bilirubinate stones because of their distinctly different origin, although they are composed of calcium bilirubinate deposited on the carcass of parasites such as ascaris lumbricoides or liver fluke etc invaded into biliary tract. When a layer consisting of bile pigment, cholesterol and calcium carbonate is deposited on cholesterol stone, they are called combination stones.

# Gallstone analysis

A quantitative microanalytical technique for gallstones has been developed, based on the preliminary separation of gallstone constituents into subgroups with solvent partition and column chromatography followed by gas-liquid chromatography (Figure 2) (Nakayama, 1968, Yamashita et al, 1988). This is very useful in the classification of gallstones, especially when macroscopic inspection fails. Recently, methods of gallstone analysis have been reviewed extensively (Soloway and Wu 1994).

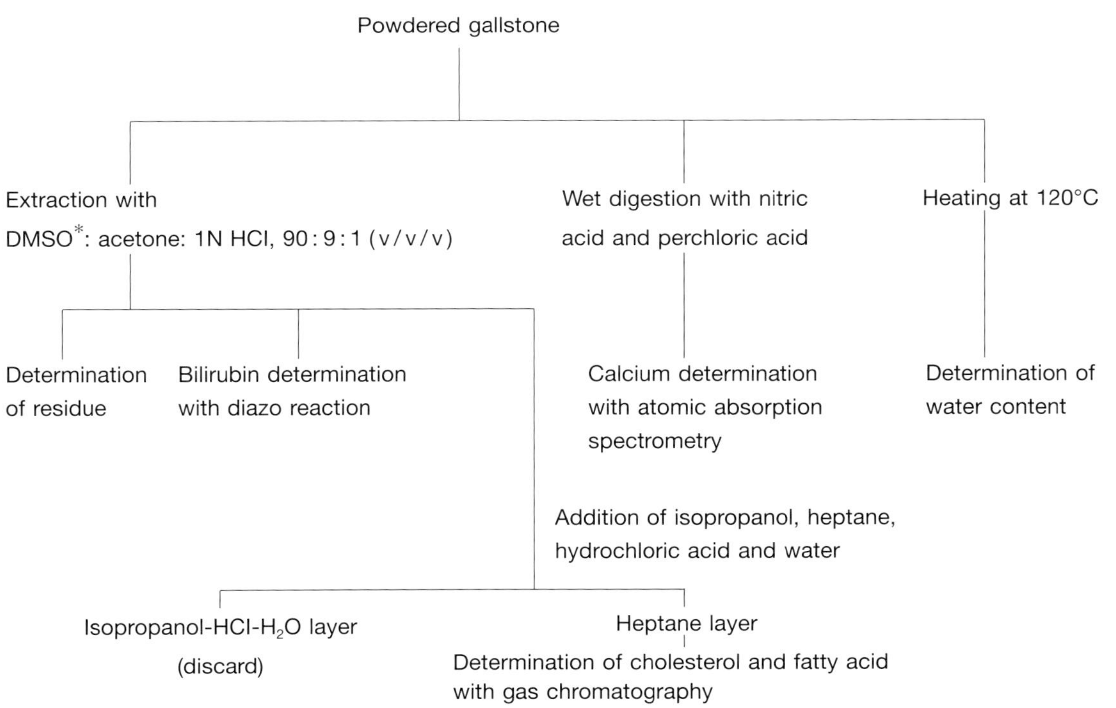


**Figure 2**

Chemical analysis of gallstone.

*Dimethylsulfoxide

Source: (Yamashita et al., 1988)

# CHAPTER TWO

# Pathology

Gallstones are defined as concrements present in the biliary tract. They occur anywhere in the gallbladder, extrahepatic and intrahepatic ducts. When stones are present in the gallbladder, the disease is called cholecystolithiasis; in the common bile duct it is called choledocholithiasis; and in the intrahepatic bile ducts it is called hepatolithiasis and the stones are called intrahepatic calculi. Gallstones differ considerably in chemical composition. They are classified according to their composition as cholesterol stones, black pigment stones or black stones, brown pigment stones or calcium bilirubinate stones, fatty acid calcium stones, inorganic stones, porphyrin-containing stones, and stones of parasitic origin as discussed in the preceding section (Chapter I). The presence of gallstones need not produce clinical manifestations, but it may induce chronic or acute cholecystitis (Mentzer, 1926). Chronic cholecystitis almost always occurs when gallstones are present, with occasional mild inflammatory cell infiltration and fibrosis; the epithelium is intact. With chronic cholecystitis the wall of the gallbladder is occasionally increased to several times its usual thickness, with mucosal diverticula (Rokitansky-Aschoff sinus) penetrating the muscular layer to varying depths. The perimuscular layer becomes dense, with many coarse collagenous bundles. The mucosal folds are coarse and, in the advanced stage, are obliterated, with the surface being trabeculated. Ulceration of the mucosa may result from the pressure exerted by gallstones. When gallstones originally present in the gallbladder migrate into the bile duct, they produce symptoms and signs such as jaundice. However, de novo formation of gallstones in the common bile duct may also occur (Hoerr, 1962). An internal biliary fistula may result between the gallbladder and duodenum or colon from the formation of an inflammatory adhesion between the gallbladder and adjacent organs and subsequent migration of a gallstone from the gallbladder or common duct into the gastrointestinal tract. When the cystic duct is obstructed by gallstones, it produces gallbladder hydrops or hydrops vesicae felleae when the primary insult is aseptic. With the advent of a secondary bacterial invasion, it may lead to gallbladder empyema. The presence of gallstones in the gallbladder predisposes to the development of acute cholecystitis, which is superimposed on the existing chronic cholecystitis. When severe inflammation sets in and obstruction of the cystic duct occurs, gallbladder empyema or empyema vesicae felleae is the result.

# CHAPTER THREE

# Epidemiology

The prevalence of gallstones differs from country to country and from area to area. This variation has attracted much attention, since such differences may be related to the difference in risk factors in situ—and hence may point to a specific factor(s) responsible for the difference which may eventually give a clue to the etiology of gallstones. However, the available data are fragmentary at best. Robertson and Dochat (1944), Newman and Northup (1959) Maki (1966), Heaton (1973), Burkitt and Tunstall (1975), and Brett and Barker (1976) give very good lists of references up to their date of publications.

## Methods of study

There are three ways of studying the prevalence of gallstones; namely, by autopsy, clinical studies and prospective studies.

### Autopsy study

Autopsy study has several potential pitfalls. The data exclude those not dying in the hospital and the data must, by necessity, depend on the variety of factors involved in the autopsy, such as autopsy technique, specific attention paid, and completeness of the recording, although much more detailed information could be collected which otherwise is missed by various diagnostic procedures. Although they do not provide a true estimate of gallstone frequency (Newman and Northup, 1959) in the population as a whole, autopsy studies estimate the prevalence of gallstones in populations (Newman and Northup, 1959) and frequently provide the only reliable data available.

### Clinical study

Clinical studies also suffer from the selection and lack of stratification of subject populations, lack of pertinent variables, and missing important information. The prevalence of gallstones cannot be deduced from the clinical records, since over half of gallstones are asymptomatic. However, clinical records, especially operation records, provide valuable information on gross differences in prevalence and detect large changes in incidence (Diehl 1987). McPherson et al found that the rate of cholecystectomy is related to the prevalence of cholelithiasis by postmortem examination using the same population (McPherson et al, 1985), although the presence of gallstones is not always an indication for removal and relevant symptoms occurred in as llittle as 18 % of the cases in a 15-year follow-up study (Gracie and Ransohoff, 1982). In general, cohort studies should be given more credence than case-control studies especially hospital-based case-control studies as the results of the latter heavily depend on which individuals are selected for controls (Sandler, 1993). There is an ethical problem of subjecting healthy persons to otherwise unnecessary examination. However, recently introduced ultrasonography is believed to be harmless, noninvasive, and at least as sensitive and specific as time-honored cholecystography (Cooperberg and Burhenne, 1980; Rome Group for Epidemiology and Prevention of Cholelithiasis, 1988a), and is beginning to be used widely in epidemiological studies.

### Longitudinal prospective study

Longitudinal prospective study also yields silent gallstone cases; therefore the prevalence obtained includes all gallstone cases. A geographic cross-sectional study (Janzon et al, 1985) of gallstone disease showed a prevalence of 50 % less than an autopsy study (Lindström, 1977) conducted in the same area. This is most likely due to the selection bias in autopsy studies and should not be explained by false negatives at screening, since the sensitivity of ultrasonographic examination has been found to be as high as 98 %.

Thus, a longitudinal prospective studies using ultrasonography is the best method available to obtain the prevalence of gallstone disease with greater precision. Autopsy and clinical retrospective studies also yield much valuable information, but they should be used with caution and are useful for obtaining crude difference which may give clues to the gross difference in the prevalence and large change in the incidence of gallstones (Heaton, 1973). In reviewing the literature on prevalence, one has to be aware of the possibility that the changes in different time periods makes it difficult to compare the prevalence in different countries unless large differences exist, i.e., marginal or undetectable differences become obscured.

## Geographical difference in the prevalence of gallstones

The prevalence of gallstone disease has been known to differ considerably throughout world. The highest prevalence of gallstones has been found in Indian populations throughout the Americas. For instance, Southwestern American Indians (Navajo, Pima, and

Sioux) have a high prevalence of gallstones. Thus, gallstone disease is called the American Indian's burden (Sievers and Marquis 1962). In Peru and Chile, gallstones are also quite common. In Europe, especially northern Europe, as well as the United States and Canada, the prevalence of gallstones is high but not as high as among American Indians. In Asia, the prevalence of gallstones in Japan is rapidly increasing to over 10 %. The Masai tribe of Kenya is said to be free of gallstone disease. Good reviews on the geographical difference in gallstone prevalence are available (Newman and Northup, 1959; Grosse, 1966; Heaton, 1973; Burkitt and Tunstall, 1975; Brett and Barker, 1976; Lowenfels, 1980; Strom and West, 1985; Diehl, 1991).

## Africa

Little information is available on the prevalence of gallstones in Africa, either at autopsy or clinically. The prevalence is generally low, especially in Subsaharan Africa (Adedeji et al, 1986)—usually less than 1 % except in South Africa. For instance, Owor (1964) quotes the experience of Vint, who found only one case of gallstones in 1,000 postmortems in Kenya in 1960. In the same article, Trowell mentioned Luigi's record that four gallstone cases were encountered in 600 autopsies in Leopoldville (Kinshasa), the Congo (Zaire) in 1960. Becker and Chatgidatis (1952, 1959) reported a great difference in the prevalence of gallstones in Caucasoid (15 %) versus Negroid (3 %) populations in South Africa. Differences in the kind of gallstones in African populations have also been reported (Onuigbo, 1977; Owor 1971). Unfortunately some are based on a qualitative analysis at best and therefore may be misleading.

### Egypt

Zaki and Kamel (1967) conducted a clinical study on the prevalence of gallstones, finding a rate of only 1 % symptomatic gallstones among patients admitted to the surgical ward at Ein Shams University Hospital in Cairo. The male : female ratio was 1 : 2. Cholesterol stones accounted for 96.0 % (72/75 cases). The prevalence of gallstones in Egypt is considered to be between those of Europe and Subsaharan Africa.

### Ghana

In Accra only 0.4 % of general admission patients were turned out to have symptomatic gallstones (Archampong, 1969). No gallstones were found in a series of 4,395 autopsies performed in Ghana from 1923 to 1955 (Edington, 1957).

### Kenya

Masai living in southern Kenya and northern Tanzania are said to have no gallstones (Biss et al, 1971), and their bile is very unsaturated for cholesterol. Indeed, at Makerere, Kenya, only three gallbladders contained gallstones in 18,000 necropsies 25 years ago (Loefler, 1988). However, this situation is rapidly changing. Formerly, operations of the biliary tract on Africans were rare. Over the past 10 years, they have been gradually increasing.

In Nairobi alone, more than seven cholecystectomies per month are performed on Africans. These stones occur in the upper and middle socioeconomic classes, predominantly in fertile, obese women who are often in their twenties and thirties. The middle-class population of Kenya is large and its economic success is expressed, among other things, by obesity. An increased intake of fat and oil, as well as sugar and meat from a mixed diet (traditional food items and European dishes) in recent years, is thought to be responsible. Loefler mentions that gallstones also occur among the smaller upper-class African populations in neighboring countries (Loefler, 1988).

### Nigeria

Parnis (1964), working in Ibadan, had only 27 gallstone patients admitted over a 5-year period. Onuigbo used the number of cholecystectomies to assess the prevalence of gallstones. As the author states, this method is not accurate (Onuigbo, 1977), but, it seems to be the only feasible one under the circumstances prevailing there. He found only seven gallstone cases in 7,500 surgical specimens in Nigerian Igbos. In a study based on the patients admitted to Lagos University Hospital from 1980 to 1984 confirmed by operation, Adedeji et al. found clinical evidence of an increasing incidence of cholecystitis or gallstones in Lagos in recent years (Adedeji et al., 1986). Increased admittance to the university hospital, increased incorporation of Western food items in the diet of urbanized Nigerian women in the last 20 years and the use of contraceptive pills are thought to be contributing factors. The male : female ratio was 1 : 5.3.

### Uganda

The prevalence of gallstones is very low. A clinical study conducted in Kampala revealed only 22 cases in 61,000 admissions (Shaper and Patel, 1964). Owor (1964, 1971) states that the overall autopsy prevalence of gallstones in Mulago Hospital, Kampala, Uganda from 1950 to 1962 was 0.87 %.

## The Americas

A longitudinal prospective study (Friedman et al., 1966) was conducted in Framingham, Massachusetts, based on the medical records of 5,209 patients between ages 30 and 62 (Framingham study). Definite gallbladder disease was found in 427 persons (8.2 %). These patients had cholecystectomy, had positive results on cholecystography for clinical reasons, and had symptoms of gallbladder disease. Since no attempt has been made to identify silent gallstones, the lower prevalence rate was expected. At present, 26 years of follow-up medical data are available, and all cohort members have passed through the peak period of risk for gallstones (Bortnichak et al., 1985) and await further study. Wilbur and Bolt found gallstones in 11 % of 1,233 men aged 35–55 years during periodic health examinations in Michigan (Wilbur and Bolt 1959). In Canada 16.7 % prevalence of gallstones was reported for women at 15 to 50 years of age (Williams et al., 1980). Recently, Ratner et al. studied very old institutionalized persons in Canada and found the prevalence of gallstones to be 61.5 % (Ratner et al., 1991). American blacks have lower prevalence rates than whites (Newman and Northup, 1959; Sichieri et al., 1990).

## American Indians

In contrast, the extremely high prevalence of gallstones in American Indian populations is well known. At least 23 different tribes are said to have a high prevalence of gallbladder disease (Shaheb, 1990); hence it has been called the American Indian's burden (Sievers and Marquis 1962). Salisbury is said to have been the first to report the high prevalence of biliary tract disease among Southwestern American Indians, i.e., Navajos (Salisbury, 1947). Lam studied 596 Pima Indians from age- and sex-stratified random samples of persons 15 to 74 years of age and found the prevalence of gallbladder disease to be as high as 48.6 % (Lam, 1954). The prevalence was significantly higher in females and increased with age in both sexes. Pima Indians aged 15 to 20 years are found to be at high risk of early development of gallbladder disease (Hesse, 1959). Age-specific prevalence of gallbladder disease in females demonstrated an extremely sharp rise between 25 and 29 years of age. Hesse commented on the high prevalence of gallbladder disease and low incidence of arteriosclerotic heart disease among Southwestern American Indians. He found the prevalence of cholelithiasis in Navajo Indians to be 24.4 % compared to about 10 % in non-Indian populations. The prevalence was markedly greater in all age groups based on the autopsy findings in those over 20 years of age (Hesse, 1964). Reichenbach reports an average prevalence of 29.9 % compared to non-Indian prevalence of 12 %. The prevalence of gallstones is also high in other Indian tribes such as the Sioux (Lam, 1954), Pima (Hesse, 1959; Comess, 1967; Reichenbach, 1967), Apache (Reichenbach, 1967) and Papago (Reichenbach, 1967) and many other Southwestern American Indians (Sievers and Marquis, 1962). The male : female ratio is 1.0 : 2.5. A cholecystographic survey showed that over 70 % of Pima Indian women over 25 years of age are expected to have gallstones (Sampliner et al., 1970). As many as 40 per cent of all adult Indian women had stones at postmortem examination compared to 21.7 % of non-Indian women; the rate was 11.6 % in Indian men against 9.7 % in non-indian men (Reichenbach, 1967). Chippewa Indians of northern Minnesota have been studied retrospectively from the medical records of the local hospital where virtually all persons living on the reservation received medical service (Thistle et al., 1971). A total of 197 cases were reviewed. The prevalence of gallbladder disease was found to be 8.8 % in the population over 20 years of age. The male : female ratio was 1 : 4. It is interesting to note that women with stronger Indian heritage were found to have a higher prevalence of gallbladder disease; this pattern did not hold in men. Micmac Indian women aged 15 to 50 living in Nova Scotia, Canada, were examined by cholecystography (Williams et al., 1977a). The prevalence of cholelithiasis was found to be 21.1 %. Glenn mentioned the high prevalence of gallstones in Alaskan Eskimos (Yamase and McNamara 1972). Recently, the prevalence of gallstones in Mexican-Americans has been much greater than in other Hispanic groups. Mexican-Americans, Cuban-Americans, and Puerto Ricans living in the United States, aged 20–74, were compared (Maurer et al., 1990). Of a total of 3,981 persons, 2,299 were subjected to ultrasonography.

The age-adjusted prevalence rate of gallstones (gallstone plus cholecystectomy) was 7.2 % for Mexican-American men (1.7 times that of Cuban-Americans and 1.8 times that of Puerto Ricans) and 23.2 % for women (1.5 times that of Cuban-Americans and 1.7 times that of Puerto Ricans). The prevalence rate reached 44.1 per cent in Mexican American women of 50–74 years of age. It was concluded that Mexican-American women have gallstones 2.1 times more frequently than Danish women and 1.5 times more often than Italian women, while Mexican-American men have gallstones only 1.4 times more often than Danish men and 1.0 times more often than Italian men. Among men, the risk of gallstone disease increases with age, education, and subscapular skinfold thickness. Among women, the risk increases with age, body mass index, four skinfold measures, diabetes, impaired glucose tolerance, and oral contraceptive usage but not with parity. Mexican-Americans are at increased risk of gallstone disease even when other risk factors are controlled in multiple logistic regression analysis. In Chile, the prevalence of gallstones is one of the highest in the world (Covarrubias et al., 1984; Nervi et al., 1989). Munizaga reports two cases of cholelithiasis in pre-Columbian mummies – both cholesterol stones and comments that in Chile gallstones are more commonly found in mummies than in present Peruvian populations (Munizaga et al., 1978). Gallstones from Alaskan-American Indians (Athapaskan Indians), Eskimos (Inuit), and Aleuts in Alaska have been analyzed and found to be mostly cholesterol stones (Figure 3) (Nakayama, unpublished).

### Hawaii

On the Pacific island of Hawaii, the prevalence of gallstones among eight ethnic groups was compared, i.e., Caucasoids, Chinese, Filipinos, Hawaiians, Japanese, Portuguese, and Puerto Ricans from the hospital admission records of 1,274 patients with gallbladder disease. The incidence of gallbladder disease decreases from Chinese to Puerto Rican, Portuguese, Caucasoids, Korean, Japanese, Filipinos, and Hawaiians, in this order (Yamase and McNamara 1972)

## Asia

The pattern of gallstone disease in Asia differs greatly from east to west. In East Asia, although the proportion of cholesterol stones is steadily increasing, a predominance of brown pigment stones or calcium bilirubinate stones still persists. In contrast, in West Asia, cholesterol stones have long been predominant. The demarcation line seems to lie roughly on the longitude passing through the eastern part of the Indian subcontinent.

### China

There seems to be a great divergence in the prevalence and kind of gallstones as China covers a very wide geographic area and has over 1.2 billion people, i.e. almost one fourth of the world population. In addition, there are many ethnic divergencies in the population, with 55 officially recognized ethnic minorities in addition to the main Han nationality (Ma, 1989). The prevalence of gallstones in China has so far not been well

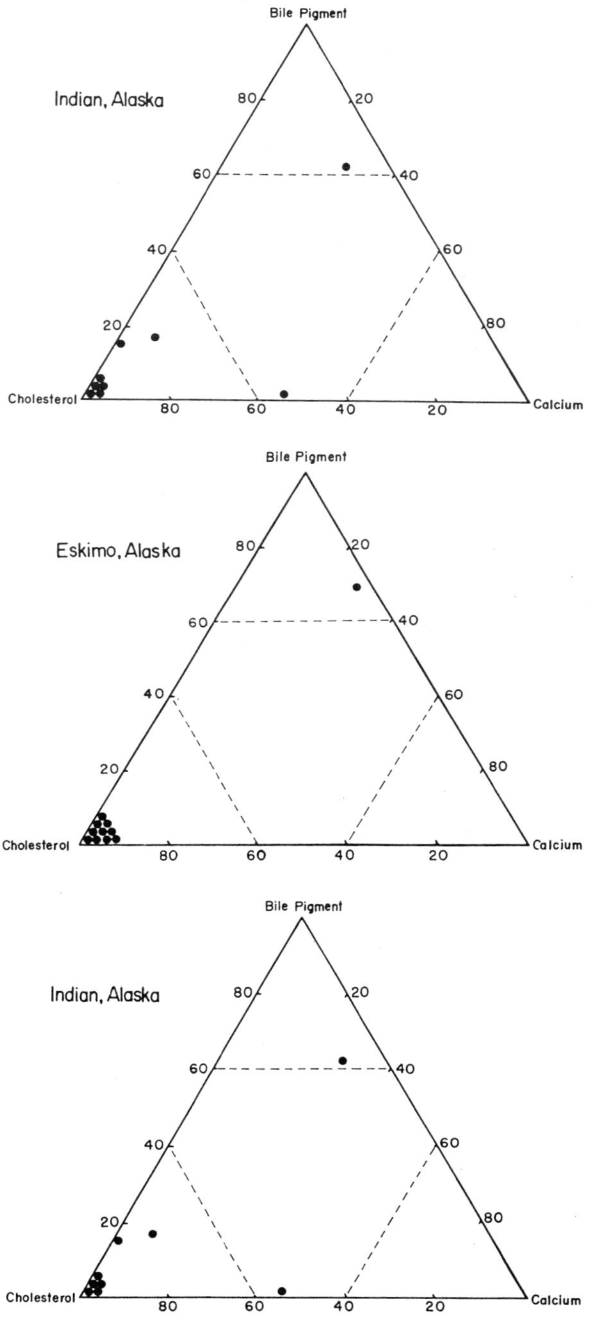


**Figure 3**

Gallstone Composition in Aleut, Eskimos, and Athapaskan Indians of Alaska

Triangular coordinates showing major constituents of gallstones, i.e., cholesterol, bile pigment and calcium.

Source: Nakayama unpublished

documented. In 1987 Huang Zhi Qiang organized the Third National Congress of Cholelithiasis and collected 11,342 cases of gallstones operated on from 1983 to 1985 at 146 institutions all over China (Huang, 1987). He reports the prevalence of gallstones in Tianjin, in northern China, to be 8.2 % (2,325/28,519 cases) of the general population examined by ultrasonography (Huang et al., 1987). In Beijing the prevalence was reported to be 4.3 % (277/6,416 cases) (Yang et al., 1987), in Shanghai 4.2 % (468/10,589 cases) (Shi et al., 1987) and in Kunming 5.9 % (330/5,588 cases) (Wen et al., 1987). The mean prevalence of gallstones collected from nine reports was 6.6 %. Xinjiang province in north-western China is of great interest. As the population there consists mainly of Uygurs (3/5), with several other ethnic groups such as Han, Kazak, Hui, Mongols, Kirgiz, Tajik, Xibe, Uzbek, Manchu, Daur, Tatar, and Russians (Ma, 1989), the pattern of gallstone disease differs greatly. Wang and Yao studied 166 cases of cholelithiasis in Xinjiang (Wang and Yao 1983) and found that cholesterol stones comprised 91.6 % (152/166 cases). When the cases were divided into Han, Uygur, and others (11.4 % consisting of Kazak, Hui, and Mongols), gallstones in 66 cases of Uygur were comprised of cholesterol stones (98.5 %) as well as in 88 cases of Han (85.2 %). Wang and Yao compiled a comprehensive list of the prevalence of different types of gallstones in different parts of China (Wang, personal communication). Xia studied 1,202 cases of cholelithiasis in Guiyang province in southwestern China, where many minority groups live in isolated areas. The proportion of cholesterol stones was found to be 58.6 %, brown pigment stones 10.5 % and black pigment stones 4.2 %. The average percentage of cholesterol stones in the western, northern and central parts of the province was about 60 % (Xia, 1987).

The proportion of gallstones found solely in the gallbladder also varies considerably from area to area. According to Wang and Yao, it varies from 89.4 % in the Uygur population of Xinjiang to 3.3 % in the Qingdao population of Shangdong province on the east coast, averaging 35.6 % of 2,846 cases reported. (Wang and Yao 1983)

## India

Rogers found the prevalence of gallstones in the general population of India to be 5.4 % (Rogers, 1925). Later Malhotra reported the prevalence of gallstones in northern Indian railroad workers and their families to be 0.14 % against a rate in southern Indian railroad workers of 0.02 % (Malhotra, 1968). Thus cholelithiasis is seven times more common in northern than in southern India. The disease is more common in women than in men in the north, but this situation is reversed in the south. Sarin, examined 201 consecutive cases of gallstone patients undergoing cholecystectomy, found that 94 % were cholesterol stones (Sarin et al., 1986). Ultrasonographic examination was carried out to detect symptomatic and silent stones in free-living urban populations in Srinagar, Kashmir (Khuroo et al., 1989). The prevalence of gallstones was 6.1 % with a male : female ratio of 1 : 3. The prevalence rose with age in both sexes, reaching peak of 29.1 % in the sixth decade in females. The prevalence is higher in parous women than in nulliparas after age adjustment.

## Israel

In spite of an earlier report (Kleeberg, 1960, 1961), Yemenite Jews (from Yemen) and Ashkenazi Jews (from Europe) were found to have a similar prevalence of gallstones (3.1 % over the age of 20 (Weingarten et al., 1990).

## Japan

The overall prevalence of gallstones in Japan has been reported to be 4.4 % based on the autopsy findings of 35,028 cases collected from 48 institutions in 1964 (Maki et al., 1964). A considerable increase was noted from the period before World War II (2.8–3.7 %) (Miyake Sr, 1913, 1930). Kameda (Kameda et al., 1980) cites a figure of 8.2 % based on the autopsy records of 18,307 cases from 1944 to 1977. When the figure is broken down on an annual basis, the rate is found to have risen dramatically from 3.0 % in 1950 to 8.0 % in 1961 and then 16.0 in in 1977, with the overall prevalence of 8.2 %. Cholelithiasis is rare below 20 years of age but increases after 30. The prevalence is 10 % at the age of 50 and reaches 22.2 % after the age of 80. The male : female ratio was 1.0 : 1.5. The proportion of silent stones is thought to be around 50 % retrospectively (Kameda, 1980). In a follow-up report based on 23,326 autopsy cases from 1949 to 1986, Kameda gives an average prevalence of gallstones in Japan of 9.6 % (Kameda et al., 1981). A prospective study with ultrasonography was conducted in Okinawa, the southernmost island of Japan (Nomura et al., 1988) giving an overall prevalence of 3.2 % and a male : female ratio of 1.0 : 1.6.

There seems to be a change in the kinds of gallstones found in Japan, especially cholesterol stones versus brown pigment stones (calcium bilirubinae stones). Miyake Sr (Figure 4), returning from the famous surgery clinic of Professor Johann von Mikulicz-Radecki of the University of Breslau, Germany noted in his classical paper that a difference existed not only in the prevalence but also in the composition of gallstones between Germany and Japan (Miyake Sr, 1913). His son, Miyake Jr (Figure 5), has clearly shown the transition from predominantly brown pigment stones (calcium bilirubinate stones) to predominantly cholesterol stones in the postwar period of 1947 to 1965 (Miyake Jr and Johnston, 1968). Maki gave a proportion of cholesterol stones of 25.8 per cent and that of brown pigment stones of 72.8 % in 1961 (Maki, 1961). In 1964 Kameda cited the prevalence of cholesterol stones to be 46.6 % and that of brown pigment stones to be 41.5 % based on infrared spectrometry analysis (Kameda, 1964). Later, in 1981, he reported that cholesterol stones increased to 71.7 % in 1981 and brown pigment stones decresed to 22.3 % (Kameda et al., 1981). By that time, the proportion of cholesterol stones had increased markedly in urban areas, while the predominance of brown pigment stones persisted. Cholesterol stones were on the rise even in remote rural areas (Kameda et al., 1981). This long-held impression that the compostion of gallstones in Japan has been gradually changing from the once predominantly brown pigment stones to cholesterol stones, approaching that of the West, was confirmed by the chemical analysis, using the same analytical technique with gallstone samples collected 40 years apart in the same institution: in 1927 by Professor Miyake Sr and in 1967–1968 by his son, Professor Miyake Jr (Nakayama and Miyake Jr, 1970) (Figure 6). Presently, younger patients have predominantly cholesterol stones in the gallbladder

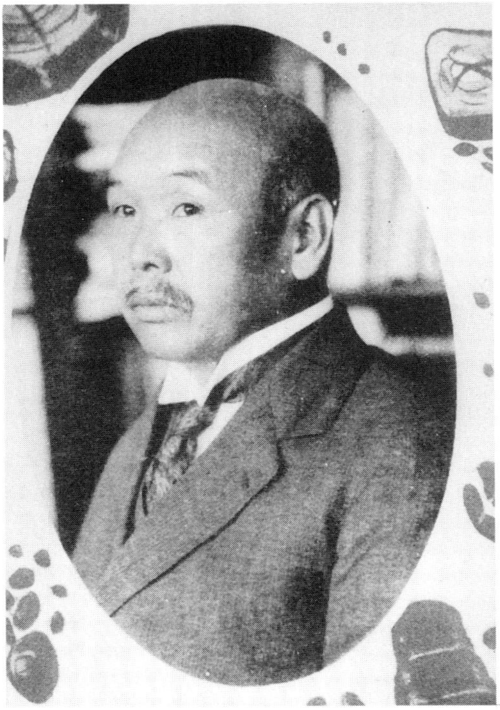

**Figure 4**

Prof. Hayari Miyake, Sr

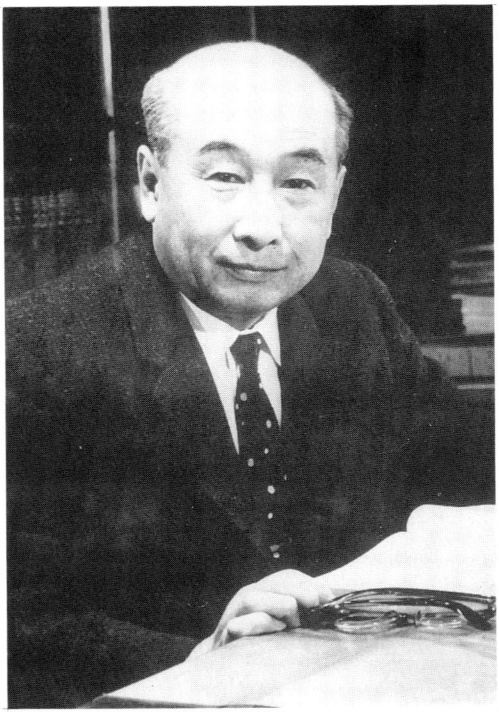

**Figure 5**

Professor Hiroshi Miyake, Jr

only (Nagase et al., 1978). Kameda found that the proportion of cholesterol stones is also very high in Okinawa (Kameda et al., 1981).

## Korea

Ludlow cites the autopsy prevalence of gallstones in Korea to be 2.9 % (Ludlow 1930). Hur, Rice, and Hong, working at Severance Hospital in Seoul, as did Ludlow 40 years before, give a figure of 1.1 % which rises 3.9 % when only those over 10 years old are counted (Hur et al., 1963). These studies may suffer from a low autopsy rate because of the strong antipathy of Koreans to postmortem examination. However, Ringsted, based on the autopsy cases at the National Medical Center (Scandinavian teaching center) in Seoul with an autopsy rates as high as 90 % gives a prevalence of gallstones of 3.8 % (Ringsted 1963). When the rate for those over 15 years of age is taken, the figure becomes 5.0 %. Min did a clinical study of 100 consecutive cases between 1963 and 1965 in Seoul, and found that half of the stones in the gallbladder contained predominantly cholesterol, while the other half contained bilirubin as a major component—probably brown pigment stones or calcium bilirubinate stones (Min et al., 1966). The bilirubin content is highest in intrahepatic duct stones; the bilirubin content of common duct stones is between that of stones in the gallbladder and intrahepatic duct. Those in the common duct without accompanying gallbladder stones are composed of cholesterol 3–10 % (average 12.2 %), calcium, and

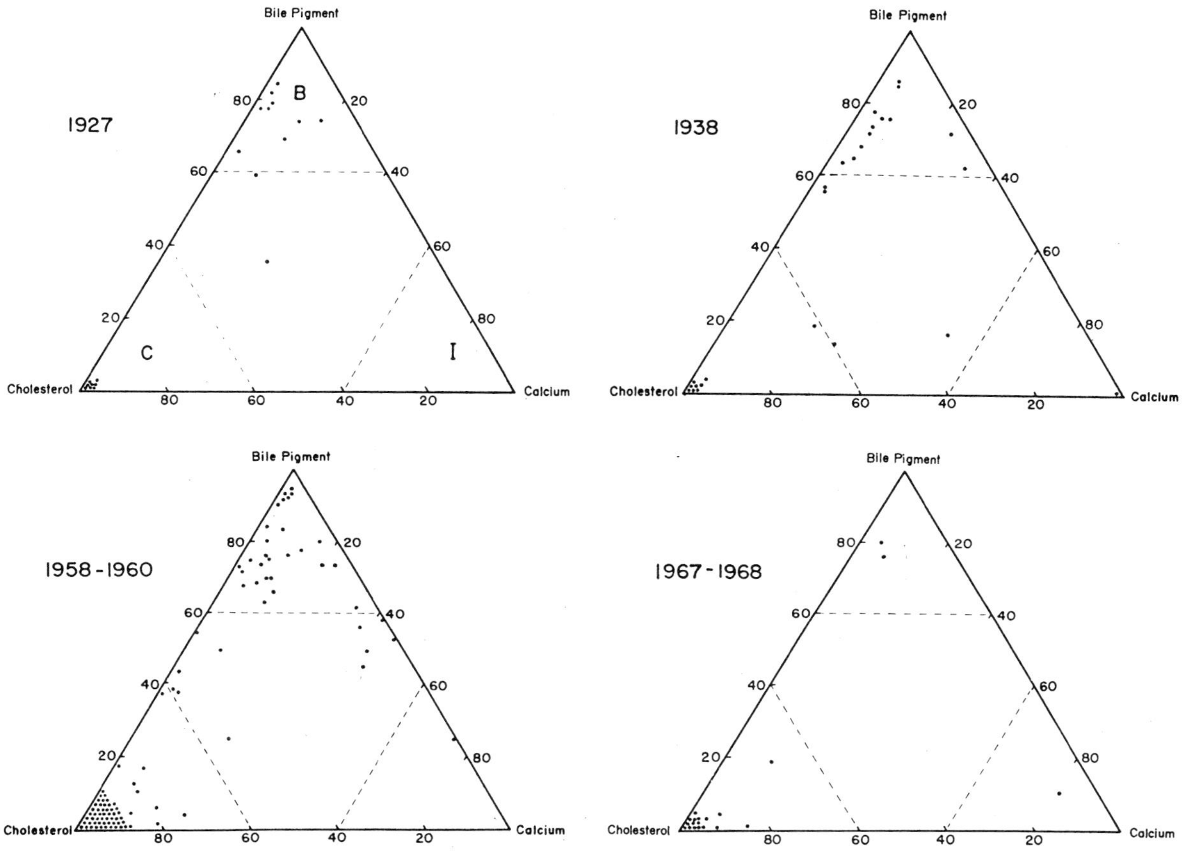


Figure 6

Chronological Changes in Gallstones in Japan (Operated Cases)

The proportion of cholesterol stones increased dramatically after World War II.

Triangular coordinates showing major constituents of gallstones i.e. cholesterol, bile pigment and calcium.

Source: Nakayama and Miyake Jr 1970

bilirubin (55.6%) – apparently brown pigment stones or calcium bilirubinate stones. There is a distinct difference between stones in the gallbladder and those in the common duct. In Min's series in 1966, such stones occurring only in the common duct were encountered in 20% of the cases; this rate is now said to be steadily declining. Gallstones occur in Korea in younger patients. Extracholecystic stones also occur more commonly in younger patients, though the incidence of common duct stones now decreased from 68% (1961–1965) to 42% (1976–1980) (Kwon et al., 1982). The female preponderance of gallstones in Korea is not as pronounced as in the West. The female : male ratio was found to be 1.0 : 1.5 (Hur et al., 1963), 1.0 : 1.2 (Min et al., 1966) and 1.0 : 1.5 to 1.0 : 1.0 (Kwon et al., 1982).

### Malaya

A comparative study of the incidence of operations for biliary disease by King (1971) disclosed that two third are ordinary cholelithiasis and one third are so-called Oriental cholangitis. The latter is the synonym for intrahepatic calculi or hepatolithiasis and is also known as recurrent pyogenic cholangitis (Cook et al., 1954; Ong, 1962), cholangiohepatitis (Fung, 1961) and Chinese biliary obstructive syndrome (Harrison-Levy, 1962). The disease is known to occur frequently in Malaya (Balasegaram, 1972) and is found not only in the Chinese population there but also in Malay, and Indians, as well as in Dayaks in Kalimantan (Borneo) (Ong, 1962). The male : female ratio for ordinary cholelithiasis is reported to be 1.0 : 2.0 and that of Oriental cholangitis to be 1.8 : 1.0 (King, 1971).

### Singapore

A study of 5,957 autopsy cases (1962–1966) in Singapore, mostly of Chinese descent, revealed an overall prevalence of gallstones of 3.1 %. In those over 20 years old it was 6.6 % (Hwang 1970). The sex ratio was about unity.

### Thailand

The prevalence of gallstones in Thailand, based on 1,427 autopsy cases has been reported to be 1.4 % (Stitnimankarn, 1960). When calculated for the two major racial groups, the prevalence for Thais was l.3 % and for Chinese 1.7 %. Male : female ratio of 1.0 : 2.0 was noted. The prevalence in women aged 40 to 49 was 3 %. Clinical cases of cholelithiasis at Siriraj Hospital in Bangkok were analyzed by Pausawasdi et al. (1979). A total of 534 cases were collected from 1970 to 1974. Cholelithiasis constituted 1.7 to 2.1 % of the admissions. A male : female ratio of 1.0 : 1.5 was apparent.

Cholelithiasis in East Asia is characterized by the near equal involvement of both sexes, a high percentage of brown pigment stones or calcium bilirubinate stones, and frequent occurrence of common duct stones, sometimes complicated by recurrent pyogenic cholangitis. However, the situation has changed rapidly in recent years in several countries, such as Japan and Korea.

## Europe

A high prevalence of gallstones, especially in northern Europe, is well known. Autopsy as well as clinical surveys have been carried out since the end of the last century. Therefore, the changing state of gallstone prevalence is well documented. Prospective studies using ultrasonography on general populations have recently been planned and successfully carried out.

### Britain

The prevalence of gallstones was variously reported to be 8.6 % (Cooke et al., 1953), 8.6 % (Horn, 1956), and 15.5 % (Bouchier, 1969). There seems to be a geographical difference within Britain. A national autopsy survey in 1956 showed gallstones to be twice as common in elderly subjects in Glasgow, Scotland as in England (Watkinson, 1967). A prospective study on weighted random samples of a specially enumerated population aged 45 to 69 years in a South Wales industrial town was done with the use of cholecystography (Bainton et al., 1976). The overall prevalence of gallstones was found to be 7.7 % (6.2 % for males and 12.1 % for females). No age-related increase in prevalence was noted probably because of the narrow age range studied.

### Denmark

An autopsy study on 7,974 cases in Copenhagen revealed the crude prevalence of gallstones to be 29.6 % (Teilum and Olsen 1988) and a male : female ratio of 1.0 : 1.6. A significant decrease in the prevalence of gallstone was noted in spite of the increase of elderly persons in the autopsy cases. After a possible peak during the period from 1920 to 1960, the prevalence of gallstones seems to have leveled off. Thus the present prevalence has become similar to the levels of 1889, 1911 and 1920–1921 (Teilum and Olsen 1988). Using newly developed real-time ultrasonography, Jørgensen studied random samples of 4,807 people aged 30–60 years, with a response rate of 78.8 % in Copenhagen. The overall prevalence of gallstones (cases with gallstones and cholecystectomized cases) was 8.5 % (Jørgensen 1987). In a follow-up study, Jørgensen's group used ultrasonography to assess an age- and sex-stratified random Danish population aged 30, 40, 50, and 60 years. They found a mean incidence of gallstones to be 2.1 % for males and 2.5 % for females over a 5-year period (Jensen and Jørgensen 1991). The incidence seems to be higher among adult women before menopause than in men of the same age. The sex difference in the gallstone incidence decreased with increasing age. The incidence is lower before 40 years and subsequently increases to a steady level.

### Finland

Based on the 1,850 autopsy cases representing 70 % of all autopsies in Finland in 1979, Domellof et al. found the prevalence of gallstones for males to be 15.3 % and that of females to be 34.5 % (Domellof et al., 1984). Age-adjusted prevalences were 8.7 % for males and 15.9 % for females. Therefore, the prevalence of gallstones is significantly lower than in Sweden.

### Germany

The prevalence of gallstones, based on the autopsy series of 11,840 cases from 1940 to 1975 at the University of Essen, was described (Balzer et al., 1986). The overall prevalence found was 20.7 % (males 13.1 % and females 33.7 %). The male : female ratio was 1.0 : 2.6. A significant rise in the prevalence was noted in this period, is partly due to the increase in the age group over 60; the authors suspect that no real increase has occurred in the last 30 years. The autopsy prevalence of gallstones in Marburg was reported to be 37.5 % (26.2 % for males and 55.1 % for females) based on the autopsy record of 3,842 cases from 1969 to 1977 (Massarrat et al., 1982).

### Italy

The prevalence of gallstones (with gallstone plus cholecystectomy) in the town of Sirmione (compliance rate of 70.6 %) was examined by Barbara and his colleagues with the use of ultrasonography (Barbara et al., 1987). The crude overall prevalence of gallstones was calculated to be 11.0 % (210/1,092 cases) (6.7 % for males and 14.6 % for females). An age-related increase of gallstones is noted in both sexes. Male (1,739 persons) and female (1,911 persons) civil servants in Rome were subjected to real-time ultrasonography (the participation rate was 71.5 % for males and 75.9 % for females) (Rome Group for Epidemiology and Prevention of Cholelithiasis, 1984, 1988a). The overall prevalence of gallstones was calculated to be 8.2 % for males and 9.4 % for females. An age-related increase in prevalence was apparent in both sexes. Since the populations studied are from the more or less upper socio-economic groups, extrapolation of the results to the general population warrants caution.

### Norway

The autopsy prevalence of gallstones has been studied by Torvik and Høivik using 11,129 cases in Oslo city hospitals from 1952 to 1957, representing 45 % of all deaths in the city of Oslo during this period (Torvik and Høivik, 1960). The overall prevalence of gallstones, including cholecystectomized cases, was 19.5 %. A male : female ratio of 1.0 : 2.1 was noted. The prevalence was found to increase progressively after age 40. A later prospective study on the prevalence of gallstones by ultrasonography, carried out by Glambek et al. on 2,464 persons between ages 20 and 70 with a response rate of 55.6 % showed the crude prevalence of 21.9 % (Glambek et al., 1987). The total age adjusted prevalence was 17.7 % for males and 21.2 % for females. The prevalence increased progressively with age, to as high as 41.3 % in the 60–69 range for females. It is noted that the prevalence found was considerably higher than that in the previous autopsy survey conducted in 1960.

### Romania

The autopsy prevalence of gallstones was reported to be 11.3 % (Acalovschi et al 1987). A recent ultrasound survey of the general population revealed the overall prevalence of gallstones to be 10.9 % and the male : female ratio to be 1 : 2 (Sporea et al., 1993).

### Sweden

Based on the autopsy record of 6,575 cases from 1925 to 1934 and the population census available, Martensson reports that the prevalence of gallstones in the Stockholm area was 10.5 % (Martensson, 1937). He found that gallstones occur more frequently in the rich and fertile district of southern Sweden and less frequently in northern Sweden, with its poorer and more barren areas. According to Zahor et al. the overall prevalence of gallstones in Malmö, in southern Sweden, over 10 years of age, with an autopsy rate of 80–85 % was 37.8 %. The male : female ratio was 1.0 : 1.4 (Zahor et al 1974). In 1977 Lindström carried out an excellent prospective autopsy study on most of the 2,218 residents over 20 years of age in the city of Malmö by personally examinig the hepatobiliary region. He found an overall prevalence of 44 % with 30 % for males and 57 % for females (Lindström,

1977). The highest prevalence was reached in males (57 %) in the 90–99 year range and in females (63 %) above 70. A declining prevalence of gallstones was noted after many years of continuing increase from the decreasing number of cholecystectomies in Sweden. Norrby et al. state that the proportions of cholecystectomies decreased to 57 % during the 10-year period from 1972 to 1980, although the frequency of cholecystectomy is a poor indicator of gallstone prevalence and should only be considered as circumstantial evidence (Norrby et al., 1986). The proportion of symptomatic gallstones also decreased, as evidenced by the decrease in pathological cholecystograms to 35 %. An older group (77–78) of women in Goetheborg, in eastern Sweden, was examined by ultrasonography, with a compliance rate of 91 % (Mellström et al., 1988). The prevalence of gallstones, including previous cholecystectomy, was 51 %. Thus ultrasonography gave a lower figure (51 %) than the autopsy study (63 %) on a similar population in the same district (Lindström, 1977).

# Geographical divergence of gallstone composition

There seems to be a wide variation in the composition of gallstones in different areas. Cholesterol stones have predominated in the West since ancient times (Rains, 1964). In contrast, in the East, brown pigment stones (calcium bilirubinate stones) predominated in the past (Miyake Sr, 1913); however, this situation is rapidly changing with brown pigment stones being replaced by cholesterol stones (Miyake Jr and Johnston, 1968; Nakayama and Miyake Jr, 1970). This difference has generally persisted to the present (Table 5) (Kaufman et al., 1989; Kameda, 1991). Even in predominantly cholesterol stone countries, there is subtle difference in gallstone composition, as revealed by Sutor and Wooley (1971). There is also a great difference within countries such as China and India (Huang, 1987b; Malhotra, 1968)

Table 5

Types of Gallstones in Japan and the United States

| | Japan* | United States† |
|---|---|---|
| Cholesterol stones | 66.9‡ | 66.7 |
| Pigment stones | | |
| Black pigment stones | 9.5 | 25.3 |
| Brown pigment stones | 21.0 | 8.0 |

* Kameda (1991): operative cases from 1969 to 1988.
† Kaufman et al. (1989): operative cases from 1987 to 1988.
‡ Expressed in percent.

# Chronological changes in prevalence

The prevalence of cholesterol stones in Japan has steadily increased especially in the postwar period (Nakayama and Miyake Jr, 1970; Kameda et al., 1980). In Scandinavia there is a decreasing prevalence of gallstones. For instance, the rate of cholecystectomy has been falling in Sweden (Ahlberg et al., 1984; Norrby et al., 1986). Teilum examined the autopsy records in Denmark since 1914 and found that the prevalence of gallstones increased up to 1955 but started to fall after 1959 (Teilum, 1989). The autopsy prevalence of gallstones was compared in Cluj-Napoca, Romania, 100 years apart (Acalovschi et al., 1987). The autopsy records of 1,538 cases in 1873–1882 and of 6,275 cases in 1973–1982 showed that the crude prevalence of 1.2 % in the earlier period increased to 11.3 % in the later period. In the United States, the rate of cholecystectomy changed little between 1970 and 1985, but when the rates are broken down by age group, the prevalence steadily declined under 45 years of age but increased markedly after 65 years (Diehl, 1987). The long-held impression that the composition of gallstones in Japan is gradually changing from the once predominantly brown pigment stones or calcium bilirubinate stones to cholesterol stones, thus approaching that of the West, was confirmed by chemical analysis in the same laboratory on gallstone samples collected in the same department 40 years apart (Figure 6) (Miyake Jr and Johnston, 1968; Nakayama and Miyake Jr, 1970; Nishimura, 1938). Therefore, not only the prevalence but also the composition of gallstones may change chronologically. The change in the prevalence may conceivably be the result of a true change in the incidence of discovered gallstones, as suggested by Heaton (1973).

# Emigration study

Emigration of people may have a great influence on the prevalence of gallstones if environmental factors have a large impact on etiology; by contrast, genetic factors should not change. The increased prevalence of gallstones in the immigrant population of Japanese descent in the United States has been noted (Editorial, 1973). A study on European emigrants, especially those from southern Europe, disclosed an increased risk of gallstones within 2 to 5 years after moving to Australia (Wheeler et al., 1970). A marked change in their nutrient intake on coming to Australia is probably the reason for the increasing incidence of gallstones.

# CHAPTER FOUR

# Pathogenesis of Gallstones

The term gallstone is derived from old English gealla, i.e., bile and stone, and is applied to the concrement formed in the biliary tract, including the gallbladder and bile duct. As explained earlier (Chapter I), gallstones are classified into several groups, and each group seems to have a different pathogenesis. Therefore, they will be dealt with separately, starting with the most common cholesterol stones. Many circumstances in the formation of abnormal bile have been identified, but the proximate causes of gallstones are far from clear at present. Several excellent reviews on the pathogenesis of gallstones are available (Bennion et al., 1978b; Fisher et al., 1979; Small, 1982; Holzbach, 1983a; Okuda et al., 1984; Cohen and Soloway, 1985; Wolpers, 1987; Hofmann, 1988; Bouchier, 1988; Cooper and Young, 1989; Swobodnik et al., 1990; Shaffer, 1992)

## Composition of Bile

Since gallstones are formed in bile from bile constituents, the composition of bile will be discussed first followed by the role of its constituents in gallstone formation. Total solid in bile is said to be 2–3 per cent for hepatic bile and 10–15 per cent for gallbladder bile, as hepatic bile is concentrated 5 to 10 times after entering the gallbladder. The major solid is composed of cholesterol (mostly free), phospholipids (mostly phosphatidyl choline, i.e., lecithin), bile acids, free fatty acids, calcium, carbonate, and proteins (Hofmann et al., 1982) (Table 6).

### Cholesterol

Cholesterol (Figure 7) in bile is mostly in free form with a very small portion in esterified form (Nakayama and Johnston, 1962) and is reported to be present as cholesterol monohydrate (Renshaw et al., 1983). Other sterols are also present, but only in small amounts (5–10%) (Lin et al., 1984; Miettinen et al., 1986). Their role in gallstone formation is yet to be determined (Ilias et al., 1980). Noncholesterol sterols present in human bile are cholestanol, sitosterol, lathosterol, campesterol, stigmasterol, and desmos-

Table 6

**Biliary Lipid Composition in Man—National Cooperative Gallstone Study**

| Biliary lipid class | |
|---|---|
| Bile acid* | 70.5 + 5.8 |
| Phospholipids* | 20.6 + 4.6 |
| Cholesterol* | 8.8 + 2.7 |
| Cholesterol/phospholipids | 0.45 + 0.19 |
| Cholesterol/bile acid | 0.13 + 0.05 |
| Phospholipids/bile acid | 0.30 + 0.09 |
| Cholesterol saturation, percent | 137.5 + 42.0 |

* Expressed in mol percent.

Source: Hofmann et al. (1982).

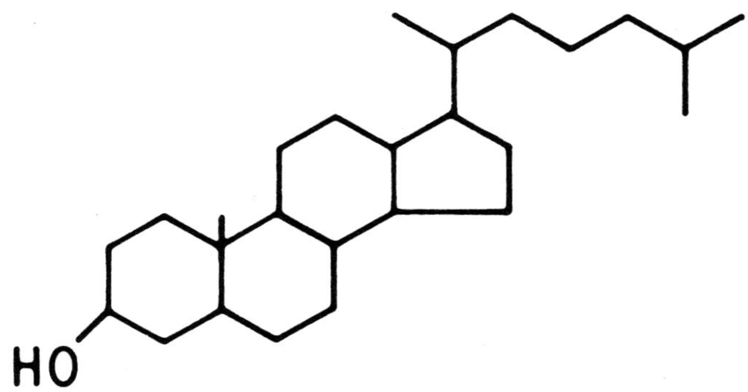

CHOLESTEROL

**Figure 7**

Cholesterol

terol, in this order of decreasing concentraton (Lin et al., 1984). The majority of biliary cholesterol is ultimately derived from plasma low density lipoproteins (LDL). LDL is taken up by the hepatocytes via hepatic membrane ligands, apolipoproteins B-100 and E receptors (Brown and Goldstein, 1984). Only 2–16 per cent of biliary cholesterol is derived from newly synthesized cholesterol (Robins et al., 1993a). It is suggested that biliary cholesterol derives from a special metabolically active pool of cholesterol within the liver and that the availability of this precursor pool determines the magnitude of biliary cholesterol secretion (Stone et al., 1985; Nervi et al., 1988). This precursor pool for biliary cholesterol may reside in the periportal hepatocytes that stain positive for 3-hydroxy-3-methylglutaryl-CoA reductase (HMG-CoA reductase) (Robins et al., 1993a).

## Phospholipids

Phospholipids in bile comprise 15–25 % of total lipids in bile and are mostly (over 95

%) composed of phosphatidyl choline (PC), i.e., lecithin (Figure 8) (Johnston et al., 1939; Philips, 1960; Nakayama and Blomstrand, 1961; Balint et al., 1965; Alvaro et al., 1986a) with small amount of phosphatidyl ethanolamine, sphingomyelin and lysolecithin (lysophosphatidyl choline) (Nakayama and Blomstrand, 1961). Lecithin is an amphiphilic molecule containing both positive and negative charges, with a hydrophilic group and two hydrophobic hydrocarbon chains. The major molecular species of lecithin in human bile are the least hydrophobic 16:0, 18:2 (40–60 %), 16:0, 18:0 (5–25 %), 18:0, 18:2 (1–16 %) and 16:0, 20:4 (1–10 %) (Alvaro et al., 1986a). Using rat liver perfusion with palmitoleic acid (16:1) and [2–$^3$H] glycerol, and then using 17:1 fatty acid and nonradiolabeled glycerol, Patton et al., found that one-third of the 16:1–16:1 and two-third of other 16:1–containing molecular species of phosphatidyl choline are synthesized by acyl remodeling of pre-existing phosphatidyl cholines, while most 16:1–17:1 phosphatidyl choline is synthesized by acyl remodeling of 16:1 phosphatidyl choline synthesized during the labeling period (Patton et al., 1994). The physicochemical properties of these different molecular species of lecithin should be taken into account when dealing with the formation of gallstones. Lysolecithin is present in human bile in a very small amount (0.5 % of total phospholipids), but a small degree (less than 2 %) of hydrolysis takes place even in a frozen state at −20°C to form lysolecithin (Hay et al 1993).

## Bile acids

Bile acid (Figure 9) in human bile constitutes two-third of biliary solids (Carey and Cahalane, 1988a) and is present with a side chain, mostly in conjugated or amidated form, with glycine or taurine at the terminal carboxyl group in a ratio of 3:1 (Sjövall, 1959), which supplies pH-resistant carboxyl and sulfonic groups. Only a very small proportion (0.1–0.2 % of total bile acids) appears as free, unconjugated bile acid in bile (Matoba et al.,

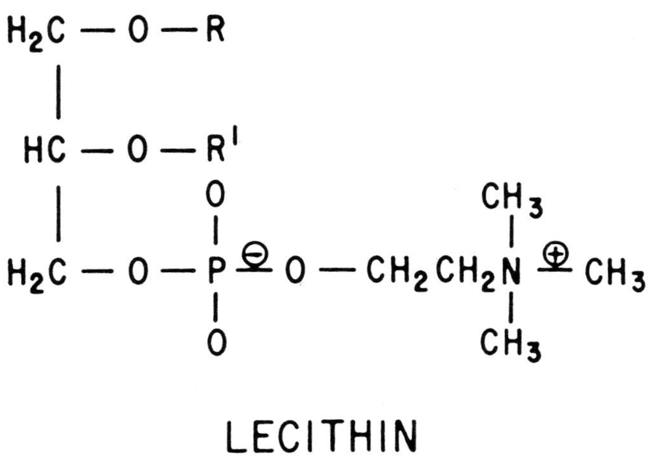


**Figure 8**

Phosphatidyl choline (Lecithin)

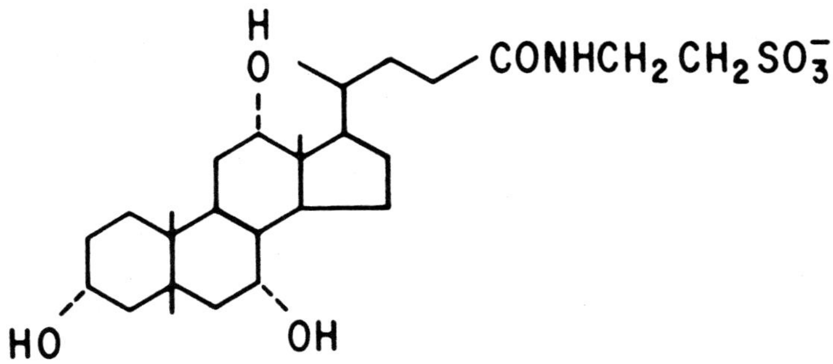


CONJUGATED BILE ACID
*(TAUROCHOLATE)*

**Figure 9**

Bile Acid (Taurocholate)

1986). On a Stuart-Briegleb model, hydroxyl groups and charged side chain lie contiguously on the hydrophilic surface of the molecule, and the bulky hydrophobic steroid hydrocarbon part lies on the opposite side. The amino acid moiety is deconjugated by bacterial conjugated bile acid hydrolase in the intestinal tract before modification of the steroid nucleus. The unconjugated (free) bile acid formed is well absorbed by passive membrane diffusion mainly in the colon (Fujii et al., 1988). The bile acid part is composed of primary bile acid (formed in liver), i.e., cholic acid ($3\alpha$, $7\alpha$, $12\alpha$-trihydroxycholanoic acid) and chenodeoxycholic acid ($3\alpha$, $7\alpha$-dihydroxycholanoic acid) and secondary bile acid (bacterial products of primary bile acid formed by $7\alpha$-dehydroxylation in the intestinal tract), i.e., deoxycholic acid ($3\alpha$, $12\alpha$-dihydroxycholanoic acid) formed from cholic acid, lithocholic acid ($3\alpha$-hydroxycholanoic acid) formed from chenodeoxycholic acid, and 7-oxolithocholic acid (Hofmann et al., 1982) (Table 7). Ursodeoxycholic acid, $3\alpha$, $7\beta$-dihydroxycholanoic acid (the $7\beta$-epimer of chenodeoxycholic acid), present in small amounts in human bile, is considered a tertiary bile acid, as it is formed mainly by intestinal flora from

**Table 7**

**Bile Acid Composition in Human Bile***

| Bile acid | Value (%)* |
|---|---|
| Cholic acid ($3\alpha$, $7\alpha$, $12\alpha$) | 32.4 + 8.8 |
| Chenodeoxycholic acid ($3\alpha$, $7\alpha$) | 39.4 + 9.6 |
| Deoxycholic acid ($3\alpha$, $12\alpha$) | 25.4 + 11.6 |
| Ursodeoxycholic acid ($3\alpha$, $7\beta$) | 1.7 + 1.92 |

* Expressed in weight percent.

Source: Hofmann et al. (1982).

7-oxolithocholic acid (3$\alpha$-hydroxy-7-ketocholanoic acid), which, in turn, is formed from chenodeoxycholic acid by 7$\alpha$-dehydrogenation. Bile acid sulfated (bile acid sulfate ester) at positions 3 (mostly), 7, and 12 has been known to be excreted in bile but only in a small amount. In healthy men only lithocholic acid is extensively sulfated; it can be considered a detoxication mechanism of otherwise hepatotoxic lithocholic acid. Its role in gallstone formation is considered to be small. Other occasionally present bile acids are allocholic acid (3$\alpha$, 7$\alpha$, 12$\alpha$-trihydroxy-5$\alpha$-cholan-24-oic acid), ursocholic acid (3$\alpha$, 7$\beta$, 12$\alpha$-trihydroxy-5$\beta$-cholan-24-oic acid), and glycosylated bile acid especially glucose conjugated bile acid. However, these acids are present in bile in only minute amounts, and their role in gallstone formation is yet to be determined. Conversion of cholesterol to bile acids starts with nuclear transformation, followed by shortening of the steroid side chain. An alternate pathway, though minor, may exist where some or most of the changes in the steroid side chain precede the changes in the nucleus; this has been reviewed recently (Björkhem, 1992). Bile acids are synthesized in peripheral cells of hepatic acini; transported to periportal cells, inducing bile acid-dependent flow and biliary lipid secretion; and then enter bile canaliculi via the canals of Hering. There is said to be a bile acid transport pathway in hepatocytes directly to bile canaliculi. Most bile salt is secreted as a monomer but forms simple micelles in bile canaliculi. Bile acid-independent flow is nearly or completely absent in man (Erlinger, 1988). The physicochemical state of bile acid is influenced by its aqueous solubility, critical micellar concentration, critical micellar temperature, aggregation number, and cholesterol and lecithin solubility, as well as by the number, position, orientation, sulfation of hydroxyl groups and by conjugation at the side chain and the state of ionization. The physicochemical properties of commonly occurring bile acids have been reviewed recently (Hofmann and Mysels, 1992). Taurine conjugates are soluble at strongly acidic pH, and glycine conjugates are poorly soluble at moderately acidic pH; unconjugates are insoluble in water medium at neutral pH. In vivo conjugated bile acids are present in micellar form in the biliary tract and in the intestinal tract, while unconjugated bile acids formed in the large intestine remain at low monomeric concentration because of the acidic pH of the proximal colon, binding to bacteria and/or being removed by passive absorption across the intestinal mucosa. Precipitation of the calcium salt of common natural conjugated bile acids usually does not occur in healthy persons.

## Bilirubin

Bilirubin in bile is mostly conjugated with glucuronic acid. It is present as bilirubin diglucuronide (BDG) and, in much smaller amounts, as bilirubin monoglucuronide (BMG), as well as glucoside and xyloside conjugates (Spivak and Yuey, 1986, Keida et al., 1991). No internal hydrogen bond is formed. These conjugates are much more soluble in bile at physiological pH than is unconjugated bilirubin (UCB), which is usually present only in small amount. In contrast, carboxyl groups in UCB molecules are, when protonated, are internally hydrogen bonded to the pyrrol rings (Schmid, 1978; Yang et al., 1993) and not exposed to the aqueous environment and therefore are not water soluble (Figure 10).

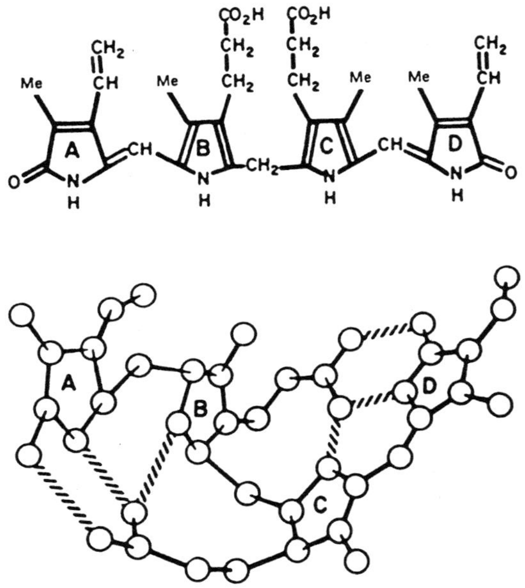

Figure 10

Intramolecular Hydrogen Bonding in Bilirubin Molecule (Schmid, 1978)

(From Schmid R: Bilirubin metabolism: state of the art. Gastroenterology 74: 1307–1312, 1978 with the kind permission of the author)

## Calcium

Calcium is a major divalent cation present in bile. It binds calcium-sensitive anions such as carbonate, phosphate, unconjugated bilirubin, and fatty acid.

## Proteins

Apolipoproteins, the protein constituents of plasma lipoproteins, are secreted into bile. Apolipoproteins A-I and A-II, the major apoproteins of high density lipoproteins (HLD), apolipoproteins C-I and C-II, major apoproteins of very low density lipoproteins (VLDL) and apolipoprotein B, a major apoprotein of low density lipoprotein (LDL) are identified in human gallbladder and hepatic bile using radioimmunoassay (Sewell et al., 1983). Their concentrations are found to be up to 10 % of their plasma levels.

# Physiology of the gallbladder

The gallbladder concentrates calcium and bile acid in parallel and acidifies bile by hydrogen ion secretion (Marteau et al., 1990; Shiffman et al., 1990). Bicarbonate is absorbed indirectly as a consequence of hydrogen secretion by the gallbladder via $Na^+$-$H^+$ exchange. The pH is lower in gallbladder bile than in hepatic bile (6.96 vs. 7.30), total

$[CO_2]$ is lower (14.1 vs 21.6 mmol/L), $P_{CO_2}$ is higher (53.8 vs 40.2 mm Hg) and $[CO_3^{2-}]$ is lower (2.52 vs. 6.11 × 105 mol/L) (Gleeson et al 1992). Gallbladder bile has a lower $[Ca^{2+}] \times [CO_3^{2-}]$ ion product (1.88 vs. $4.74 \times 10^{-8}$ mol/L) than hepatic bile (Gleeson et al., 1992). The pH of gallbladder bile correlates positively with total $[CO_2]$, $[CO_3^{2-}]$, and $[Ca^{2+}] \times [CO_3^{2-}]$ but negatively with $P_{CO_2}$.

Gallbladder contraction is regulated by diverse neurohormonal mechanisms, i.e., neural regulation via the parasympathetic pathway, causing contraction of the gallbladder, and via the sympathetic pathway, causing relaxation and hormonal regulation by cholecystokinin (CCK), motilin, endogenous opiates, pancreatic polypeptides (PP), and somatostatin. An excellent review of the subject is available (Everson, 1991). Ingestion of meals, especially fat, is the most potent stimulus to the intestinal release of CCK. Gastric emptying influences gallbladder contraction by regulating the pattern and rate of delivery of the meal to the upper small intestine. However, the gallbladder contracts not only in the postprandial period but also in the interdigestive or fasting period. The bile acid pool stored in the gallbladder after the overnight fast ranges from 60% to 90% (Everson et al., 1981; Lanzini et al., 1987 Lanzini and Northfield 1990). The gallbladder and sphincter of Oddi smooth muscle have unique reciprocal regulation, i.e., a stimulus which contracts the gallbladder relaxes the sphincter of Oddi to force bile into the duodenum.

# Cholesterol Stones

The concept of the pathogenesis of cholesterol gallstones has shifted between hepatogenic (identifying the liver as the primary site of derrangement) and cystogenic theory (focusing on the gallbladder). As stated earlier, Naunyn held that inflammation of the gallbladder and its sequelae is the primary event in the formation of gallbladder stones (Naunyn, 1892)—the cystogenic theory. At the beginning of the twentieth century, Aschoff and Bacmeister held that excessive secretion of cholesterol by the liver is the primary cause of radial cholesterol gallstones (Radiäre Cholesterinsteine) (Aschoff and Bacmeister 1909)—the hepatogenic theory. In the 1960s, following an investigation by Admirand and Small (1968), secretion of supersaturated or lithogenic bile by the liver and solubilization of cholesterol by mixed micelles of bile acid and phospholipids were held to be responsible. In the 1980s, the importance of choleserol rich phospholipids-cholesterol vesicles (Sömjen and Gilat, 1986) was emphasized in the nucleation of cholesterol monohydrate crystals (Halpern et al., 1986a). Now the pendulum seems to be swinging back toward cystogenic theory as the hypersecretion of mucin in the gallbladder has been found to begin long before the increase of cholesterol saturation in bile and the subsequent appearance of cholesterol monohydrate crystals (Freston et al., 1969; Lee et al., 1981b). Mucin, a high molecular weight glycoprotein, not only accelerates heterogeneous nucleation of cholesterol monohydrate crystals but also provides a trap for cholesterol monohydrate crystals to grow. Thus, the stages of cholesterol gallstone formation can conveniently be divided into (1) hepatic secretion of bile supersaturated with cholesterol; (2) accelerated nucleation and precipitation of cholesterol monohydrate crystals affected by pronucleating and antinucleating factors; and (3) agglomeration and growth of nascent cholesterol crystals to macroscopic gallstones. Gallbladder stasis provides the time necessary for these dynamic processes to occur, i.e., precipitation, retention, and subsequent growth of cholesterol monohydrate crystals into gallstones. Impaired gallbladder motility may be considered a pivotal adjunct to cholesterol gallstone formation.

# Formation of Supersaturated (Lithogenic) Bile

Ever since the discovery of the in vivo synthesis of cholesterol by the balance studies (Schoenheimer and Breusch, 1933) and by radiolabeled precursor studies (Bloch and Rittenberg, 1942) and in vivo conversion of cholesterol to cholic acid by a study using tritium labeled cholesterol (Bloch et al., 1943), cholesterol-bile acid metabolism has been thought to be of great importance in the formation of gallstones. In spite of having one hydrophilic hydroxyl group, cholesterol is practically insoluble in water because of its bulky hydrocarbon steroid nucleus. Aqueous solubility of monomeric cholesterol monohydrate is said to be $10^{-8}$ M ($2.6 \times 10^{-8}$ M at 20°C) (Lee et al., 1987a). Therefore, nature devised a mean(s) of transporting this water-insoluble compound safely to the gastrointestinal tract after it moves from the liver to bile canaliculi. However, this useful mechanism becomes disrupted under certain circumstances and cholesterol is precipitated out, leading to the formation of gallstones. First, we consider the homeostasis of major bile constituents in order to aid our understanding of the mechanism underlying the formation of supersaturated bile to consider the pathogenesis of gallstone formation on a metabolic basis.

## Homeostasis of cholesterol

Homeostasis of cholesterol, a major constituent of cholesterol gallstones, is quite important to the body and is the net result of all inputs and outputs, the former from endogenous synthesis and absorption of dietary cholesterol which are tightly interregulated and the latter by conversion to bile acid in the liver and the direct secretion of unaltered cholesterol in bile, with subsequent fecal excretion and only a small amount converted to steroid hormones followed by excretion in urine—the bulk of cholesterol loss occurring via bile. Apparently 40% of removal of cholesterol occurs by its conversion to bile acid (Vlahcevic et al., 1991). The liver synthesizes half of the body's cholesterol and plays a major role in the homeostasis of cholesterol, being quantitatively the major site of lipoprotein uptake, one of the two sites of lipoprotein formation, synthesizing bile acid from cholesterol and secreting cholesterol in bile.

### Mobilization of cholesterol

The concept of reverse cholesterol transport is invoked to explain the mechanism of cholesterol mobilization from extrahepatic sources (Tall, 1990). The free cholesterol hydrolyzed reaches the cell membranes, is removed by HDL, and is reesterified by serum lecithin-cholesterol acyl transferase (LCAT). A place occupied in the cell membrane and on HDL is freed for the removal of another molecule of free cholesterol generated from the storage pool. Cholesterol ester from HDL is transferred to LDL and VLDL and is delivered to the liver as a result of the hepatic uptake of these particles (Tall and Small 1978). The role of the liver in homeostasis of cholesterol and LDL has been reviewed recently (Dietschy et al., 1993). Uptake of LDL is regulated by the activity of the hepatic LDL receptors (Goldstein et al., 1985; Harvel 1986). Lovastatin, which enhances LDL receptor activity in the liver, has been shown to increase the hepatic uptake of LDL in men (Kervinen et al., 1993). In the liver, the receptor is located along the basolateral membranes and is internalized after binding lipoproteins (Pathak et al., 1990). About 70% of LDL degradation takes place in the liver—of which 80% depends on the LDL receptor (Spady et al., 1985a). LDL receptors are regulated by the cholesterol flux. The primary response to a change in cholesterol availability in hepatocytes is an alteration in cholesterol synthesis. When the capacity of this compensatory mechanism is exceeded, changes in receptor-dependent LDL occur (Spady et al., 1985b). Coordinate regulation of LDL receptor uptake and cholesterol synthesis is demonstrated by the tissue culture technique. Transcription of the LDL receptor gene regulates synthesis of the LDL receptor, which, in turn, controls the number of LDL receptors expressed by a hepatocyte to meet the cholesterol requirement. The half-life of LDL receptor is said to be 24 hours, but cholesterol synthesis responds over a much shorter period. Lipoproteins are rapidly dissociated from the receptor and brought to lysosomes, where their constituents are degraded. Choelsterol ester, the primary constituent of LDL, is hydrolyzed to free cholesterol, to be utilized further. Excess cholesterol is reesterified and stored as cholesterol ester. Thus, cholesterol exists in the liver both in free unesterified form and as fatty acid ester, with the majority being free cholesterol. The level of free cholesterol in the liver is also a function of the rate of cholesterol esterification. Storage of excess cholesterol in a form of cholesterol esters is regulated by acyl:CoA cholesterol-acyl transferase (ACAT) and neutral cholesterol hydrolase.

## Synthesis of cholesterol

Cholesterol is synthesized from a single functional compartment inside hepatocytes (Figure 11). HMG-CoA reductase, a rate-limiting enzyme of the synthesis of cholesterol from acetate, is regulated by the enzyme synthesis, by its degradation, and possibly by a rapid activation/inactivation mechanism (Beg et al., 1987). The short-term stability of HMG-CoA reductase is affected by the sterol, i.e., the half-life of the enzyme protein is greatly shortened by an increased sterol load to reduce cholesterol synthesis (Bell et al., 1976). Long-term changes are regulated by the enzyme synthesis controlled by the rate of transcription of mRNA for the enzyme (Nakanishi et al., 1988), which, in turn, is regulated by binding of the transcription factors to the regulatory region of the HMG-CoA reductase gene (Osborne et al., 1987). Human liver seems to respond to an enhanced demand for cholesterol by expressing more LDL receptors and increasing cholesterol synthesis. The capacity of the response is larger for the synthesis of HMG-CoA reductase than for the synthesis of LDL receptors. Cholesterol content in the liver is controlled by

Acetyl-CoA
|
β-Hydroxy-β-methyl-glutaryl-CoA
| HMG-CoA reductase
Mevalonate
|
Squalene
|
Cholesterol

**Figure 11**

Synthetic Pathway of Cholesterol

homeostatic mechanisms with up- or down-regulation of LDL receptor number, cholesterol synthesis through HMG-CoA reductase, and storage of excess cholesterol as ACAT-generated cholesterol ester. The coordination of lipoprotein uptake and cholesterol synthesis maintains a constant supply of cholesterol and avoids acute overloading or shortage, and is said to be based on the common regulatory region of the gene encoding (Esser et al., 1988).

### Secretion of cholesterol

Part of the cholesterol in the liver is secreted into bile as such, a process coupled with secretion of bile acids, and part is converted to bile acid. The latter constitutes approximately 40 % of total cholesterol removal (Vlahcevic et al., 1991). Expansion of hepatic cholesterol pool for biliary secretion is effected by the increased input from de novo synthesis of cholesterol and lipoprotein uptake and decreased disposition from de novo bile acid and cholesterol ester synthesis. In older studies, both obesity and administration of chenodeoxycholic acid result in parallel changes in cholesterol synthesis and biliary cholesterol secretion (Bennion and Grundy, 1975; Key et al., 1980). However, the majority of biliary cholesterol is preformed and is not from de novo intrahepatocyte synthesis (Turley et al., 1981, 1983; Robins and Brunengraber, 1982; Robins et al., 1993a). The rate of biliary cholesterol secretion is determined both by the species and by the rates of bile acid and biliary phosphlipid secretion (Robins and Armstrong, 1976; Turley et al., 1979; Carulli et al., 1984; Bilhartz and Dietschy, 1988). Diurnal cycling influences the contribution of newly formed cholesterol. In mid-light, when cholesterol synthesis is at a low point, biliary cholesterol is more dependent on bile salt and phospholipid secretion than in mid-dark, when cholesterol synthesis is high, biliary cholesterol secretion is not significantly related to bile salt secretion, and is less significantly related to phosphlipid secretion (Robins et al., 1993b). Increased cholesterol secretion at mid-dark occurs in response to increased cholesterol synthesis. It is suggested that biliary cholesterol derives from a special metabolically active pool of cholesterol within the liver (Stone et al., 1985; Nervi et al., 1988). Availability of free cholesterol in this precursor pool regulated by intrahepatic cholesterol synthesis, plasma lipoproteins, and esterification rates also determines the magnitude of biliary cholesterol secretion (Stone et al., 1985). The site of this precursor pool seems to be the periportal hepatocytes that stain positive for HMG-CoA reductase (Robins et al., 1993a). With an increase in hepatic cholesterol synthesis, the specific activity of cholesterol in bile remains constant. In vivo radiolabeled preformed cholesterol injected into the rat appears in bile, rapidly bypassing the intrahepatic compartment (Robins and Brunengraber, 1982). A more recent study in the rat in which newly synthesized cholesterol and preformed cholesterol were separately labeled and traced separately showed that newly synthesized cholesterol is not evenly distributed throughout the liver but is preferentially secreted into bile (Robins et al., 1985). Newly synthesized cholesterol in bile originates from the interior of the hepatocyte. Increased levels of total (Kawata et al., 1991) and free cholesterol in liver microsomes (Sahlin et al., 1992) and cytosol (Smith et al., 1990) and nonspecific lipid transfer protein concentration (Kawata et al., 1991) are noted in cholesterol stone patients. Preformed cholesterol, in near-complete equilibrium in the whole liver and bile, seems to be transported directly from blood through the plasma membrane of the hepatocytes and secreted from the canalicules without first entering the interior of hepatocytes and mixing with newly synthesized cholesterol. Therefore, hepatic cholesterol synthesis and biliary cholesterol secretion may be independently regulated. In fact, large changes in cholesterol synthesis fail to produce any change in the magnitude of biliary cholesterol secretion (Turley and Dietschy, 1979; Ahlberg et al., 1981a). Cholesterol secretion was virtually unchanged after the acute lowering of cholesterol synthesis by a single dose of lovastatin, an inhibitor of HMG-CoA reductase, but fell considerably only during chronic lovastatin treatment (Mitchell et al., 1991a). Cholesterol synthesis seems to affect biliary cholesterol secretion, but the effect is not immediate and therefore may be indirect. Unlike human subjects with an interrupted enterohepatic circulation (Schwartz et al., 1978b), there appears to be little if any preferential secretion of newly synthesized cholesterol in normal human subjects (Mitchell et al., 1991b). No precursor-product relationship between hepatic synthesis of cholesterol and biliary cholesterol can be elicited (Gregory et al., 1975). Only 20–30% of biliary cholesterol input is derived from the newly synthesized cholesterol (Schwartz et al., 1978b). Hepatic cholesterol esterification is suggested to be one of the major intrahepatic determinant of the size of the biliary cholesterol precursor pool (Nervi et al., 1984). In the rat, cholesterol secreted in VLDL and biliary cholesterol are derived from a common pool regulated by hepatic cholesterol synthesis and esterification (Stone and Evans., 1992). This common bile/VLDL cholesterol secretory pool may be functionally distinct from the cholesterol pool for bile acid synthesis or availability of free cholesterol in this common biliary cholesterol, and the VLDL cholesterol precursor pool is not a major determinant of bile acid synthesis. Smith et al. maintain that an increase in hepatic HMG-CoA reductase activity and a decrease in ACAT activity in patients with cholesterol stones result in an increase of the biliary cholesterol precursor pool of free cholesterol (Smith et al., 1990). The reported negative correlation beween serum cholesterol and the presence of cholesterol stones may be explained by a common pool of cholesterol available for excretion into either plasma or bile (Thijs et al., 1990). Progestational agents inhibiting cholesterol esterification (Nervi et al., 1983) may be lithogenic. In the rat, biliary cholesterol output is well correlated with the ACAT activity in a reciprocal manner.

## Homeostasis of bile acid

Homeostasis of bile acid is maintained by enterohepatic circulation and regulation of the rate of synthesis.

### Enterohepatic circulation of bile acid

Enterohepatic circulation of bile acid consists of hepatic and intestinal phases (Figure 12). Bile acids secreted in bile are almost entirely conjugated either glycine or taurine with amide linkage (Matoba et al., 1986) which reduces pK and thereby increases their solubility at physiological pH of intestinal tract. When bile salts are not ionized, they become lipophilic and undergo passive absorption in the intestinal tract. Ionization depends on the pKa of bile salt and the pH of the environment. Taurocholate, with the highest pKa of 2.2, is almost entirely ionized and actively absorbed, while the least polar glycodeoxycholate undergoes passive absorption to a considerable extent. Bile salts not absorbed in the small intestine are subjected to bacterial degradation by intestinal flora and are subsequently absorbed (Fujii et al., 1988). Overall efficiency of the enterohepatic circulation is over 95 % per pass. The bile acid pool of around 2.5 g, cycling two times per meal and more than six times per day, is well preserved. Thus, total hepatic secretion amounts to 15 g, with a loss of 0.5 g/day. The increased loss is compensated for by the increase in bile acid synthesis up to 5 g/day (Dowling et al., 1970). Bile salts in portal blood are bound to albumin and brought to the liver. Uptake in the liver takes place in the periportal area and is active,

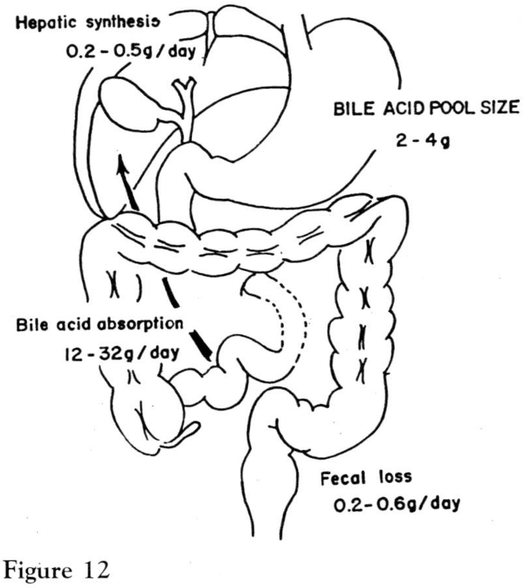


**Figure 12**

Enterohepatic Circulation of Bile Acid

sodium-dependent, and perhaps catalyzed by proteins (Von Dippe et al., 1982).

## Synthesis of bile acid

In hepatocytes, bile salt is bound to a variety of bile salt-binding proteins (LeBlanc and Waxman, 1990). The bile salt-protein complex may control the rates of bile acid synthesis and vesicle formation. Bile salt is secreted by an active, energy-requiring process. Transit of bile salt via hepatocytes is quick and quite efficient. The liver is the sole site of bile acid synthesis and bile salt is the major solubilizer of cholesterol in bile. Bile acid synthesis consists of three steps: (1) nuclear transformation, i.e., hydroxylation at the $7\alpha$ and $12\alpha$ positions, followed by (2) hydroxylation at the 26 or 27 positions and (3) shortening of the side chain of cholesterol by mitochondrial enzymes – this last step has been reviewed recently (Björkhem, 1992). The major synthetic pathway from cholesterol to bile acid begins with hydroxylation at the $7\alpha$ position, which is the rate-limiting step controlled by cholesterol $7\alpha$-hydroxylase belonging to cytochrome P-450 enzymes (Figure 13). Subsequent $12\alpha$-hydroxylation by cholesterol $12\alpha$-hydroxylase determines whether cholic acid or chenodeoxycholic acid is synthesized. Obligatory intermediates in the major pathway for the biosynthesis of cholic acid and chenodeoxycholic acid are $3\alpha$, $7\alpha$, $12\alpha$-trihydroxy-$5\beta$-cholestanoic acid (THCA) and $3\alpha$, $7\alpha$-dihydroxy-$5\beta$-cholestanoic acid (DHCA). Oxidative cleavage of the side chain of these intermediates entails $\omega$-oxidation followed by $\beta$-oxydation to yield C-24 carboxylic acid, and side chain cleavages in cholic acid and chenodeocycholic acid are found to be identical (Une et al., 1994). Alternate pathway for cholic acid synthesis involves a microsomal 25-hydroxylation and accounts for less than

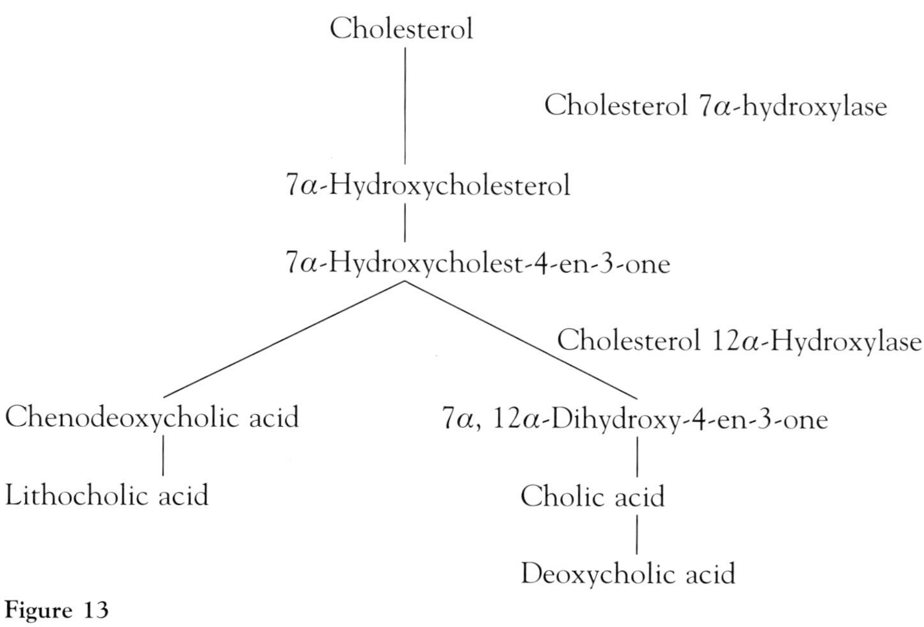


**Figure 13**

Key Enzymes in Bile Acid Synthesis

5 % of cholic acid synthesis in man (Duane et al., 1988b). The other minor mitochondrial pathway operates first by hydroxylation at the 27 position (Fredrickson and Ono, 1956; Anderson et al., 1972), followed by hydroxylation at the $7\alpha$ position controlled by 27-hydroxycholesterol $7\alpha$-hydroxylase, which is said to be distinctly different from the more familiar cholesterol $7\alpha$-hydroxylase (Martin et al., 1993). In man, $7\alpha$-hydroxycholesterol and 27-hydroxycholesterol are metabolized to preferentially cholic and chenodeoxycholic acids respectively (Anderson et al., 1972).

### Feedback control

A rate-limiting enzyme for the synthesis of bile acid from cholesterol, cholesterol $7\alpha$-hydroxylase, representing a major control point for removal of cholesterol from the body, is dynamic and has a very short half-life belonging to a member of the P-450 group with a very short half-life of 2 to 3 hours (Danielsson and Wikvall, 1981). It has recently been purified and its DNA sequence determined (Noshiro and Okuda, 1990). The enzyme is controlled by several factors, i.e., feedback control by bile acid, mainly by hydrophobic bile acids (Heuman et al., 1988, 1989), a cholesterol substrate pool, a protein regulator (Coleman, 1987), and a phosphorylation reaction (Sanghvi et al., 1981). Negative feedback control of bile acid synthesis by hepatic bile acid flux is known to be present. A recent study on the activity, mass, and catalytic efficiency of hepatic cholesterol $7\alpha$-hydroxylase in a rat with bile fistula, a key microsomal enzyme for the conversion of cholesterol to bile acid, showed that bile acid infusion at a rate of hepatic bile acid flux, after temporary interruption of the enterohepatic circulation of bile acid, lowered the enzyme activity and mass, thus providing clear evidence that bile acid synthesis is modulated by the catalytic efficiency and mass of hepatic cholesterol $7\alpha$-hydroxylase (Shefer et al., 1991). Hepatic bile acid depletion increases bile acid synthesis mainly by activating cholesterol $7\alpha$-hydroxylase, with only a small rise in enzyme mass. When cholesterol is available, as in a case of mevalonolactone supplementation, the infusion of taurocholate results in the formation of catalytically less active cholesterol $7\alpha$-hydroxylase. In a follow-up study from the same laboratory using rabbits, Xu et al. found that glycocholic or glycodeoxycholic acids inhibit bile acid synthesis as much as 40 %, the amount of inhibition depending on bile acid flux, not on the toxicity (Xu et al., 1992; 1993). Feedback regulation of cholesterol $7\alpha$-hydroxylase involves control of mRNA levels and activation or inactivation of the enzyme protein. Both cholesterol (Spady and Cuthbert, 1991; Pandak et al., 1991; Shefer et al., 1992) and bile acid flux (Jelinek et al., 1990; Shefer et al., 1991; Pandak et al., 1992) control mRNA levels of cholesterol $7\alpha$-hydroxylase. Hepatic alpha-hydroxy bile acid flux modulates cholesterol $7\alpha$-hydroxylase activity, which is also related to the change in mRNA levels controlled by the hepatic cholesterol substrate supply (Shefer et al., 1991, 1992). Alpha-hydroxy bile acid not only suppresses cholesterol $7\alpha$-hydroxylase activity but also inhibits production of HMG-CoA reductase mRNA, which interrupts the supply of the newly synthesized cholesterol for the formation of cholesterol $7\alpha$-hydroxylase. Thus, cholesterol $7\alpha$-hydroxylase mRNA levels decrease. Cholesterol $7\alpha$-Hydroxylase mass and steady-state mRNA levels increase following bile diversion, and decrease following duodenal infusion of taurocholate into a bile fistula in the rat providing evidence that taurocholate regulates choleserol 7$\alpha$-hydroxylase, either directly or indirectly, at the level of gene transcription, not via down-regulation of HMG-CoA reductase (Pandak et al., 1991, 1992). When cholesterol is present in excess, cholesterol 7$\alpha$-hydroxylase transcriptional activity is upgraded and removal of cholesterol from the hepatocytes is facilitated by the increase in bile acid synthesis (Jones et al., 1993). Conversely, when the cholesterol supply is decreased, cholesterol 7$\alpha$-hydroxylase transcriptional activity is down-regulated and elimination of cholesterol via bile acid synthesis is decreased. Glycocholic acid inhibits both HMG-CoA reductase and cholesterol 7$\alpha$-hydroxylase activity, while glycodeoxycholic acid depresses cholesterol 7$\alpha$-hydroxylase without reducing HMG-CoA reductase activity. Glycocholic acid produces greater and more complete suppression of bile acid synthesis by inhibiting HMG-CoA reductase activity and limiting the input of newly synthesized cholesterol – a preferred substrate of cholesterol 7$\alpha$-hydroxylase (Schwartz et al., 1978a, Turley and Dietschy, 1981, Robins et al., 1982a). However, no significant changes in the activities of both enzymes occur following the infusion of glycoursodeoxycholic acid. Thus, negative feedback regulation of hepatic bile acid synthesis depends on the hepatic flux of normally present bile acids such as cholic, chenodeoxycholic, and deoxycholic acid conjugates. Heuman et al. observed in rat that the relatively hydrophilic bile acids (ursocholate, ursodeoxycholate, hyocholate, hyodeoxycholate) did not alter cholesterol 7$\alpha$-hydroxylase or HMG-CoA reductase activities. In contrast, more hydrophobic bile acids (cholate, chenodeoxycholate, deoxycholate) down-regulate cholesterol 7$\alpha$-hydroxylase and HMG-CoA reductase activities in order of increasing hydrophobicity (CA$<$CDCA$<$DCA) (Heuman et al., 1988). A highly significant negative correlation was observed between the hydrophobicity index of the bile acid pool after bile acid feeding and the activities of cholesterol 7$\alpha$-hydroxylase and HMG-CoA reductase (Heuman 1989, Heuman et al., 1989). On the other hand, depressed bile acid synthesis in cultured hepatocytes fails to be down-regulated by the presence of bile acid; other factors, such as substrate availability, may well be important (Davis et al., 1983). Liver histology remains normal during bile acid replacement in the rat (Shefer et al., 1991) and rabbit (Xu et al., 1992). Therefore, the inhibitory effect of infused bile acid is not attributable to hepatotoxicity, as suggested by Davis et al. (1988). Thus, bile acid synthesis seems to be mediated by both the availability of cholesterol substrate and the activity of the rate-determining enzymes for bile acid synthesis, i.e., cholesterol 7$\alpha$-hydroxylase, although recent studies indicate that bile acid synthesis is not substrate-limited except in circumstances where cholesterol availability is sharply reduced (Björkhem and Åkerlund, 1988; Einarsson et al., 1989). The presence of definitive hepatic cholesterol precursor sites associated with the synthesis of bile acids and secretion of biliary cholesterol has been shown (Schwartz et al., 1975, 1978a). Specific activity of biliary cholesterol is usually in near equilibrium with the cholesterol pool used for bile acid synthesis (Schwartz et al., 1978a). In an elegant study using labeled mevalonic acid and [$^{14}$C]cholesterol, Schwartz et al. developed a multicompartmental model to describe and quantitate the metabolism of cholesterol in these hepatic compartments based on the metabolic and kinetic interrelationships of bile acids, biliary cholesterol, and plasma cholesterol. They found that the peak specific activity of bile acid reached after 100 minutes and was higher than that of biliary cholesterol, which was higher than that of plasma free cholesterol (Schwartz et al., 1978a). The specific acitivity of plasma free cholesterol became higher than that of other lipids after 12 hours and remained higher throughout the study. These sites derive 70 % of cholesterol from plasma, 60 % of which is free cholesterol. About 30 % and 20 %, respectively, of the cholesterol input into bile acid and biliary cholesterol precursor sites are derived directly from the newly synthesized hepatic cholesterol. The major portion of cholesterol aimed at bile acid synthesis and biliary cholesterol secretion appears to be derived from plasma lipoprotein free cholesterol (Schwartz et al., 1982).

### Bile acid and biliary cholesterol

Next, the possible link between hepatic uptake of plasma lipoproteins and biliary cholesterol and bile acid production should be considered. The relationship between disorders of lipoprotein metabolism and gallstone disease has been documented. HDL cholesterol is found to be negatively associated with gallstone formation (Gordon et al., 1977), while Portman et al. report a relation between $HDL_2$ and gallstones (Portman et al., 1980). Hypercholesterolemia type II, or familial hypercholesterolemia, with inefficient removal of LDL by the liver, does not have an increased incidence of gallstones; by contrast hypertriglyceridemia or hyperlipoproteinemia, type IV, is accompanied by a higher incidence of gallstones (Ahlberg et al., 1980). Two explanations have been offered. One is that more lipoproteins are required to carry the increased amount of triglycerides, which predisposes to cholesterol hypersecretion because of a possible link between cholesterol synthesis and secretion. The other alternative is that cholesterol is diverted from bile acid synthesis to lipoprotein formation, with a decrease in the bile acid pool (Angelin and Einarsson, 1988). Bile acid synthesis may exert a net regulatory effect on the quantity of cholesterol transported to bile. During bile formation, simple leaching of lipid from the canalicular membrane apparently does not occur. Transcellular flux of bile salt and secretion may promote lipid vesicle formation. Different coupling ratios between different bile salts and lipid influence cholesterol solubilization in bile.

### Interrelationship of biliary secretion of cholesterol, phospholipids, and bile salt

Secretion of bile supersaturated with cholesterol occurs in cholesterol gallstone patients but also in some persons who do not form gallstones (Nakayama and Miyake Jr, 1970; Holzbach et al., 1973). Bile acids stimulate the synthesis (Balint et al., 1971; Young and Manson, 1972) and secretion (Nilsson and Scherstén, 1969; Wheeler and King, 1972) of phospholipids. Transport and secretion of cholesterol and phospholipids into bile are closely linked to each other (Wheeler and King, 1972) and, in turn, to secretion of bile acids (Carey et al., 1984). The coupling between bile acids and lipid output appears to occur at the level of the bile canaliculus (Verkade et al., 1990). The relationship between the hydrophobicity of different bile acid species and their capacity to induce biliary lipid secretion has been investigated (Gurantz and Hofmann, 1984; Carulli et al., 1984; Bilhartz and Dietschy, 1988). The basic abnormality in most gallstone patients is in the coupling of cholesterol to bile salt secretion. A low bile salt secretion rate leads to a higher cholesterol : bile salt ratio and secretion of supersaturated bile; a high secretion rate of cholesterol also leads to the formation of supersaturated bile by raising the cholesterol : bile salt ratio. At a high bile salt flux rate, less lipid is secreted per molecules of bile salt than at a low bile salt flow rate (Wheeler et al., 1968). Cholesterol/phospholipid secretion is constant over a broad range of flow rates except at the lowest flow rate of bile salt, with relatively more cholesterol secretion (Wagner et al., 1976). Most of the lecithin in bile is not newly synthesized (Robins and Brunengraber 1982). Therefore, like cholesterol, it is not likely to be formed in membranes within the interior of the hepatocytes where de novo synthesis takes place.

Between meals, the majority of bile acids remain more or less in the gallbladder, especially during the overnight fast, and the secretion of bile acids becomes quite low. Cholesterol and phospholipids secretion also decrease yet remains relatively high with respect to bile acids. In the postprandial period, secretion of bile acids in bile recovers and the saturation of bile by cholesterol again becomes low.

## Production of supersaturated bile

In order for the production of supersaturated bile with cholesterol to take place, three possible circumstances must be considered: hypersecretion of cholesterol-enriched vesicles in the face of normal bile salt flux or normal secretion of cholesterol-enriched vesicles in the face of hypoflux of bile salt through the liver or combined excessive secretion of cholesterol-enriched vesicles and hypoflux of bile salts. The first can be seen in obese patients, northern Europeans, Chilean women, and in persons on a high-calorie diet, high-cholesterol diet, or slimming diet. The second is seen in nonobese patients and in patients with loss of function of the distal ileum, either by the disease process or resection, in pregnancy, and in cerebrotendinous xanthomatosis. The third can be seen in American Indian populations, with an extremely high incidence of gallstones (Bell et al., 1973), during pregnancy, in the postnatal period, and with administration of clofibrate. The mechanism underlying discoordination of secretion of cholesterol, phospholipids, and bile acids cannot be explained adequately at present. Hofmann and others proposed that biliary lipid secretion is best described by linkage coefficients, i.e., the ratio of phospholipids to bile acid secretion or the ratio of cholesterol to bile acid secretion (Gilmore et al., 1982; Danzinger et al., 1984). The cholesterol : phospholipids ratio should, in principle, indicate the cholesterol : phospholipids ratio of the vesicles whose secretion was induced.

In rats, feeding of diosgenin has been known to increase cholesterol secretion in bile (Nervi et al., 1988). Addition of simvastatin to the diet induces the hepatic secretion of a human-like highly cholesterol-supersaturated bile (Rigotti et al., 1993). After feeding for 1 week, biliary cholesterol in rats rose 500 %, bile acid decreased by 50 % and phospholipid levels remained unchanged.

## Hypersecretion of biliary cholesterol

Increased hepatic receptors may play a role in the hypersecretion of biliary cholesterol. In obese individuals, cholesterol hypersecretion seems to be the major abnormality (Shaffer and Small, 1977). More recent studies show that even in nonobese patients with gallstones, cholesterol hypersecretion is the most common abnormality (Grundy et al., 1974; Valdivieso et al., 1979; Nilsell et al., 1985). Cholesterol secretion in gallstone patients is 50% higher than in controls, whereas the rate of bile acid secretion is normal (Nilsell et al., 1985). The extent of saturation of bile with cholesterol seems to be related to food intake. Administration of mevalonolactone, a precursor of cholesterol synthesis, moderately increases the activity of cholesterol $7\alpha$-hydroxylase and the enzyme mass. Apparently the enterohepatic flux of $7\alpha$-hydroxylated bile acid and hepatic cholesterol formation control hepatic choleterol $7\alpha$-hydroxylase. Mevinolin, a cholesterol synthesis inhibitor, decreases biliary cholesterol secretion both acutely in rats (Stone et al., 1985) and chronically in man (Duane et al., 1988a), indicating direct control of cholesterol synthesis over biliary secretion of cholesterol. Thus, the following hypothesis for regulation of biliary cholesterol secretion is proposed (Cooper, 1991): a small, metabolically active free cholesterol pool determining the rate of biliary cholesterol secretion is located in the endoplasmic reticulum or Golgi region, where cholesterol synthesis, cholesterol $7\alpha$-hydroxylation, cholesterol esterification, and the initial steps of VLDL assembling take place. The site of the formation of phospholipids-cholesterol vesicles, ultimately destined for biliary secretion, is located in this region of the hepatocytes. The formation or translocation of these vesicles is in some way regulated by the rate of bile salt flux through hepatocytes. Progressively lower fractional conversion of cholesterol to bile acid may contribute to the increased hepatic secretion of cholesterol. Reduced activity of cholesterol $7\alpha$-hydroxylase to decrease the bile acid pool and to increase the cholesterol pool has not been found in man with any consistency. Secretion of phospholipids is more closely linked to the secretion of bile acid (Nilsson and Schersten, 1969) or to the bile acid pool size (Swell et al., 1971) than that of cholesterol in man. Persons with a decreased bile acid pool have greatly decreased secretion of phospholipids and only slightly decreased secretion of cholesterol (Swell et al., 1971; Bell et al., 1972), leading to the formation of supersaturated bile. Pima Indians show hypersecretion of cholesterol and enterohepatic circulation of bile acid deficiency before the actual formation of cholesterol stones occurs (Bell et al., 1973). In young Chilean men, heavy consumption of legumes decreases lecithin secretion, favoring stone formation (Nervi et al., 1989). The breaking point in bile acid pool size with and without gallstones is estimated from the regression line to be around 1.6 to 1.8 g. Therefore, the secretion of biliary phospholipids and cholesterol per bile acid pool seems to be the most critical factor in determining the state of saturation of cholesterol in bile.

## Change in bile acid

### Bile acid pool size

In 1970 Vlahcevic and his colleagues showed that, in cholelithiasis patients, the bile acid pool is decreased as much as 50% compared with normal controls (Vlahcevic et al., 1970a); this was later confirmed by others (Swell et al., 1971; Bell et al., 1972). Subsequently, it was found that the bile acid pool is reduced before the actual formation of gallstones (Bell et al., 1973; Einarsson et al., 1985). Bell et al. found a marked increase in the fractional catabolic rate of the primary bile acids and suggested that lowered efficiency of reabsorption of bile acids in the terminal ileum is responsible for the decreased bile acid pool size (Bell et al., 1973). However, in a later study, no correlation was found by Einarsson et al. between saturation level of bile and fractional catabolic rate (Einarsson et al., 1985). A negative correlation is found to be present between supersaturation of bile and bile acid synthesis, suggesting that the diminished size of the bile acid pool may be due to reduced bile acid synthesis. This conclusion is quite compatible with the altered rate of hepatic secretion of bile acids found, since an inverse relation between recycling frequency and bile acid pool size has been demonstrated (Low-Beer and Pomare, 1973; Northfield and Hofmann, 1975; Mok et al., 1977). An increase in enterohepatic circulation results in an increased turnover rate. Reduction of the bile acid pool may ensue until a new steady state is achieved, in which synthesis equals secretion. If bile acid secretion exceeds a certain level, synthesis may not increase sufficiently to compensate for the loss. This is especially so since the human liver has a limited capacity to adjust bile acid synthesis. Thus cholelithiasis may be considered as a disease of "inappropriate repression" (Schoenfield., 1972), since there seems to be no compensatory increase in bile acid synthesis in the presence of a decreased bile acid pool. However, the earlier belief of deficient bile salt secretion from a contracted bile acid pool in gallstone patients has been criticized (Carey and Cahalane, 1988a) because of the subnormal CCK release during formula perfusion of duodenum with diversion of bile into the gallbladder, and the presence of gallstone(s) in the gallbladder results in an apparent contraction of the bile salt pool when measured by the isotope-labeled bile salt dilution technique. Furthermore, biliary lipid secretion seems to be entirely normal regardless of pool size (Northfield and Hofmann, 1975) except lowest pools (Mok et al., 1977). Hypoflux of bile salt does not seem to occur in most of cholesterol stone patients (Carey and Cahalane, 1988b).

### Change in bile acid species

Bile salt plays a major role in bile formation; therefore, a disturbance in the homeostasis of bile salt predictably influences bile formation. Chenodeoxycholic acid is less lithogenic than cholic acid, because it carries less cholesterol into bile. This may be a critical determinant of the propensity to stone formation (Cooper, 1991). Women taking oral contraceptives (Bennion et al., 1976), pregnant women, and men taking estrogen (Henriksson et al., 1989) are said to have higher cholic : chenodeoxycholic acid ratios, leading to the formation of supersaturated bile, with an increased incidence of gallstones. There is increasing evidence showing that the level of deoxycholic acid in bile is related to cholesterol saturation in bile and hence to the risk of formation of cholesterol gallstones (Pomare and Heaton, 1973a; Arnesjo et al., 1975; McDougall et al., 1976; Marcus and Heaton, 1986a, 1988). Only 10 % of the bile acid pool reaches the colon, where cholic acid is rapidly converted to deoxycholic acid by anaerobic 7$\alpha$-dehydroxylation. About one-third to one-half of the newly formed deoxycholic acid is absorbed by passive diffusion, enters the enterohepaic circulation, and is transported to the liver (Hepner et al., 1972), together with any previously formed or recyled deoxycholic acid entering the colon. The amount of circulating deoxycholic acid is about 500 mg and constitutes 10–40 % of bile acid in bile. Marcus and Heaton extensively reviewed the current literatures and found that a raised level of deoxycholic acid was frequently encountered in cholesterol gallstone patients in 19 out of 20 comparisons (Marcus and Heaton, 1988). They concluded that excess deoxycholic acid in the bile of gallstone patients is not secondary to their gallstones; rather, it antedates gallstone formation and favors the formation of supersaturated bile. Types IIb and IV hyerlipoproteinemia patients have higher deoxycholic acid proportions and generally have bile saturated with cholesterol (Ahlberg et al., 1980). A correlation between the proportion of deoxycholic acid in the bile acid pool and the cholesterol saturation index is also recognized (Van der Linden and Bergman, 1977a, Hofmann et al., 1982; Alvaro et al., 1986a; Jazrawi and Northfield, 1986). Feeding of deoxycholic acid in physiological amounts raises the molar percentage of cholesterol in bile (Low-Beer et al., 1975), and that of cholic acid, a precursor of deoxycholic acid, a proportion of deoxycholic acid, and also the cholesterol saturation index of bile (Carulli et al., 1981). Reducing deoxycholic acid in bile is done by various means, such as administration of antibiotics, i.e., metronidazole and ampicillin (Low-Beer and Nutter 1978; Pomare et al., 1976), by ingestion of live Streptococcus faecium-displacing anaerobes in the colon (Salvioli et al., 1982), by feeding bran (Pomare et al., 1976; Watts et al., 1978; Marcus and Heaton, 1986b) and lactulose, synthetic unabsorbable disaccharide and an inhibitor of bacterial 7$\alpha$-dehydroxylase (Thornton and Heaton, 1981) and is always accompanied by a decrease in the cholesterol saturation index of bile. Since deoxycholic acid is absorbed slowly and incompletely, slowing the colonic transit may increase its absorption, cause expansion of its circulating pool, and increase the cholesterol saturation of bile, as in constipation (Marcus and Heaton, 1986a), which may increase the chance of supersaturation of bile and hence of gallstones. Whole gut transit time, deoxycholic acid pool size, and cholesterol saturation are correlated with each other. Because of the more hydrophobic character and hence greater detergency of deoxycholic acid, it was suggested to leach out more cholesterol from the canalicular membrane (Carulli et al., 1984). Thus any regimen which alters the amount of deoxycholic acid induces changes in the cholelsterol saturation of bile, which strongly suggests that deoxycholic acid directly affects cholesterol saturation of bile. Marcus and Heaton concluded that the critical factor is probably the size of the circulating deoxycholic acid pool, since slowing down of intestinal transit by loperamide raises the cholesterol saturation of bile and increases the deoxycholic acid pool without changing the proportion of deoxycholic acid (Marcus and Heaton, 1986a). Deoxycholic acid increases cholesterol secretion (Marcus and Heaton, 1988), is a more potent inhibitor of cholesterol 7$\alpha$-hydroxylase (Heuman et al., 1988), and causes a slight decrease of bile acid synthesis and a slight expansion of the cholesterol pool, predisposing to gallstone formation. Increased exposure of bile salts to anaerobic bacteria in the intestine increases secondary bile acid and decreases cholic acid and to some extent chenodeoxycholic acid (Chijiiwa et al., 1990). Hydrophobic secondary bile acid down-regulate de novo bile acid synthesis by inhibiting cholesterol 7$\alpha$-hydroxylase (Vlahcevic et al., 1991) which leads to a reduced bile acid pool size that circulate more frequently to keep bile salt secretion rates within normal limits (Hofmann and Hofmann, 1974). Increased hydrophobicity and rapid recirculation of bile acid lead to cholesterol hypersecretion in bile (Marcus and Heaton, 1988), enhance secretion of more hydrophobic molecular species of lecithin (Salvioli et al., 1985) and shortened nucleation time (Donovan et al., 1989; Jüngst et al., 1993). Although the mechanism of the effect of deoxycholic acid on cholesterol saturation in bile is still to be clarified, two explanations have been offered (Marcus and Heaton, 1988). The first is that deoxycholic acid which has the strongest detergent property and is very hydrophobic, leaches out cholesterol from the cell membrane when passing through bile canaliculi. The second explanation is that deoxycholic acid may displace chenodeoxycholic acid from the bile acid pool (Pomare and Low-Beer, 1975), thus reducing the curbing effect of chenodeoxycholic acid on cholesterol saturation. Chenodeoxycholic acid exerts an inhibitory effect on cholesterol saturation, while deoxycholic acid may inhibit chenodeoxycholic acid synthesis, or deoxycholic acid conjugates compete with chenodeoxycholic acid conjugates for absorption from the ileum.

### Parallel regulation of HMG-coenzyme A reductase, cholesterol 7$\alpha$-hydroxylase, and ACAT activities

Parallel changes of cholesterol and bile acid synthesis seems to occur as a result of parallel regulation of rate-limiting enzymes, respectively, i.e., HMG-CoA reductase and cholesterol 7$\alpha$-hydroxylase activities (Russel and Setchell, 1992), such as after treatment with up-regulators such as cholestyramine (Reihnér et al., 1989; Åkerlund et al., 1991) and thyroid hormone or such down-regulators as bile salt feeding (Shefer et al., 1973).

**Mechanism:** Under most experimental conditions, HMG-CoA reductase activity changes in parallel with the activity of cholesterol 7$\alpha$-hydroxylase (Vlahcevic et al., 1991). This linkage is important for cholesterol homeostasis, as an increase in cholesterol synthesis always causes a compensatory increase in the degradation of cholesterol. Up-regulation of cholesterol 7$\alpha$-hydroxylase may lead to increased consumption of cholesterol substrate, which, in turn, results in a compensatory increase in the activities of HMG-CoA reductase. Reduction of cholesterol synthesis results in a decrease of cholesterol 7$\alpha$-hydroxylase activity and bile acid synthesis (Reihnér et al., 1990b; Mitchell et al., 1991a; Sudjiana-Sugiaman et al., 1994). However, both studies were conducted after prolonged reduction of cholesterol synthesis. Therefore, direct and short-term regulation of bile acid synthesis by cholesterol synthesis is not known, although consistent reduction in bile acid synthesis after a single dose of lovastatin, an inhibitor of HMG-CoA, has been observed. In rat the mRNA levels of HMG-CoA reductase is controlled by the hepatic taurocholate flux, while the mRNA levels of cholesterol 7$\alpha$-hydroxylase is regulated by the substrate supply (Shefer et al., 1992). The end products, cholesterol and bile acids, control posttranscriptional regulation of HMG-CoA reductase and choelsterol 7$\alpha$-hydroxylase, respectively, thus demonstrating the steady-state feedback regulation of the rate-controlling enzymes of cholesterol and bile acid synthesis. Apparently these two regulators modulate each enzyme at specific but different locations. Since the preferred substrate pool for cholesterol 7$\alpha$-hydroxylase is newly synthesized cholesterol (Schwartz et al., 1975, 1978b), bile acid synthesis is indirectly regulated by the cholesterol synthesis via HMG-CoA reductase. Inclusion of cholic acid and chenodeoxycholic acid reduces HMG-CoA reductase activity, mRNA level and transcriptional rate (Björkhem et al., 1993). Cholic acid markedly suppresses HMG-CoA reductase activity, with relatively modest effects on transcription rate and mRNA level. Dietary cholesterol seems to down-regulate HMG-CoA reductase predominantly by a posttranscriptional mechanism (Ness et al., 1991). Apparently, bile acid regulates HMG-CoA reductase at both the transcriptional and posttranscriptional levels. Cholesterol feeding up-regulates cholesterol 7$\alpha$-hydroxylase, which is also mediated by the increased level of mRNA (Björkhem et al., 1991). Cholesterol 7$\alpha$-hydroxylase activity and corresponding mRNA levels are decreased by bile acid feeding. However, the transcription level of cholesterol 7$\alpha$-hydroxylase is not significantly reduced by chenodeoxycholic acid but rather by cholic acid (Björkhem et al., 1993). The majority of the down-regulation of cholesterol 7$\alpha$-hydroxylase by bile acid in the bile fistula rat is due to the effect on mRNA level and transcription rate (Pandak et al., 1991). The work on the lymph fistula rat, in which no transport of absorbed cholesterol reaches the liver, established that the effect of bile acid on cholesterol 7$\alpha$-hydroxylase is not due to its effect on cholesterol absorption (Åkerlund and Björkhem, 1990). Thus bile acid suppresses HMG-CoA reductase and cholesterol 7$\alpha$-hydroxylase but with different mechanisms.

Recently, both enzymes were purified sufficiently to permit complete elucidation of DNA sequences, and probes became available to quantitate mRNA levels for each enzyme (Simonet et al., 1988; Noshiro et al., 1990; Li et al., 1990). In man, administration of single dose of lovastatin, a competitive inhibitor of HMG-CoA reductase, which inhibits the rate-limiting enzyme for synthesis of cholesterol directly and primarily, reduces cholesterol synthesis and biliary cholesterol secretion. At the same time, it promptly decreases bile acid synthesis and its secretion (Mitchell et al., 1991a), which may affect biliary cholesterol independently, as biliary cholesterol secretion is to a great extent dependent on biliary secretion of bile acid. Thus, cholesterol synthesis seems to be an immediate regulator of bile acid synthesis, presumably serving to offset the partially acute alteration in cholesterol input. However, the underlying mechanism of this regulation remains uncertain.

**Relation to cholelithiasis:** Numerous attempts have been made to determine whether the increased or decreased activity of 3-hydroxy-3-methylglutaryl CoA reductase, HMG-CoA reductase – a key enzyme for the synthesis of cholesterol from acetate – and cholesterol $7\alpha$-hydroxylase activity – a key enzyme for the conversion of cholesterol to bile acid – is present in gallstone patients. However, these studies produced only controversial results and subsequent confusion (Table 8). Almost simultaneously in 1970s Nicolau et al., (1974), Salen et al., (1975), Northfield and Hofmann, (1975), Coyne et al., (1976), and, later, Key et al., (1980) and Carulli et al., (1980) reported that, in cholesterol gallstone patients HMG-CoA reductase activity is increased and cholesterol $7\alpha$-hydroxylase activity is decreased. Recently, gas chromatography-electron capture mass spectrometry has been applied to the quantitation of plasma mevalonic acid, providing a simpler and more practical way of assessing human cholesterol synthesis than the conventional sterol balance study (Scoppola et al., 1991). For determination of cholesterol $7\alpha$-hydroxylase activity, the serum free $7\alpha$-hydroxycholesterol concentration was assayed using isotope dilution-mass spectrometry with deuterium-labeled $7\alpha$-hydroxycholesterol, and was found to be positively correlated with cholesterol $7\alpha$-hydroxylase activity (Einarsson et al., 1986, Björkhem et al., 1987). Subsequently, serum esterified and/or total $7\alpha$-hydroxycholesterol was found to have a significant positive correlation by capillary gas-liquid chromatography-selected ion monitoring (GLC-SIM) using $5\alpha$-cholestane-$3\beta$,$7\beta$-diol as the internal standard (Yamashita et al., 1990; Oda et al., 1990; Okamoto et al., 1994). Serum $7\alpha$-hydroxy-4-cholestane-3-one, an intermediate on the bile acid synthetic pathway, was determined by isotope dilution-mass spectrometry and found to reflect the activity of cholesterol $7\alpha$-hydroxylase (Axelson et al., 1991). However, recent studies using these more accurate and sophisticated methodologies failed to show such parallel changes in both HMG-CoA

**Table 8**

**Bile Acid Pool Size, Bile Acid Synthesis, Cholesterol $7\alpha$-Hydroxylase and Metabolism of Cholesterol and Bile Acids in Cholelithiasis**

| Author | Year | HMG-CoA reductase | Bile acid pool | Bile acid synthesis | Cholesterol $7\alpha$-hydroxylase | ACAT |
|---|---|---|---|---|---|---|
| Vlahcevic | 1970a | | ↓ | ↓ | | |
| Swell | 1971 | | ↓ | → | | |
| Bell | 1972 | | ↓ | | | |
| Nicolau | 1974 | ↑ | | | ↓ | |
| Salen | 1975 | ↑ | | | ↓ | |
| Northfield | 1975 | | → | → | | |
| Coyne | 1976 | ↑ | | | ↓ | |
| Einarsson | 1989 | → | | | → | |
| Oda | 1990 | | | | → | |
| Kawata | 1991 | | | | ↓ | |
| Reinhér | 1991 | → | | | → | → |
| Stahlberg | 1991 | | | | | → |
| Honda | 1992 | → | | | ↓ | |
| Berr | 1992a | | ↓ | → | | |

reductase and cholesterol 7$\alpha$-hydroxylase activities, and their activities seem to be unaltered in cholelithiasis patients (Oda et al., 1990; Reihnér et al., 1991). The previous methods used for determination of cholesterol 7$\alpha$-hydroxylase activity are criticized, as they are based on the conversion of exogenously added, radiolabeled cholesterol with a very low conversion rate (less than 0.1%) and difficulty in getting the added cholesterol equilibrated with endogenous cholesterol (Einarsson et al., 1986). The best method for the assay of cholesterol 7$\alpha$-hydroxylase should be the measurement of the actual mass of the product, i.e., 7$\alpha$-hydroxycholesterol (Björkhem, 1985; Oda et al., 1990). A highly sensitive and specific method for the simultaneous determination of mevalonate and free 7$\alpha$-hydroxycholesterol in plasma has been developed which is well correlated with the activities of HMG-CoA reductase and hepatic cholesterol 7$\alpha$-hydroxylase respectively (Yoshida et al., 1993). However, the latter finding is at variance with that of Oda et al., who found that cholesterol 7$\alpha$-hydroxylase activity is more closely correlated with the serum level of esterified 7$\alpha$-hydroxycholesterol (Oda et al., 1990).

Yoshida et al. utilized dimethylethylsilyl ether derivatives of mevalonyl benzylamide and 7$\alpha$-hydroxycholesterol for gas chromatography-mass spectrometry with high resolution selected-ion monitoring in higher-mass regions permitting the simultaneous determination of trace amounts of mevalonate and 7$\alpha$-hydroxycholesterol present in plasma (Yoshida et al., 1993). Using this high-resolution gas chromatography-mass spectrometry, Honda et al. determined HMG-CoA reductase and cholesterol 7$\alpha$-hydroxylase in liver biopsy specimens obtained surgically from gallstone patients and controls (Honda et al., 1992). Cholesterol saturation of hepatic bile is found to be considerably higher than that of controls, and total bile acid concentration in hepatic bile is increased. Honda et al. found a positive correlation between HMG-CoA reductase and cholesterol 7$\alpha$-hydroxylase activities. However, both activities did not differ significantly irrespective of the presence of gallstones. Only mean activity of cholesterol 7$\alpha$-hydroxylase tended to be lower in cholesterol stone patients. The authors concluded that the high degree of saturation in hepatic bile found in cholesterol stone patients in the study was not due to the increased hepatic cholesterol synthesis but rather to inappropriate feedback inhibition of cholesterol 7$\alpha$-hydroxylase activity induced by increased hepatic bile acid concentration. Recently Shoda et al. using gas chromatography-mass spectrometry with high resolution selected-ion monitoring (Yoshida et al., 1993) report that plasma mevalonate levels are lower in cholesterol stone patients than in controls suggesting higher cholesterol saturation of bile is not due to the increased cholesterol synthesis in the liver but rather by the secretion of excess cholesterol from extrahepatic (dietary) sources (Shoda et al., 1994). As the method of assay of HMG-CoA reductase and cholesterol 7$\alpha$-hydroxylase activities improves, more accurate information is expected. A significant correlation was recently established between cholesterol 7$\alpha$-hydroxylase, on the one hand, and both HMG-CoA reductase and LDL receptor expression, on the other, during stimulation of bile acid synthesis (Reihnér et al., 1990a). No elevation of hepatic cholesterol concentration in patients with gallstones was found (Reihnér et al., 1991). Hypersecretion of cholesterol in bile may be due to reduced esterification of cholesterol in the hepatocyte (Smith et al., 1990) catalyzed by microsomal enzyme, acyl-CoA : cholesterol acyltransferase (ACAT) (Suckling and Stange, 1985). However, ACAT activity is not lower in patients with gallstones (Reihnér et al., 1991; Stahlberg et al., 1991). The proportion of esterified cholesterol is similar to that in the previous studies (Maton et al., 1980; Nervi et al., 1981; Reihnér et al., 1991). No correlation was found between the cholesterol saturation index (CSI) of bile and hepatic HMG-CoA reductase, cholesterol 7$\alpha$-hydroxylase, and ACAT activities (Reihnér et al., 1991). Therefore, Reihnér et al. concluded that distinct abnormalities in cholesterol-metabolizing enzymes are not of major importance for the development of gallstones and that the etiology of gallstones is multifactorial. Inverse correlations beween ACAT and HMG-CoA reductase activities are found in gallstone patients (Reihnér et al., 1991). An alternate pathway of bile acid synthesis via 27-hydroxycholesterol which preferentially leads to the synthesis of chenodeoxycholic acid has been studied (Mitropoulos and Miyant, 1967; Anderson et al., 1972; Martin et al., 1993; Shoda et al., 1993b). However, the role played by this pathway in the pathogenesis of gallstones is not well understood at present.

# Nucleation

The overall state of solubilization of cholesterol or the solute-solubilizer relationship in bile can conveniently be described by the triangular coordinate phase diagram of bile salt-phospholipids-cholesterol (Admirand and Small, 1968) (Figure 14), which greatly increases the understanding of the underlying mechanisms and describes the phase relationship at equilibrium. Each point within the triangular diagram represents the relative composition of bile in terms of the molar ratio of three major components, i.e., bile salt, phospholipids, and cholesterol. When the cholesterol concentration is low, simple bile salt micelles and mixed bile salt-phospholipids-cholesterol micelles coexist in various proportions in the micellar zone below the solid line i.e. equilibrium solubility limit – equilibrium cholesterol solubility (Hegardt and Dam, 1971; Holzbach et al., 1973; Carey and Small, 1978). When the point representing the composition of bile occurs in the metastable-labile zone between the solid line and the dashed line i.e. metastable-labile limit – effective cholesterol solubility (Admirand and Small, 1968), unilamellar or multilamellar vesicles and cholesterol crystals may also be present in addition to simple bile salt micelles and mixed bile salt-phospholipids-cholesterol micelles. When the point falls outside the dashed line, cholesterol precipitates out, leading to the formation of cholesterol stones. The cholesterol saturation (the saturation index or lithogenic index) can be calculated by the use of rectangular coordinate (Thomas and Hofmann, 1973), critical tables (Carey 1978) or personal computer (Kuroki et al., 1986). As native bile is far more complex, the static equilibrium represented by the triangular phase diagram may be far from the actual physiological state of bile.

## Nucleation time

Supersaturation of cholesterol in bile is an important but not necessarily sufficient pre-

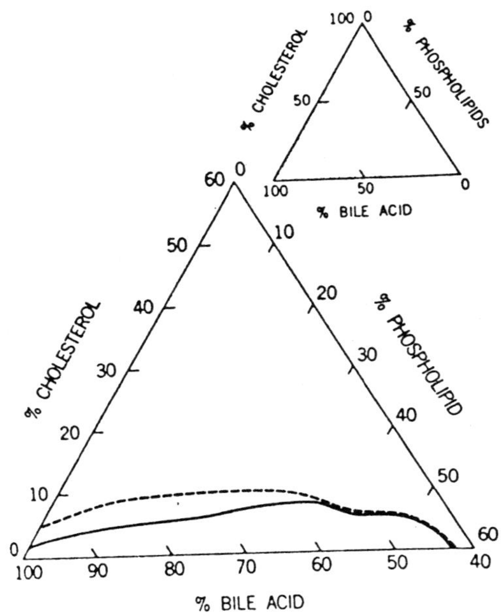


**Figure 14**

Triangular Coordinate Phase Diagram of Biliary Lipid Composition

Each side of the triangle represents the percentage of the total number of moles of bile salt, phospholipids (lecithin) and cholesterol. Since the sum of bile salt, phospholipids (lecithin), and cholesterol equals 100 %, the composition of any bile containing these compounds can be represented as a single point within triangular phase diagram (Admirand and Small, 1968). When the cholesterol concentration is low, simple bile salt micelles and mixed bile salt-phospholipids-cholesterol micelles coexist in various proportions in the micellar zone below the solid line i.e. equilibrium solubility limit (Hegardt and Dam, 1971; Holzbach et al., 1973; Carey and Small, 1978). When the point representing the composition of bile is located in the metastable-labile zone between the solid line and the dashed line i.e. metastable-labile limit (Admirand and Small, 1968), unilamellar or multilamellar vesicles and cholesterol crystals may be present in addition to simple bile salt micelles and mixed bile salt-phospholipids-cholesterol micelles. When this point falls outside the dashed line, cholesterol precipitates out, leading to the formation of cholesterol stones.

requisite for the formation of cholesterol gallstones, since supersaturated bile has been recognized to occur not only in gallstone bearers but also occasionally in those without gallstones (Figure 15) (Nakayama and Van der Linden, 1970; Holzbach et al., 1973; Bennion and Grundy, 1978). However, most do not go on to form gallstones and the frequency of supersaturated bile correlates with the prevalence of gallstones (Figure 16) (Nakayama and Van der Linden, 1971, Redinger and Small, 1972). Up to 80 % of persons with supersaturated bile do not have gallstones (Holzbach et al., 1973; Carey and Small, 1978; Holan et al., 1979; Busch et al., 1990). Therefore, it was thought that some additional condition(s) is necessary for gallstones to form. In 1979 Holzbach and his colleagues (Holan et al., 1979

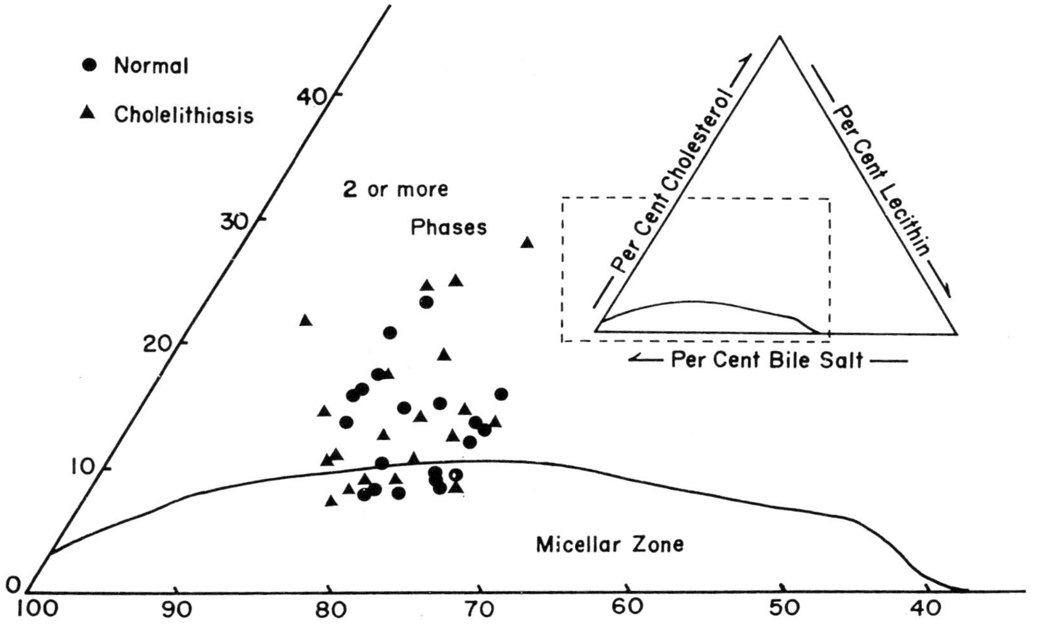


Figure 15

Bile Composition: Normal and in Cholelithiasis

Only the line of metastable-labile limit of cholesterol solubility (Admirand and Small 1968) is shown. Lecithin being a major phospholipid in bile.

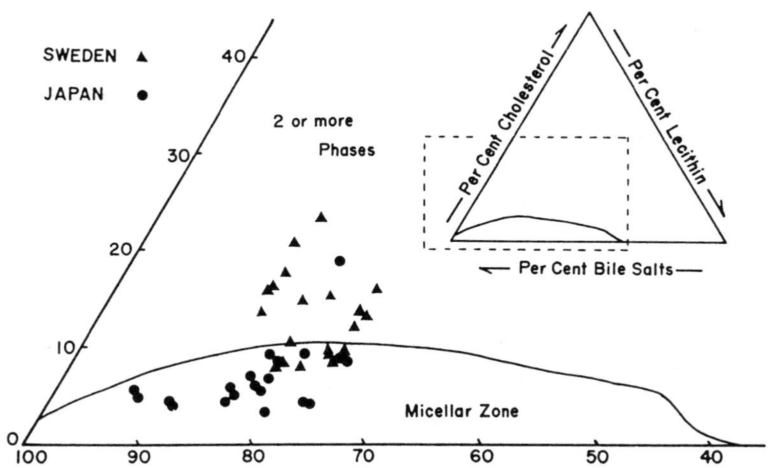


Figure 16

Bile Composition: Sweden versus Japan

Only the line of metastable-labile limit of cholesterol solubility (Admirand and Small 1968) is shown.

coined the term nucleation time to denote such a condition, i.e., the interval required for the initial appearance of microscopically detectable cholesterol monohydrate crystals from isotropic bile maintained in vitro at the physiological temperature of 37°C. The newer term crystal observation time has been proposed recently, as what one observes is in fact the end product of nucleation (Strasberg et al., 1990). Holzbach and his colleagues (Holan et al., 1979) found that cholesterol monohydrate crystals appear much more rapidly from bile of gallstone patients, i.e., rapid nucleators (2.9 days) than from the controls, i.e., slow nucleators (15 days) and that nucleation time more reliably distinguishes stone formers from nonformers. Subsequently, the presence of this difference was confirmed by others (Sedaghat and Grundy, 1980; Burnstein et al., 1983; Gollish et al., 1983). The possible presence of residual microcrystals left after ultracentrifugation (Holan et al., 1979), which may, if present, be responsible for the rapid nucleation time, has been excluded by adding a filtration step (Pattinson and Willis, 1991a). It was found that nucleation time is extended after the ultracentrifugation-filtration step but it is still significantly different, confirming an intrinsic difference between bile from gallstone patients and normal controls.

## Course of nucleation of cholesterol crystals and growth

The course of nucleation of cholesterol crystals and growth consists conceptually of micellation, aggregation, fusion, nucleation, crystal type conversion and crystal growth. Nucleation of crystals may be either homogeneous or heterogeneous. The former takes place in the medium completely devoid of impurities or foci around which certain molecules aggregate and form crystals. The latter takes place when impurities or foci are present. Nucleation consists of two processes, i.e., formation of nuclei and their growth. The thermodynamic threshold for nucleation in the former case is far greater than in the latter. It is believed that the latter type of nucleation occurs in native bile, since it occurs rapidly and at relatively low cholesterol supersaturation, and bile usually contains a variety of impurities or foci in a form of bilirubin precipitates, exfoliated epithelial cells, or bacteria, as described in detail by Juniper and Burson (1957). Multilamellar cholesterol-phospholipids vesicles aggregate and fuse into a critical cluster which provides for cholesterol monohydrate crystal nuleation and growth.

The nucleation of cholesterol crystals in bile represents three combined and overlapping processes: (1) formation and appearance of free cholesterol nuclei; (2) the formation of primitive microcrystals; and (3) a certain amount of growth in the size of these precipitate forms, permitting them to reach the microscopically detectable range (200 nm). Nucleated cholesterol crystals are said to consist of only four to eight molecules (Konikoff et al., 1992). First, flexible hair-like structures 90–100 nm wide and several microns in length are observed under polarizing phase contrast and video-enhanced microscopy. These are replaced in sequence by needle, ribbon, spiral and tube-like cholesterol monohydrate crystals and finally reach the stage of the commonly known plate-like crystals. Since the original test for nucleation time by Holan et al. is based on light microscopy to detect cholesterol monohydrate crystals, it is well beyond the nucleation stage (Holan et al., 1979). Nucleation should be observed not only by the first appearance of crystals but, more importantly, by the number of crystals formed over the observation time. Recently, a novel, facile, and highly reproducible serial spectrophotometric turbidometric technique has been devised in Holzbach's laboratory for semiquantitative assay of nucleation time and construction of a cholesterol monohydrate crystal growth curve which permits a quantitative estimate of the potency or comparative abundance of a given kinetic effector substance (Busch et al., 1990). Two assay modes are used, i.e., a crystal-seeded mode for estimating the effects of an effector on crystal growth alone and an unseeded mode for variable effects on the onset time for nucleation and rate of cholesterol crystal growth. The extinction coefficient ($\varepsilon$) is determined up to 10 times during the assay and is read at any wavelength ($\lambda$) where interference from the chromophore (e.g., pigment) is negligible. The effect of an individual effector can be assessed by comparing the result from the crystal-seeded mode and the unseeded mode. The widely accepted term nucleation time repesents in fact only one point on a crystal growth curve, whereas the onset time, crystal growth rate and maximal final crystal concentration can be calculated from the crystal growth curve obtained (Busch et al., 1990). The sigmoidal pattern of the growth curve indicates the transition from a metastable to a stable or pseudostable state. Unfortunately, this newer method cannot be applied to native bile (Busch et al., 1990). The nucleation time measured with duodenal bile is prolonged (Van Erpecum et al., 1988; Janowitz et al., 1990) but still be a reliable indicator (Van Erpecum et al., 1990). The usefulness of duodenal bile for studying the sequence of biliary events is emphasized by its easier accessibility.

## Secretion of biliary cholesterol, phospholipids, and bile acid and vesicle formation

### Mechanism of biliary lipid secretion

The mechanism of the secretion of biliary lipids is poorly understood. Lipids enter bile canaliculi as unilamellar vesicles composed mostly of phospholipids and cholesterol which are probably formed within or adjacent to the Golgi apparatus, such as in the smooth-surface endoplasmic reticulum (Marzolo et al., 1990; Cohen and Carey, 1990a). Microtubules are probably involved in the movement of lipids from the Golgi complex to bile canaliculi as colchicine, which interferes with microtubule polymerization, seems to reduce cholesterol and phospholipid secretion in bile (Barnwell et al., 1984; Crawford et al., 1988; Andreini et al., 1994). All phospholipids and cholesterol entering bile canaliculi are in vesicles (Ulloa et al., 1987). Different theoretical modes of transport of biliary lipids through the canalicular membrane, including exocytosis, membrane shedding, and fusion budding, have been proposed (Marzolo et al., 1990, Coleman and Rahman, 1992). Selected domains of the canalicular membrane are shed by a specific topographically restricted budding process contributing in part to biliary lipid secretion (Marzolo et al., 1990; Coleman and Rahman, 1992). Canalicular membrane microdomains composed of

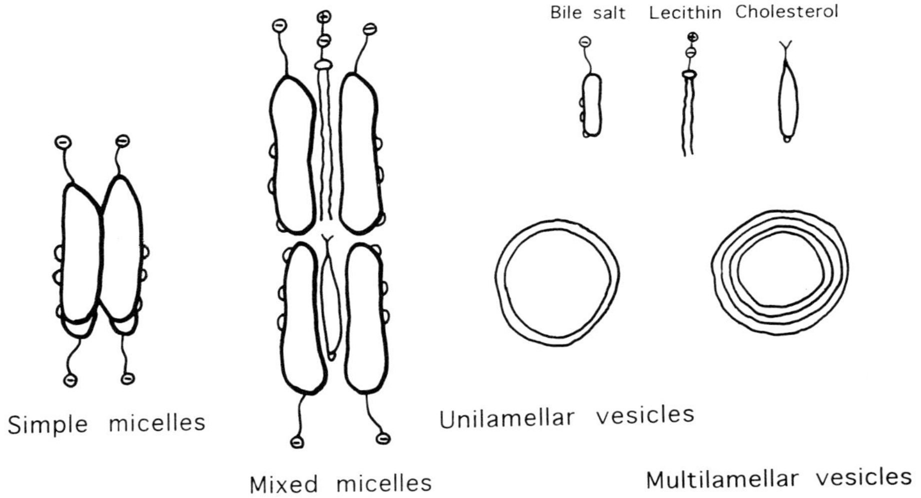


**Figure 17**

Unilamellar and Multilamellar Vesicles

biliary lipids and selectively segregated, membrane-bound proteins are pinched off in a vesicular form into the canalicular lumen, where the unilamellar vesicles yield secondary structures such as multilamellar vesicles and mixed micelles (Figure 17).

## Structure of vesicles

The fine structure of vesicles has been studied using a variety of techniques such as transmission electron microscopy, freeze fracture electron microscopy, fast-freeze cold-stage transmission electron microscopy (Falls et al., 1982), video-enhanced microscopy (Halpern et al., 1986a), quasi-elastic light scattering spectroscopy (QLS) (Mazer and Carey, 1983), and nucleomagnetic resonance (NMR) spectroscopy (Stark et al., 1985). However, because of the inherent formation of artifacts by the sample preparation when applied to the study on the particles in aqueous media, the images observed may be quite different from what is actually present. Bile salts are secreted as monomers by a carrier-mediated mechanism (Ruetz et al., 1987), and, in turn, mediate vesicle formation (Nilsson and Schertén, 1969) in the repository for phospholipids and cholesterol derived from the exchangeable pool – so-called bile acid-dependent vesicular transcytosis. Some vesicle secretion into bile is said to be bile acid independent (Coleman, 1987) and originates from pericentral cells. Bile salts are not associated with the vesicles at the time of secretion but enter the canaliculi by a separate carrier-mediated transport process (Ruetz et al., 1987). Once secreted, these three lipids – cholesterol, phospholipids, and bile salt – interact with each other. The vesicles entering bile canaliculi are solubilized by bile salts to more thermodynamically stable, so-called mixed micelles. This process continues and is completed in the gallbladder.

## Cholesterol transport in bile

Biliary lipids have hydrophobic and hydrophilic surfaces. Hydrophobic surfaces bind together and exclude the aqueous environment, while hydrophilic surfaces face toward the surrounding aqueous environment, forming micelles (Mazer et al., 1979). Thus, cholesterol present in high concentration in bile is solubilized in thermodynamically stable bile salt and polymolecular aggregates, i.e., mixed bile salt-phospholipids micelles 1 to 6 nm in diameter. Micellar constituents amplify the capacity of bile salt to solubilize and transport cholesterol. The molar ratio of phospholipids to bile salt is often only 1 : 3. Cholesterol is also dispersed in thermodynamically, metastable, closed, spherical, unilamellar phospholipids-cholesterol vesicles 40 to 100 nm in diameter consisting of a single bilayer (McLean and Philips, 1982; Mazer and Carey, 1983; Sömjen and Gilat, 1983; Nichols, 1988), which is said to be the main vehicle of secretion of phospholipids and cholesterol from the liver and is driven by the transhepatic flux of bile salts. When secreted cholesterol exceeds the solubilization limit of bile salt-phospholipids micelles, excess cholesterol is dispersed in much larger lipid vesicles. Vesicles are an aqueous suspension of a lamellar liquid crystalline phase reduced to its smallest molecular dimensions (Carey and Cahalane, 1988a). The existence of such two distinctly separate cholesterol-containing fractions in human hepatic and gallbladder bile has been suggested by earlier studies using gel filtration (Thureborn, 1963; Nakayama and Miyake Jr, 1965; Bouchier and Cooperband, 1967; Pattinson, 1985), by quasi-elastic light scattering spectroscopy (Mazer and Carey, 1983), and video-enhanced contrast microscopy (Sömjen and Gilat, 1983; Halpern et al., 1986a). Vesicles contain practically no bile salt (Lee et al., 1987a) and may have a protein coating (Pattinson, 1985). A distinct and constant protein profile is associated with vesicles (Rigotti et al., 1993). Amino acid sequencing of the amino terminus of a 130-kDa protein also isolated and detected in the canalicular membrane demonstrated a complete identity with aminopeptidase N, a canalicular transmembrane hydrophobic glycoprotein, suggesting involvement of the canalicular membrane in the secretory mechanism of biliary lipids. Other 114- and 68-kDa proteins associated with biliary vesicles are also found to be hydrophobic glycoproteins (Miquel et al., 1993). The cholesterol content of vesicles determines their stability. Unstable vesicles aggregate to form much larger multilamellar vesicles (Mazer et al., 1980) or liquid crystals (Holzbach and Corbusier, 1978, Olszewski et al., 1973), or phospholipid lamellae (Sömjen et al., 1990) (500 to 1,000 nm) consisting of multiple concentric lipid bilayers, i.e., lamellar vesicles or mesophase (Holzbach and Marsh, 1974). The ratio between biliary vesicles and micelles ranges widely and is comparatively larger in dilute systems such as hepatic bile (Burnstein et al., 1983; Sömjen and Gilat, 1986; Ulloa et al., 1987). The transition between the carriers in bile is a function of bile salt concentration (Sömjen and Gilat, 1985), i.e., bile salt, the most abundant biliary lipid, strongly affects the balance between the aggregational forms of phospholipids, and thus the distribution of biliary cholesterol among the carriers. The ratio depends on the degree of supersaturation of cholesterol, major bile acid species, the ratio of bile salt to phospholipids, total lipid concentration in bile, and state of the enterohepatic circulation of bile salt, i.e., in the fasting and postprandial periods (Pattinson and Chapman, 1986).

Vesicles are of particular importance as transport components in human bile (Pattinson and Chapman, 1986; Sömjen et al., 1990). Nonmicellar cholesterol has been shown to be physiologically the predominant and sometimes the exclusive form of cholesterol transport in bile by column chromatography, density gradient ultracentrifugation, transmission electron microscopy, and quasi-elastic light scattering spectroscopy (QLS) (Lee et al., 1987a). With low bile salt secretions such as during fasting, cholesterol is transported exclusively by vesicles. In gallbladder bile, more cholesterol is present in micelles than in hepatic bile. Gallbladder bile is more stable in terms of solubilization of cholesterol (Nakayama and Van der Linden, 1974, 1975; Harvey et al., 1988). If bile is unsaturated, all vesicular lipids are micellized (micellar excess) and do not form cholesterol monohydrate crystals. However, when bile is supersaturated with cholesterol, all the cholesterol present cannot be soublilized in mixed micelles. In supersaturated bile, simple bile salt micelles coexist with mixed bile salt-phospholipids-cholesterol micelles and cholesterol/phosphlipids vesicles (Donovan et al., 1991). Equilibrium dialysis revealed that the total lipid concentration, and the bile salt : lecithin (a major phospholipid in bile) ratio but not cholesterol content influences intermixed micellar/vesicular (non-lecithin-associated) concentrations (IMC) of bile salts (Donovan et al., 1991). Vesicles are responsible for metastable supersaturation or prolonged stability of cholesterol in supersaturated bile, as in hepatic bile (Gollish et al., 1983), in which the vesicles present are relatively unsaturated with cholesterol (Kibe et al., 1984; Ulloa et al., 1987). Thus, a significant proportion, over 60 %, of cholesterol in bile is carried by the vesicles. Vesicles, both unilamellar and multilamellar (Figure 17), are identified as major vehicles of biliary cholesterol transport. Their presence is demonstrated in bile even by a nondisturbing, independent physical method such as small angle X-ray diffraction (Sömjen et al., 1990). Recently, even with conventional electron microscopy of hepatic tissues, morphological evidence of the intracanalicular multilamellar bodies and unilamellar vesicles was obtained (Rigotti et al., 1993). A distinct, constant, and similar protein profile was associated with lamellar carriers in both rat and human bile. The hepatic localization and distribution of the 130-kDa lamellar protein, identified as aminopeptidase N, reveal a distinctive pattern in the canalicular plasma membrane domain. The gallbladder provides a recess where maturation of the solubilization process takes place and reaches equilibrium. Recently, Sömgen et al. (1990) provided evidence by electron microscopy, after negative staining and small angle X-ray diffraction study, that multilamellar vesicles, devoid of bile salt and protein, formerly recognized in model systems (Holzbach and Corbusier, 1978) are also present in human gallbladder bile. Most biliary cholesterol is carried by multilamellar vesicles, followed by unilamellar vesicles and mixed micelles in this order. Cholesterol crystallizes from multilamellar vesicles. Bile salt regulates the equilibrium between the various forms of cholesterol carriers.

## Role of vesicles in cholesterol crystal nucleation and growth

When cholesterol is present in excess of the micellar capacity, it is solubilized in a form of cholesterol-phospholipids vesicles. Vesicles seem to play an important role in the emergence of cholesterol monohydrate crystals rather than micellar carriers (Halpern et al., 1986a, b; Lee et al., 1987a). Cholesterol and phospholipids interchange between mixed micelles and vesicles. When the cholesterol content of bile exceeds the micellar-solubilizing capacity, phospholipids are more easily transferred to the micelles than cholesterol (Harvey et al., 1987). Subsequently, residual vesicles become increasingly enriched with cholesterol and the thermodynamically labile, cholesterol-rich vesicles are formed, which coexist with fully saturated mixed micelles (micellar insufficiency) (Sömjen and Gilat, 1983, 1985; Mazer and Carey, 1983; Mazer et al., 1984). Thus vesicles become highly enriched with cholesterol (cholesterol : phospholipids ratios up to 2 or greater) and contain esssentially no bile salt (Mazer and Carey, 1983; Cohen and Carey, 1990b), while mixed bile salt-phospholipids-cholesterol micelles have low cholesterol content (cholesterol: phospholipids ratios less than 0.3) (Mazer et al., 1980). The greater propensity of phospholipids to be micellized results in a higher cholesterol : phospholipids ratio in the vesicles, reaching as high as 2.0 from the original 0.5 in bile canaliculi (Hofmann et al. Nat. Coop Study, 1982; Kibe et al., 1985; Harvey et al., 1987).

## Nucleation from vesicles

Nucleation from the vesicles depends on the cholesterol : phospholipids ratio. When this ratio exceeds equimolar, cholesterol may exit from the vesicles, nucleate, and grow to form macroscopic crystals of cholesterol monohydrate, leading to the formation of cholesterol gallstones (Collins and Phillips, 1982; Phillips, 1990). During the progressive micellation of vesicular phospholipids and cholesterol by the presence of bile salt, transfer of lipids occurs from vesicles to micelles through the aqueous phase and during the collision of carriers (Nichols et al., 1988). An increase in the cholesterol : phospholipids ratio reduces the stability of vesicles. When crystallization occurs, remaining vesicles devoid of excess cholesterol are probably dissolved by bile salt micelles (Carey and Small, 1978). Further crystal growth occurs not from the micelles but from vesicles supersaturated with cholesterol (Lee et al., 1987a). However, in a recent study in a cholesterol-fed prairie dog cholesterol is found to nucleate rapidly from mixed micelles and cholesterol-phospholipid vesicles are not required in this model (Ahrendt et al., 1994). Hepatic bile is frequently supersaturated, as judged from the cholesterol saturation index, but nucleation of cholesterol crystals takes place with the greatest difficulty indicating that vesicles in hepatic bile are very stable (Lee et al., 1987a). In dilute bile, interfacial energy is minimized when excess cholesterol precipitates with phospholipids, first as metastable, cholesterol-rich vesicles prior to the formation of cholesterol monohydrate crystals (Mazer and Carey, 1983). In fact, cholesterol crystals are less frequent in hepatic bile (Van der Linden and Nakayama, 1974) except after intravenous injection of fat emulsion (Van der Linden and Nakayama, 1976).

## Formation of multilamellar vesicles

Cholesterol-rich, unilamellar vesicles aggregate to form much larger multilamellar vesicles – form of lamellar liquid crystals or mesophase. The multilamellar vesicles thus formed are most likely to provide the key microscopic environment for nucleation of cholesterol monohydrate crystals and their subsequent growth, and seem to be the critical first step leading to cholesterol gallstone formation (Halpern et al., 1986a, 1986b; Harvey et al., 1987; Peled et al., 1988). Halpern, using time-lapse, video-enhanced contrast microscopy, observed that the sequence of events characterizing the process of cholesterol monohydrate crystal formation is the rapid de novo formation of unilamellar vesicles from the isotropic micellar phase followed by vesicular aggregation (Halpern et al., 1986a). These vesicles rapidly aggregate, fuse, and enlarge until cholesterol monohydrate microcrystals appear. The nucleation process for cholesterol microcrystal formation most likely occurs within multilamellar vesicles or mesophase, which is only the first of a two-step transition in a sequential series of physical ordering processes (Holzbach and Corbusier, 1978). Multilamellar vesicle formation must have a lower kinetic energy requirement, and the second step (cholesterol microcrystal formation) must be rate-limiting. This sequence of events occurs more rapidly in gallbladder bile from patients with cholesterol gallstones (Holan et al., 1979; Sedaghat and Grundy, 1980; Gollish et al., 1983). After entering the gallbladder, the total lipid concentration rises because of the concentrating activity of the gallbladder. Nucleation is also influenced by the concentration of the solutes present in bile, and when bile is more concentrated, as in the gallbladder, vesicles become more cholesterol rich and nucleation is more prone to take place (Strasberg et al., 1990; Van Erpecum et al., 1993). This is because micellation and aggregation are more likely to occur when the carriers exist more in proximity. When bile stasis is present in the gallbladder, there is a greater likelihood that nucleation will take place, leading to the formation of gallstones (Pomeranz and Shaffer, 1985). After nucleation of cholesterol monohydrate crystals, aggregation of vesicles stops (Holzbach and Marsh, 1974) as the vesicles become unsaturated for cholesterol because of cholesterol depletion. Nucleation of cholesterol crystals decreases the amount of cholesterol in vesicular phase without affecting the amount solubilized in the mixed micelles (Lee et al., 1987a). Cholesterol for crystal growth derives from biliary vesicles supersaturated with cholesterol, not from biliary micelles (Halpern et al., 1986b; Harvey el al., 1987; Lee et al., 1987a, Peled et al., 1988).

### Composition of different carriers

Using model bile systems, the amount of cholesterol in the vesicle and, hence, its metastability are determined by the degree of supersaturation, total lipid concentration, and bile acid : phospholipids ratio (Kibe et al., 1985; Halpern et al., 1986b). The relationship between the percentage of cholesterol carried by vesicles and/or their composition and their propensity to form cholesterol monohydrate crystals, i.e., nucleation time, has been studied by gel filtration chromatography, which resolves three peaks—of void volume vesicles, of smaller vesicles, and of the mixed micelles (Nakayama and Miyake Jr, 1965; Pattinson et al., 1991). Void volume vesicles are occasionally present in gallbladder bile with gallstones but not in those without gallstones. No correlation was found between nucleation time with either the percentage of cholesterol carried by vesicles or cholesterol : phospholipids ratio of the void volume vesicles (Pattinson et al., 1991a). Nucleation time is found to correlate with the composition of the smaller vesicles. However, no significant differences in the composition or percentage of the smaller vesicular form or combined vesicular forms are found between gallbladder bile with or without gallstones. These rather confusing results are partly due to the fact that cholesterol-supersaturated bile is in a metastable state and not in thermodynamic equilibrium. Biliary mixed micelles and vesicles coexist with a common intermediate, monomer or monomer plus a simple micellar concentration of bile salt. The composition of different carriers changes depending on the intermixed micellar/vesicular (non-lecithin-associated) bile salt concentration (IMC). Recently, classic equilibrium dialysis has been modified to correct for dialysant dilution and the Donnan effect (Donovan et al., 1991). Micelles and vesicles are separated from cholesterol-supersaturated model bile using high-performance liquid chromatography, with an eluant containing IMC of bile salt usually substituted for by equivalent sodium cholate to avoid a change in the composition of mixed micelles and vesicles. Subsequently, rapid centrifugal ultrafiltration is added (Donovan and Jackson, 1993). Only by keeping correct values of the monomer (plus micellar) concentration of bile salt, i.e., IMC constant, can different cholesterol carriers, such as micellar, vesicular, and potentially other cholesterol-carrying particles, be separated unchanged and accurately quantitated. IMC increases with the increase in total lipid concentraton and bile salt : phospholipids ratio but decreases appreciably as the overall bile salt composition becomes more hydrophobic (Donovan et al., 1993). Hydrophilic bile salts are preferentially distributed in the IMC, while hydrophobic bile salts are preferentially associated with phospholipids in the mixed micelles and vesicles. Thus bile salt composition, in addition to total lipid composition and bile salt : lecithin ratio, is a critical determinant of the relative and absolute concentration of bile salt species in the IMC. Nucleation occurs rapidly after exposure of vesicles to hydrophobic bile salt, i.e., deoxycholic acid and chenodeoxycholic acid with a concomitant decrease in the vesicluar cholesterol : phospholipids ratio and increased precipitation of cholesterol crystals (Van de Heijning et al., 1994). With ursodeoxycholic acid, most hydrophilic bile salt, no nucleation occurs and the cholesterol : phospholipids ratio is kept constant. Thus the kinetics of cholesterol crystallization is governed by the hydrophobicity of bile salt. Recently, a method of quantitative estimation of the hydrophilic-hydrophobic balance of mixed bile salt solutions has been devised using reversed phase, high-performance liquid chromatography (HPLC) (Heuman et al., 1989).

## Role of molecular species of lecithin

Supplementation of bile with phosphatidyl choline (lecithin), a major phospholipid in bile, is shown to cause marked prolongation of the nucleation time, shift of cholesterol from vesicles to mixed micelles and lowering of the cholesterol : phospholipids ratio in bile (Jüngst et al., 1993). The distribution of lecithin molecular species between vesicles and micelles, in cholesterol-supersaturated bile has been studied (Cohen and Carey, 1991). The descending rank order of lecithin molecular species, present in bile, as represented by fatty acid in the sn-1 and sn-2 positions is 16 : 0–18 : 2, 16 : 0–18 : 1, 16 : 0–20 : 4, and 18 : 0–18 : 2 (Hay et al., 1993). Thus as much as 30 identifiable molecular species are present in human bile. Lecithin species of bile represent the most hydrophilic hepatic phospholipids and other tissues. With binary lecithin mixtures, vesicles are enriched with lecithin containing the most saturated sn-1 or sn-2 chains i.e., 16 : 0–16 : 1, 16 : 0–18 : 1, 18 : 0–18 : 1 as much as 2.4-fold, while mixed micelles with the more unsaturated lecithins, i.e., 16 : 1–18 : 2, 18 : 1–18 : 2, and 8 : 1–18 : 3 in model bile (Cohen and Carey, 1991), as well as in human gallbladder bile (Booker et al., 1992). Since molecular species of lecithins adsorbed onto filamentous cholesterol crystals are more saturated than in whole bile and all essentially identical to those in biliary vesicles, this finding provides chemical evidence for a vesicular origin of the critical cholesterol nucleus (Konikoff et al., 1994). Partitioning between vesicles and micelles is determined by sn-1 chain length and degree of unsaturation at both the sn-1 and sn-2 positions (Booker et al., 1992). Gel filtration, lipid analysis, and quasi-elastic light scattering revealed that apparent micellar cholesterol solubilities and metastable vesicle cholesterol : lecithin molar ratios are as much as 60 % and 100 % higher, respectively, in bile composed of unsaturated lecithins. The kinetics of bile salt-vesicle interaction is most rapid with unsaturated lecithin-rich vesicles (Cohen et al., 1990a). Acyl chain packing constraints imposed by distinctly different particle geometries may explain the asymmetric distribution of lecithin molecular species between vesicles and mixed micelles, as well as variations in apparent micellar cholesterol solubilities and vesicle cholesterol : lecithin molar ratios. Lecithin containing more saturated fatty acid chains, particularly those with saturated fatty acyl chains, pack more tightly and therefore partitions better into cholesterol-rich vesicles with highly ordered bilayer structures (Cohen and Carey, 1991). Lecithin with more highly unsaturated fatty acid chains partitions more favorably in mixed micelles with loosely associated packing. Therefore, fewer cholesterol-rich vesicles form with higher cholesterol : phospholipids ratios. An increase of apparent cholesterol solubility by lecithin with more unsaturated fatty acid is observed (Cohen and Carey, 1991). Thus micellar solubility and vesicular cholesterol : phospholipids ratio depend on the molecular species of lecithins. Phospholipid molecular species influence crystal habits and transition sequences or metastable intermediates during cholesterol crystallization from bile salt-rich model bile (Konikoff et al., 1994). Cholesterol can crystallize from model and native biles as filamentous crystals covered by a surface layer of lecithin molecules (Konikoff et al., 1992). During growth, filamentous crystals are transformed via metastable intermediates into classical plate-like cholesterol-monohydrate crystals. The surfaces of filamentous crystals are enriched preferentially with lecithin molecular species having longer and more saturated sn-1 and sn-2 acyl chains compared to mixed lecithin species of whole bile (Konikoff et al., 1994). Time sequences and transformations between metastable crystalline intermediates are altered markedly by specific phospholipid species: saturated short-chain, medium-chain, and polyunsaturated long-chain lecithins induce rapid precipitation of short, filamentous crystals which slowly become plate-like by "arborization". Long-chain saturated lecithin and natural sphingomyelins, shown to be present in bile although in small amount (Nakayama and Blomstrand, 1960), markedly retard cholesterol crystallization. Thus, modification of biliary lecithin species may have a profound influence on the physical chemistry of bile and subsequently on gallstone formation and prevention.

Dietary fish oil alters the composition of various phospholipids, which, in turn, affect gallstone pathogenesis (Magnuson et al., 1989a; Booker et al., 1990). Fish oil may reduce the availability of arachidonic acid, the precursor for prostaglandin synthesis in the gallbladder. In human bile, 16:1–18:1 (1-palmitoyl-2-linoleoyl-phosphatidyl choline [PLPC]) comprises about 55 % of biliary phosphatidyl choline (PC), while most species of PC, including 1-steatoyl-2-arachidonyl-phosphatidyl choline (SAPC), comprise a small fraction, less than 3 %, of total biliary PC (Kawamoto et al., 1980; Alvaro et al., 1986b). Human hepatocyte selectively recruits PLPC for biliary secretion and effectively excludes SAPC and other phospholipids from bile. Biliary secretion of PC increases as micelle-forming bile acid secretion increases (Swell et al., 1968). Bile acid also rapidly stimulates PC synthesis (Nilsson and Scherstén, 1970). Bile with gallstones contain a smaller proportion of lecithin (PC) 16:0–20:4, the principal arachidonyl lecithin species than controls, which is said to play an important role in gallstone formation as arachidonyl lecithin and $PGE_2$ synthesis increase in human bile prior to cholesterol nucleation (Marks et al., 1992). Although some authors found increased arachidonyl lecithin in the bile of patients with gallstones (Dam et al., 1971; Cantafora et al., 1981), others found no difference (Ahlberg et al., 1981b; Berr et al., 1992b). A higher arachidonyl lecithin level was found in the bile of patients with morbid obesity, but the difference was not statistically significant (Hay et al., 1993). There is no molecular species difference between persons with cholesterol and black pigment stones (Hay et al., 1993). Selective composition of PC is said to depend on the hydrophobic-hydrophilic balance of bile acid constituents (Salvioli et al., 1985; Van Berge Henegouwen et al., 1987; Berr et al., 1992b). Hydrophobic bile acid stimulates secretion of arachidonic and stearic acid- rich PCs, implying the physical-chemical mechanism for selectivity. However, Shamburek et al. found that hydrophobicity of bile acid has no effect on PC selectivity but that selectivity decreases moderately as total PC secretion increases (Shamburek and Schwartz, 1993). When the hydrophobic index is prepared for lecithin, those for bile acids (Heuman et al., 1989) and lecithin are correlated positively, i.e., more hydrophobic bile acids are associated with biliary secretion of hydrophobic lecithins. Further, Hay et al. found that most hydrophobic major lecithin species 18:0–18:2 are present in greater proportions in bile with cholesterol monohydrate crystals in their sediments and in those with cholesterol saturation index greater than unity (Hay et al., 1993). Biliary PLPC is derived largely from hepatic preformed PLPC but partially from the newly synthesized PLPC as well (Shamburek and Schwartz, 1993).

## Pro- and antinucleating factors

Formation of supersaturated bile and cholesterol-rich vesicles is a prerequisite for cholesterol nucleation but is not sufficient for the initiation of nucleation and continued crystal growth (Holzbach, 1986). Subsequently, it was noted that, even with the same degree of supersaturation, cholesterol monohydrate crystals appear much more rapidly in bile from gallstone bearers (abnormal) than from those without gallstones (normal). Therefore, it seems likely that there are factors working against nucleation in normal bile or its absence in bile of gallstone bearers, i.e., antinucleating factor(s) (Holzbach et al., 1984). However, it was also found that the tendency for rapid nucleation can be transferred from abnormal to normal bile (Burnstein et al., 1983) and the existence of a heat-labile, nonmucin glycoprotein with a molecular mass of 300 kDa was proposed. Later studies showed that the effectors considered are in fact immunoglobuins (Harvey et al., 1991). Therefore, there seem to be factor(s) acting for nucleation, i.e., pronucleating factor(s). However, the presence of pronucleating factor(s) in the bile of cholesterol gallstone patients would not explain the prolonged metastability of bile from healthy controls. When the factor hinders traversal of the energy barrier to reach crystal nucleation, it is said to inhibit crystallization (i.e., the antinucleating factor), while overcoming the barrier is said to promote crystallization (i.e., the pronucleating factor). Antinucleating factors prevent events of the thermodynamic pathway, slowing the growth of submicroscopic crystals and possibly inhibiting initiation of the nucleation process (Holzbach et al., 1984). The criteria for a pronuceating substance were proposed by Strasberg et al. (Harvey and Strasberg, 1993): (1) The substance should be present in abnormal bile and, if present also in normal bile, there must be quantitative and qualitative differences. (2) Its removal from abnormal bile alters the nucleation of cholesterol from rapid to slow. (3) Addition of the substance to slow nucleating control or model bile alters the nucleation of cholesterol from slow to rapid. The promoting effect is indicated by the shortened crystal detection and increased crystal growth, while the inhibitory effect is indicated by a decrease in crystal growth rate and a reduction in the final crystal concentration, as determined by the growth assay.

### Identification of pro- and antinucleating factors

Although the patients with cholesterol stones cannot be separated clearly from those with pigment stones and controls on the basis of total protein concentration in bile, in concordance with the previous study (Yamazaki et al., 1988), high biliary protein concentrations are frequently associated with the presence of cholesterol crystals and may be related to the pathogenesis of cholesterol stones (Jüngst et al., 1991). In fact, almost all subjects having bile with total protein levels over 10g/L were found to have cholesterol crystals in bile. The existence of lipoprotein complexes in bile has been suggested by paper electrophoresis (Verschure, 1956; Verschure and Mijnlieff, 1956), by gel filtration (Thureborn, 1963; Nakayama and Miyake Jr, 1965,1966; Bouchier and Cooperband, 1967; Pattinson, 1985), by zone electrophoresis (Lafont et al., 1977), and by double immunodiffusion and sodium dodecyl sulfate polyacrylamide gel electrophoresis (Martigne et al., 1988). Strasberg and his colleagues showed that high biliary protein concentrations are closely associated with the reduced metastability of bile in the early stage of cholesterol crystal formation (Strasberg et al., 1988) in concordance with the findings in prairie dogs (Lee et al., 1981b) and ground squirrels (Smith et al., 1987). Total lipids, total bile acids, phospholipids, and pH of bile are not significantly different (Jüngst et al., 1991). Quantitative abnormalities in total biliary protein (Gallinger et al., 1987; Li and Luo, 1990a) and different biliary proteins ( Levy et al., 1984; Gallinger et al., 1985; Groen et al., 1988,

1989b) may promote cholesterol nucleation and cholesterol stone formation. On the other hand, some biliary proteins consistently exhibit the inhibitory effect. Apolipoproteins A-I and A-II have been shown to slow nucleation (Kibe et al., 1984) and to strikingly inhibit the growth rate and number of crystals formed in both seeded and unseeded modes of cholesterol nucleation and crystal growth assays (Sewell el al., 1983). In disease the nucleation inhibitor could be either absent, blocked, or inactivated.

The initial stage of cholesterol gallstone formation, i.e., nucleation of cholesterol monohydrate crystals, occurs in mucus gel adherent to gallbladder mucosa (Hultén, 1968b) which may offer a quite different environment for cholesterol crystal nucleation and growth than in bile. Marked hypersecretion of mucin, resulting in the accumulation of mucus gel in the gallbladder lumen, is noted prior to the appearance of cholesterol monohydrate crystals in every animal model (Freston et al., 1969; Lee et al., 1981b; Lee and Scott, 1982; Pemsingh et al., 1987), and mucin is found within the central nidus region of cholesterol stones (Smith and LaMont, 1985). Gallbladder mucin and densely glycosylated macromolecules secreted by the gallbladder are major constituents of gallbladder mucus, and its protein core contains two structurally and functionally different domains (Smith et al., 1989), i.e., a densely glycosylated domain is possibly responsible for vesicoelastic and gel-forming properties and a sparsely glycosylated binding domain for hydrophobic ligands such as cholesterol and bilirubin (Smith and LaMont, 1983, 1984; Afdhal et al., 1990). Mucous glycoprotein secreted by gallbladder epithelium accelerates the nucleation of cholesterol monohydrate crystals (Lee et al., 1981b; Levy et al., 1984; Smith and LaMont, 1985) and crystal growth in unseeded assay mode. The growth rate is proportional to the mucin concentration. Addition of mucin purified from human hepatic bile at as low a concentration as 100 $\mu$g/ml was found to shorten significantly nucleation time (Yamasaki et al., 1993). However, mucin as a promotor has been challenged (Harvey et al., 1986; Gallinger et al., 1987). Mucus glycoprotein forms viscous gel on the surface of the gallbladder lumen (Levy et al., 1984, Gallinger et al., 1985; Smith, 1987) where nucleation and growth of cholesterol monohydrate crystals take place. Hypersecretion of mucin may be induced by an increase in phospholipids containing arachidonic acid (Ahlberg et al., 1981b; Cantafora et al., 1981). Arachidonic acid, a precursor of prostaglandin, stimulates mucin secretion. An antiprostaglandin agent, aspirin, inhibits mucin release, cholesterol nucleation, and gallstone formation in the prairie dog (Lee et al., 1981a, 1981b), and indomethacin, a potent cyclooxygenase inhibitor, suppresses mucin hypersecretion and gelation in the gallbladder explant (LaMont et al., 1983b). However, other investigators found that the addition of aspirin to a lithogenic diet failed to reduce the incidence of gallstones in the hamster and the prairie dog (Cohen et al., 1991). A significant correlation between the proportion of deoxycholic acid in the bile acid pool and the amount of arachidonic acid in phospholipids is found to be present (Van Berge Henegowen et al., 1987). Therefore, an increase in deoxycholic acid in bile is suggested to lead to gallstone formation by promoting nucleation through an increase in mucin. However, it has been shown that the concentrations of both apolipoproteins which act as detergent molecules (Smith et al., 1978) and mucous glycoprotein are similar in normal and abnormal bile (Sewell et al., 1983;

Harvey et al., 1986; Gallinger et al., 1987).

**Analysis of biliary glycoprotein**

Purification of protein from bile has been difficult because of the presence of a variety of proteins (up to 4.5 % of solid) in bile (Holan et al., 1979) and various other biliary constituents. Although albumin is a dominant protein in bile, it has no significant effect on nucleation (Holzbach, 1984; Fukudome et al., 1987; Gallinger et al., 1987). The presence of putative protein-promoting factors has been proposed (Burnstein et al., 1983; Gollish et al., 1983; Martigne et al., 1988). In 1985 Gallinger et al. found that removal of mucin has no siginficant effect on nucleation time (Gallinger et al., 1985). Later they isolated non-mucous protein from the bile of patients with and without gallstones (Gallinger et al., 1987). Subsequently, Groen et al. subjected T-tube bile to concanavalin A (Con A) lectin-affinity column chromatography (Groen et al., 1988). Biliary protein isolated from the same bile sample by Con A lectin-affinity column chromatography contained both anti- and pronucleating activities, i.e., one antinucleating factor which does not bind to Con A (flow-through fraction) and is unstable and one pronucleating factor which binds to Con A but is stable and can be eluted by $\alpha$-d-methylmannopyranoside (eluted or bound fraction). There is no correlation between the lipid or protein content of T-tube bile and its nucleation-influencing activity. Apparently, nucleation of cholesterol crystals depends on a balance between antinucleation and pronucleation factors present in the same bile. The nucleation-promoting factor isolated is heat labile and insensitive to proteases. It is thought to be a glucose-containing and mannose-containing glycoprotein, as activity is found in the bound fraction of con A lectin-affinity column chromatography (Groen et al., 1988, 1989b, 1990). The protein isolated is different from that in mucin which does not contain glucose or mannose. It consists of two components of 150 kDa and 5 kDa (Groen et al., 1988). The sugar group seems to be important for activity, as treatment with a mixed glucosidase preparation decreases the nucleation-promoting activity. As this factor is present in bile from patients both with and without gallstones, and is present not only in gallbladder bile but also in hepatic bile, the authors concluded that this is a normal constituent of bile, and is of hepatic or from the bile duct epithelium origin. It affects solubilization of cholesterol in bile by inducing a shift of cholesterol and phospholipids from micelles to vesicular phase and also by interacting directly with cholesterol-phospholipids vesicles. This nucleation-promoting activity is greatly increased in bile from patients with multiple gallstones. After subjecting bile to a molecular sieving column to remove soluble mucin glycoproteins as well as high molecular weight proteins (>200 kDa), the remaining low molecular weight protein (<200 kDa), and other biliary components are applied to lectin affinity column with four different types of lectin and a newly devised, sensitive cholesterol crystal growth assay (Busch et al., 1990). Busch et al. in Holzbach's laboratory found that the bound protein fractions (presumably glycoprotein) obtained apparently have both promoting and inhibitory activities, even in the absence of gallstones, in definitely different relative concentrations (Busch et al., 1991). Therefore, a balance between the coexisting effectors seems to be important.

Recently, using an array of chromatographic procedures, including gel filtration chromatography, HP (Helix pomatia) affinity chromatography, and reverse-phase HPLC, Holzbach and his colleagues isolated and purified biliary glycoprotein fractions, one having inhibitory (Ohya et al., 1993) and the other promoting (Abei et al., 1993b) activities, which were characterized by activity analysis with cholesterol crystal growth assay, electrophoresis, and deglycosylation. Promoting and inhibitory factors seem to coexist. Only a small amount of these proteins is necessary to produce an effect. The antinucleator needs only to attach itself to the most rapidly growing microdomains on a submicroscopic crystal surface (Holzbach and Busch, 1991). Isolated antinucleating biliary glycoprotein (Ohya et al., 1993) consists of a heterodimer, (Mr of 120 kDa) with two subunits of similar size. Each subunit is characterized by an isoelectric point of 6.6 and shows comparable inhibitory activity. The subunits share a similar polypeptide backbone based upon a highly similar amino acids profile, suggesting that the differential subunit glycosylation alone may account for the apparent heterodimeric structure. This biliary glycoprotein (Ohya et al., 1993) was recently identified as belonging to the cytokeratin family of proteins (Schwarzendrube et al., 1992). Pronucleating biliary glycoprotein (Abei et al., 1993a) has an Mr of 42 kDa, with a concentration-dependent cholesterol nucleation-promoting activity. It consists of an extensively glycosylated monomer with an acidic isoelectric point probably based on the sialic acid content of the carbohydrate moiety. Abei et al. found that $\alpha_1$-acid glycoprotein (AAG) accounts for the greatest portion of a net biliary Con A-bound promoting activity derived from the currently defined and well-identified glycoproteins (Abei et al., 1993b). The amino acid sequence and immunochemical data identified this 42-kDa glycoprotein as a biliary form of AAG (Abei et al., 1994). Glycans in this extensively glycosylated protein play an important role in its potent promoting activity. However, the AAG concentration in human gallbladder bile is about 5 $\mu$g/ml, and its level is significantly higher in cholesterol gallstone patients than in gallstone-free patients (Nuutinen et al., 1992). However, more than 60% of total Con A binding promoting activity remains unaccounted for, suggesting the presence of other important and still unidentified promotors in human bile. Comparson of the effects of immunoabsorptive removal of each of the putative promotors, IgM, IgA, IgG, APN (aminopeptidase N), pcPLC (phospholipase C) and AAG shows that the promoting potency is IgM > IgA = AAG > IgG. APN and pcPLC show no effect on crystal growth at their apparent physiological concentrations. Recently, Ahmed et al. (1994) proposed that the different effects of biliary proteins modulating nucleation may be nonspecific and may be related to their hydrophobic : hydrophilic index, determined experimentally by measuring retention time on a phenyl-agarose column chromatographic ligand than their secondary structure. The most hydrophilic proteins show maximal pronuleating potency and less hydrophilic proteins show minimal or no pronuleating potency.

**Substances and conditions favoring nucleation**

They include bilirubin (Lillemore et al., 1988), calcium (Shiffman and Moore, 1987), immunoglobulin (Harvey et al., 1991), and phospholipase C present in human gallbladder bile (Pattinson, 1988; Pattinson and Willis, 1990; 1991b; Little et al., 1993) and fibronectin (Chijiiwa et al., 1991). Inflammatory changes in the gallbladder mucosa sometimes encountered in the presence of gallstones may allow an increased flux of plasma proteins into bile (Jüngst et al., 1991) and complicates the situation. The taurine conjugate of deoxycholic acid shortens the nucleation time and accelerates nucleation in artificial bile (Van Berge Henegouwen et al., 1987). Efficient fusion of vesicles occurs in the presence of very small phospholipase C activity, which may be found in human bile (1.2 nmol/min/ml) (Little et al., 1993). An immediate increase of radius of vesicles of 1 nm on addition of phospholipase C corresponds to the rapid binding of phospholipase C to the surface of vesicles. However, the level of enzyme activity is relatively low, and would have a significant effect only on phospholipid levels, and hence cholesterol solubility, in a situation of prolonged gallbladder stasis such as impairment of gallbladder emptying (Pattinson and Willis, 1990).

Thus an imbalance between biliary proteins having either inhibitory or promoting activities on nucleation and/or growth of cholesterol monohydrate crystals is important at the initial stage of cholesterol gallstone formation. However, the relative contribution of promotors and inhibitors remains to be studied. The inhibitory effect seems to be saturable, while the promoting effect is not (Busch et al., 1991). The conditions which favor nucleation include increased pH (Shiffman and Moore, 1988a), decreased gallbladder emptying (Doty et al., 1983), and enhanced gallbladder absorption (Lee, 1978; Conter et al., 1986b; Roslyn et al., 1987a).

## Role of lipid peroxidation and phospholipase in cholesterol monohydrate crystal formation

Recently, it was suggested that lipid peroxidation may play a significant role in the precipitation of cholesterol from bile and thus in the pathogenesis of cholesterol stones (Lichtenberg et al., 1988). Phospholipid peroxidation markedly reduces the stability of the mixed micellar system in bile composed of cholate, PC, and supersaturated cholesterol. Lichtenberg et al. suggest that, in view of the increased lipid peroxidation in the elderly, the increased frequency of gallstones with age may be explained by the possible peroxidation of biliary phospholipids. Recently, Groen et al. studied the influence of phospholipases $A_2$, C, and D on nucleation time using model bile (Groen et al., 1989a). While phospholipase C decreases nucleation time, phopsholipases $A_2$, and D inhibit nucleation, prolong nucleation time and influence nucleation by nonspecific protein effects, although earlier Neiderhiser showed that phospholipase $A_2$ does not influence cholesterol solubilization in bile (Neiderhiser and Roth, 1970). Cleavage products formed after incubation of native bile with different phospholipases are choline, phosphoryl choline, and free fatty acid; phospholipases present in bile do not seem to play an important role in the formation of cholesterol gallstones. However, it was suggested that phospholipase $A_2$ could modulate nucleation indirectly by releasing arachidonic acid from PC (Carey and Cahalane, 1988a;

Van Berge Henegouwen et al., 1987), probably by inducing hypersecretion of mucin in the gallbladder, as in the prairie dog (La Morte et al., 1986). Another possibility is that degradation of PC present in micelles and vesicles decreases cholesterol solubilization in bile, leading to the direct crystallization of cholesterol. Although formation of lysophosphatidyl choline reduces cholesterol solubilization in bile, addition of a stoichiometric amount of oleic acid fully restores it (Neiderhiser and Roth, 1972a). Recently, phospholipase C has been identified in bile free from bacterial infection in cholesterol stone patients (Pattinson, 1988; Pattinson and Willis, 1990). Phospholipase C activity is measured by the release of phosphoryl[$^3$H]choline from the substrate 1, 2-dipalmitoyl-sn-glycero-3-phospho[N-methyl-$^3$H]choline. Addition of phospholipase produces cholesterol precipitation (Neiderhiser et al., 1966). Using phospholipase C purified by a Con A affinity column and incubating with pronase, Pattinson et al. found that incubation of phospholipase C in model bile induces a transfer of cholesterol and phospholipids from micellar to vesicular phase and accelerates the nucleation time concomitant with phospholipid hydrolysis (Pattinson et al., 1991). As little as 7% of phospholipid hydrolysis is necessary for lipid transfer from micelles to vesicles. These effects are prevented by incubating phospholipase C activity with EDTA, resulting in reduced transfer of lipid and extended nucleation time. Bacterial phospholipase C produces the same effect. It was found that pronase digestion does not diminish phospholipase C activity and, hence, phospholipid hydrolysis. This is in contrast to the finding by Groen that pronase digestion of a Con A-bound fraction prevented phospholipid breakdown without affecting lipid transfer (Groen et al., 1989b). Whether or not phospholipase C is one, if not the specific, component in the Con A nucleation-promoting fraction has been contested. Using quasi-elastic light scattering spectroscopy, Little et al. found that phospholipase C from Clostridium perfringens induces rapid aggregation and fusion of phospholipids-cholesterol vesicles – a prerequisite for cholesterol monohydrate crystal formation (Little et al., 1993). Vesicle growth can be sustained for days in the absence of $Ca^{2+}$ once diacylglycerol is generated. The hydrolysis product of phospholipase C leads to destabilization and fusion of cholesterol-saturated biliary vesicles. However, the activity of phospholipase necessary to influence nucleation seems to be high, and different phospholipases may have opposite effects. Therefore, the question of the role of biliary phospholipase C in the pathogenesis of gallstones is far from settled.

## Role of calcium and magnesium

Calcium participates in gallstone formation as the structural part of the gallstones, promoting fusion of acidic phospholipid vesicles (Kibe et al., 1985; Holzbach, 1986), accelerates cholesterol monohydrate crystal growth (Neithercut, 1989), and enhances the ability of mucin to bind both hydrophobic compounds (Smith and LaMont, 1984) and bilirubin (Niu et al., 1989).

**State of calcium in bile**

Calcium exists as either free $Ca^{2+}$ ions or as bound/complexed calcium. Only free ion, $Ca^{2+}$, is available to participate in chemical reactions and enter into solubility relationships (Moore, 1984). Most calcium in bile (70 to 80%) is bound to calcium-binding ligands, including macromolecules such as bile acid micelles and mucous glycoprotein, as revealed by ultrafiltration (Sutor and Wilkie, 1977a) and equilibrium dialysis (Williamson and Percy-Robb, 1980), but the former accounts for only 20–30%. Calcium affinity for biliary lipid aggregates in model bile has been studied by Donovan et al., (1994) using calcium electrode. Calcium binding increases with increasing bile salt concentration and PC content and varies with species (dihydroxy and trihydroxy bile salt) and with conjugation (glycine and taurine conjugates). Most calcium is bound to mixed micelles, with minor contributions by bile salt monomers, simple micelles, and vesicles. Bile salt-induced binding of calcium to mixed micelles and vesicles may be important in the nucleation of cholesterol and bilirubin from native bile.

**Calcium precipitation in bile**

Calcium probably binds to mucin, an anionic polymer involved in the initial stages and growth of gallstones. Such binding provides a buffering effect and diminishes the rise of calcium ion. Addition of mucin was found to inhibit calcium carbonate precipitation in vitro (Yamasaki et al., 1993). Less than 20% is in the form of ionized calcium ($Ca^{2+}$) (Sutor et al., 1980; Marteau et al., 1990; Shiffman et al., 1990) and may be co-precipitated with anions present in bile such as carbonate. The most abundant calcium salt in gallstones is calcium carbonate (Bogren and Larsson, 1963; Sutor and Wooley, 1973). The gallbladder acidifies bile by secreting $H^+$ ions (Rege and Moore, 1987; Marteau et al., 1990) and offsets the decrease in calcium solubility (Shiffman et al., 1990), thereby lowering biliary carbonate concentrations and the $[Ca^{2+}] \times [CaCO_3]$ product (Gleeson et al., 1992), and potentially protecting calcium precipitation (Rege et al., 1987, 1989; Gleeson et al., 1992). Hydrogen ion secreted by the gallbladder combines with $HCO_3^-$ in gallbladder bile. Saturation of calcium salt depends on the product of both free ionized calcium and anion concentrations ($Ca^{2+} \times$ anion) in solution. Saturation can then be exceeded by increases in either anion concentration or calcium concentration (Moore, 1984). Hydrogen ion secretion by the gallbladder seems to be necessary to transform hepatic bile supersaturated with calcium carbonate to gallbladder bile unsaturated with calcium carbonate. Defective acidification of gallbladder bile in gallstone patients renders bile supersaturated with $CaCO_3$ and may lead to the precipitation of calcium carbonate, which may serve as a nidus for the subsequent formation of gallstones (Shiffman and Moore, 1988b). Alternatively, it may lead to the formation of calcium-carbonate containing gallstones or calcification of already existing gallstones (Gleeson et al., 1992). Up to 30% of gallstones are radiopaque (Rome Group for Epidemiology and Prevention of Cholelithiasis, 1987), and a considerably higher percentage is radiodense by computed tomography (CT) (Rajagopalan et al., 1989). Several cystalline forms are present, i.e., aragonite and vaterite for calcium carbonate and apatite and whitlockite for calcium phosphate. Gallstones often have concentric layers or shells of different composition, reflecting the changing bile composition during their growth (Nakayama, 1971; Sutor and Wooley, 1974b). However, calcium ions ($Ca^{2+}$) in bile are similar regardless of the kind of gallstones present and normal control bile (Gollish et al., 1983; Marteau et al., 1990). As bile becomes concentrated in the gallbladder, the solubility of calcium salt decreases and may precipitate to form a nidus for gallstone formation. The gallbladder absorbs large amounts of calcium from bile (Rege et al., 1987), reducing intraluminal free $Ca^{2+}$ and the risk of precipitation of calcium. Most gallstones contain a core of calcium around which cholesterol and bilirubin precipitate (Been et al., 1979; Smith and LaMont, 1985, Pitchumoni et al., 1987), which are suspected to play an important role in gallstone pathogenesis by serving as a nidus (Moore, 1984). This conclusion is supported by the finding that hyperparathyroidism is associated with an increased incidence of cholelithiasis (Selle et al., 1972) and by studies on canine models (Dawes et al., 1988, 1989). Prairie dogs fed a high-cholesterol diet developed cholesterol gallstones and an increased concentration of calcium in bile (Strichartz et al., 1988). Recently, adsorption of bile acid was found to occur on amorphous calcium phosphate, which may serve as a nidus for cholesterol and bilirubin precipitation (Govers et al., 1994). Glycine-conjugated and unconjugated dihydroxy bile acids have a high binding affinity for amorphous calcium phosphate. A cholesterol-rich diet in prairie dogs induces an increase in chenodeoxycholic acid, with a concomitant decrease of cholic acid in bile; the change in secondary bile acids is not significant (Abedin et al., 1989). A similar change in bile acid composition is noted with a carbohydrate-rich diet, irrespective of the iron content. Diet-induced alterations in bile acid composition may modify calcium solubility or gallbladder function, contributing to the increased calcium in gallbladder bile observed during cholesterol and pigment stone formation. Calcium, calcium ion, and bound calcium increase linearly with increasing concentrations of bile salt (Shiffman et al., 1992a). A previous report (Marteau et al., 1990) failed to detect a difference in measured $Ca^{2+}$ in bile between controls and gallstone patients. However, when $Ca^{2+}$ is examined as a function of bile salt and examined by the analysis of covariance using bile salt as the covariate, a subtle but significant increase of $Ca^{2+}$ is found in gallbladder bile from gallstone patients throughout the entire range of bile salt (Shiffman et al., 1992a). Usually bile from gallstone patients is less concentrated, but decreased calcium concentration is not observed. The free ionized calcium : total calcium ratio is unchanged. However, more than half of the bile samples were saturated or supersaturated with at least one calcium salt, such as calcium carbonate. Both gallbladder mucin and $Ca^{2+}$ were increased with gallstone formation in man following rapid weight reduction, and excess $Ca^{2+}$ in gallbladder bile increased curvilinearly with increasing mucin concentration (Shiffman et al., 1992b). Mucin may modulate $Ca^{2+}$ in gallbladder bile, and vice versa. Calcium enhances the hydrophobic binding properties of mucin (Niu et al., 1989) and the pronucleating property (Holzbach, 1986). Mucous glycoprotein may be responsible for calcium precipitaiton in bile (Maki et al., 1971, Nagashima et al., 1974). A calcium-binding protein inhibiting calcium carbonate precipitation in an in vitro model system was isolated from cholesterol stones (Shimizu et al., 1989).

**Calcium in the course of gallstone formation**

Calcium ion combines with several biliary anions such as carbonate, phosphate, bilirubinate, or palmitate to form poorly soluble salts in bile which are often present in the central region of gallstones (Sutor and Wooley, 1973; Crowther and Soloway, 1990). Bile salt inhibits precipitation of calcium hydroxyapatite or its precursor, i.e., amorphous calcium phosphate, by reducing calcium activity or poisoning nascent crystals (calcium-buffering hypothesis) (Crowther and Okido, 1994). Calcium in gallbladder bile is increased even before the actual formation of gallstones in prairie dogs (Strichartz et al., 1988), in dogs (Dawes et al., 1989), and in man (Shiffman et al., 1992a) and with the presence of gallstones (Shiffman et al., 1992a). Free calcium ions influence the kinetics of cholesterol precipitation (Toor et al., 1978). The presence of PC influences calcium binding of bile acid (Stevens et al., 1991). Calcium as free $Ca^{2+}$ ion promotes fusion of acidic phospholipid vesicles and accelerates cholesterol crystal growth independent of its effect on mucin (Toor et al., 1978; Holzbach, 1986). Biliary calcium could promote the aggregation of supersaturated vesicles by a reduction of their net negative surface charge, thereby reducing intervesicle repulsive forces (Neithercut, 1989). This may promote the formation of microscopically visible multilamellar vesicles from which initial cholesterol monohydrate crystals may precipitate. Biliary calcium does not trigger nucleation and requires the completion of the initial steps of nucleation before the promotion of crystal formation. Thus many key steps depend on the presence of both calcium and mucin.

In human bile, calcium precipitation is the requisite event in the initiation and growth of pigment stones and is postulated to initiate cholesterol gallstone formation by forming a nidus for cholesterol precipitation. Bile from patients with gallstones, either cholesterol or pigment, is often supersaturated with calcium and liable to calcium precipitation (Shiffman and Moore, 1987). Gleeson et al. found that bile of patients with surface gallstone calcification has a similar concentration of total calcium and calcium ions but higher gallbladder pH, higher carbonate ion concentration, and higher $[Ca^{2+}] \times [CO^{2-}]$ ion product than bile from patients with radiolucent stones (Gleeson et al., 1992; Knyrim and Vakil, 1992). Surface deposits rich in calcium and bile pigment are often found on gallstones with no accompanying stone obstruction of the cystic duct (Phemister et al., 1939). Feeding calcium to animals increases their biliary calcium concentration by increasing ionized calcium and biliary calcium-unconjugated bilirubin ion product ($Ca^{2+} \cdot UCB$) (Magnuson et al., 1989b). Therefore, prolonged feeding of calcium supplement may promote formation of a calcium bilirubinate, which is consistently found in the center of almost all cholesterol stones (Been et al., 1979; Pitchumoni et al., 1987). In prairie dogs on a cholesterol-rich lithogenic diet, increases in cholesterol saturation and total protein concentration precede cholesterol monohydrate crystal formation (Magnuson et al., 1990). However, changes in ionized calcium, unconjugated bilirubin concentration, and pH, decreased gallbladder emptying (Doty et al., 1983), and enhanced gallbladder absorption (Lee, 1978; Roslyn et al., 1987a, Conter et al., 1986b) are noted only after the formation of cholesterol monohydrate crystals and gallstones.

Biliary calcium and magnesium increase the number of cholesterol monohydrate crystals at lower concentrations than sodium and influence the rate of development of gallstones. Amiloride, which reduces the concentrating ability of gallbladder mucosa by inhibiting sodium-hydrogen ion exchange (Strichartz et al., 1989a), reduces the intraluminal calcium concentration and the incidence of gallstone formation in animals from 83 % to 13 % (Strichartz et al., 1989a). Calcium concentration decreases in gallbladder bile but not in hepatic bile. Therefore, altered gallbladder absorption and increased biliary calcium are important critical factors in the pathogenesis of cholesterol gallstones, as can be deduced from the presence of calcium salts in the central matrix of many, if not all, cholesterol stones.

## Growth of cholesterol monohydrate crystals into gallstones

Since it is impossible to observe the transition from cholesterol monohydrate crystals to cholesterol gallstones in man, one must extrapolates the findings in experimental animals. According to MacPherson et al., as early as 12 hours after the commencement of a high-cholesterol diet in the ground squirrel, cholesterol saturation of bile starts to rise and cholesterol crystals appear in bile after 24 hours (MacPherson et al., 1987). Aggregation of molecules to form critical clusters marks the beginning of nucleation. After 2 weeks, the cholesterol crystals thus formed aggregate to produce microliths. After 10 weeks they grow into gallstones of 1 mm and after 20 weeks of 2 mm in diameter. The growth of larger cholesterol monohydrate crystals occurs preferentially at crystal face "defects" such as spiral, step, or edge dislocations (Nakagawa et al., 1985). Nucleation and growth of crystals seem to be a continuous process. Cholesterol crystals are cemented together with matrix consisting mainly of mucin glycoprotein interspersed between cholesterol crystals shaping mature gallstones (Sutor and Wooley, 1974a; Bills and Lewis, 1975; Been et al., 1979; LaMont et al., 1984, Smith and LaMont, 1985). Calcium bilirubinate may precipitate out during formation and may be present in the core of cholesterol stones. Recently, the role of gallbladder mucin in postnucleation gallstone maturation has been studied in a novel model system (Afdhal et al., 1993). Uniformly sized cholesterol crystals are incubated in a model bile with varying degrees of cholesterol supersaturation. The average crystal area is calculated under a polarized microscope. Acceleration of crystal growth by gallbladder mucin is found to be concentration and time dependent. Concomitant decrease in cholesterol saturation, an increase in total cholesterol mass, and a decrease in the total number of crystals suggest the net transfer of cholesterol to larger crystals. As the cholesterol concentration decreases, the surface free energy of small crystals favors their release of cholesterol molecules to either solution or to larger crystals with lower free surface energy and hence more stability. Microscopic formed elements with a laminated, multicolored structure resembling miniature gallstones have long been known as microspheroliths, mostly in the German literature (Juniper et al., 1956); they are single, organized crystalline structures varying from 7 to 50$\mu$ in size (Juniper and Burson, 1957). Their shape varies from spheres to cubes, ovoid, lemons, drumbells. wheat sheaves, clubs, and multilobulated stars that may be clear, colorless, or opaque and varying shade of gray, yellow, brown, and green. Studies by phase contrast and scanning electron microscopy on the development of gallstones in squirrel monkeys fed an atherogenic diet disclosed that the shape and nature of gallstones gradually change during the period of feeding (Osuga et al., 1974). Irregular sand-like stones develop after 3 months of feeding on a lithogenic diet. Simple radial stones appear after 6 months, and complex multilobular and mulberry stones first after 9 months. Very slow growth of stones is apparent, since no visible stone is present before 3 months. Gradual transformation of simpler to more complex forms is indicated by the fact that sand-like stones are the only form present at 3 months. After 9 months, complex and simple forms may coexist. After 12 months, gallstones in squirrel monkeys vary widely in size. In fact, in gallbladders from which complex forms of stones have been removed, only fine, sand-like, and simple radial stones are noted in some animals. Monkeys with gallstones have a much higher concentration of simple and aggregated crystals in the gallbladder, as well as hepatic bile. Single euhedral crystals, most frequently seen, seem to enlarge by layer growth and aggregation with other crystals resulting in clusters. Their edges are often irregular, suggesting that dissolution of crystals is taking place. A polygonal or irregular growth layer is seen due to two-dimensional nucleation or a spiral mechanism. An alternate course of development is by assembly of round but irregular concrements, including a "wagon wheel" form, so named for the axle with radiating spokes described by Osuga et al. (1974). A somewhat rarer microcrystalline form, nearly polygonal, which may be related to the wagon wheel configuration, is also present. The platy unit or the assembly of layers of parallel crystals is the basic unit of microliths and macroscopic gallstones. Bilirubin crystals are distributed throughout in some stones. Multilobular stones are formed by the adhesion of groups of simple radial stones (Juniper and Woolf, 1956; Osuga et al., 1974). Different sizes of stones present in squirrel monkeys on long-term dietary regimens indicates that gallstones grow gradually, with new stones forming continuously (Osuga and Portman, 1971). Gallstones increase in size, number, and total mass during the period of feeding. A hypothetical sequence of events in the course of development of gallstones in squirrel monkeys is beautifully illustrated by Osuga et al. (1974).

Crystals seen in the bile of squirrel monkeys have a striking resemblance to those observed in man, described earlier in detail by Juniper and Woolf, (1956); and Juniper and Burson, (1957), who gave very detailed descriptions of three types of microliths consisting of aggregates of cholesterol crystals, of calcium bilirubinate granules, and of microspheroliths. The findings by phase contrast microscopy are fully corroborated by scanning electron microscopy. The predominant orientation of crystal bands is radiation from the center outward. No foreign body or parasite eggs or bacteria are usually found in the center of cholesterol stones. Bilirubin globules are sometimes found in the central zones, but not as a central core. They are composed predominantly of calcium salt of unconjugated bilirubin mono-anion (Womack et al., 1963) and may play a pivotal role in the initial phase of gallstone formation (Malet et al., 1986b). When cholesterol-phospholipid vesicles coalesce in the mucin-glycoprotein gel, calcium bilirubinate precipitates out, forming bilirubin globules (Smith and LaMont, 1983, 1985). Analysis of gallstones in layers reveals that, in addition to bilirubin as seen in the so-called Liesegang rings, other bile constituents such as cholesterol, bile acid, and calcium content vary considerably (Nakayama, 1971; Sutor and Wooley 1974b). Mulberry stones are composed of individual simple stones with their identity retained, but are attached to their neighbors by interlocking surface crystals.

### Speed of the growth of gallstones

Incomplete emptying of the gallbladder favors gallstone growth, as it permits retention of bile in the gallbladder containing growing gallstones. Mucin seems to be an important factor in trapping crystals for further growth to macroscopic gallstones. Crystals are often seen trapped in a mucous substance in bile, especially in the gallbladder. Hultén stressed the importance of the growth of crystals in mucin layers present in a niche between mucosal folds of the gallbladder wall (Hultén, 1970). Repeated growth and dissolution, particularly at the surface of gallstones, seem to be taking place, as suggested by the often irregular edge of the crystals (Osuga et al., 1974). Apparently, gallstones seem to be formed when the net rate of crystallization is greater than the net rate of dissolution or passage into the intestinal tract (Schoenfield, 1972). Diurnal or periodic changes in bile composition result in alternating formation and dissolution of crystals. This is in agreement with the previous study on prairie dogs with $^{14}C$-cholesterol loading and determination of specific activity. It was found that cholesterol in gallstone is equilibrated with other parts of the cholesterol pool and not sequestered as a static component, suggesting possible regression (Brennenman et al., 1972). In man, growth of cholesterol monohydrate crystals and gallstones is thought to be much slower than in experimental animals. Repeat cholecystography (Wolpers, 1974) and $^{14}C$ dating (Mok et al., 1986) revealed that the growth rate of cholesterol gallstones in man is estimated to be 0.6 mm per year. Symptoms usually appear after 5 to 20 years.

### Solitary versus multiple cholesterol stones

Cholesterol gallstones may be either solitary or multiple. Their differences have been noted in several respects, such as nucleation time and recurrence rate after complete dissolution. The nucleation time is found to be shorter in the bile of patients with multiple stones than those with solitary stones (Groen et al., 1990; Tudyka et al., 1994) due to the high titers of pronucleating factors in the former (Mok et al., 1992). The rate of recurrence is higher with multiple stones than with solitary stones after complete dissolution by adjuvant treatment, either oral cholelitholysis and/or extracorporeal shockwave lithotripsy (ESWL) (Villanova et al., 1989). Their growth patterns seem to be considerably different. In a painstaking study spanning over 36 years using cholecystography, which gives better definition of images than ultrasonography, Wolpers documented 48 cases of patients who initially had normal cholecystograms but subsequently developed gallstones in the gallbladder; 19 were solitary stones and 29 were multiple (Wolpers and Hofmann, 1993). He found that solitary stones are formed after a precursor phase of formation of free-floating crystal laminae of cholesterol. A single lamina acts as a nucleus for the development of a solitary stone shaped as an ellipsoid. About 10% of solitary stones contain a solitary pigment center. Alternatively, the laminae form aggregate loosely, and undergo extended compaction and internal remodeling into compact spheroids. Multiple stones are formed, without a precursor phase, first with the appearance of thin cholesterol crystals which aggregate to form spheres, not laminae, up to 1 mm in size. Next, these spheres develop into gallstones. When sudden aggregation of similar sheres stops at the earlier stage, sandy stones develop. When spheres continue to coalece mulberry stones are formed, which, in turn, were transformed into either faceted stones (if many are present) or barrel-shaped stones (if few are present) over a few years. The primary spheres conglomerate in one of two ways, i.e. small numbers of spheres coalesce into a large number of stones, or large numbers of spheres coalesce into a small number of stones. Temporary occlusion of the cystic duct leads to the supersaturation of bile with calcium bilirubinate and/or calcium carbonate, which, in turn, deposits on the surface of gallstones; metamorphosis of the stone center may occur. During the observation period the secondary or even third generation of stones may appear.

## Role of the Gallbladder in Gallstone Formation

Although much emphasis has recently been placed on the changes taking place in bile (biliary event), the role of the gallbladder in the formation of cholesterol gallstones (gallbladder event) should not be underestimated. The gallbladder must play an important role in the formation of cholesterol stones, since they are formed mainly in the gallbladder even though bile is more supersaturated with cholesterol in other compartments of the biliary tract and removal of the gallbladder by cholecystectomy cures the disease and cholecystectomy prevents gallstone formation in experimental animals (Van der Linden et al., 1959). The gallbladder has a pronounced effect on the composition of bile produced by the liver by regulating the enterohepatic circulation of bile acid. Obviously, knowledge of the local gallbladder event is required to understand fully the pathogenesis of gallstones. Neither the liver nor the gallbladder alone has an exclusive role in the formation of cholesterol stones, which are the end product of interactions between the liver and the biliary tract. Bile lithogenicity, nucleation in bile and bile stasis, are interdependent processes in the formation of gallstones. For instance, in experimental animals, lithogenic bile is said to induce hypersecretion of mucin by the gallbladder mucosa and impairs gallbladder motility prior to actual gallstone formation. Brief alternating excursions of filling and emptying of the gallbladder occur in both the fasting and fed states. Gallbladder filling and emptying are not monotonous during the fasting and postprandial states. Brief alternating excursions of filling and emptying would almost continually mix the concentrated gallbladder bile with fresh incoming dilute hepatic bile (Abiru et al., 1994). After ingestion of a meal, the gallbladder empties about two-third to three-quarters of its initial volume (Lawson et al., 1983). This is determined by the hydrostatic hepatic pressure and gallbladder contraction as driving forces and phasic and tonic contraction of the choledochoduodenal junction as resistance. Increased diversion of bile into gastrointestinal tract in cholesterol stone patients results in the increased recycling and turnover of bile salt and decreased bile acid pool (Roslyn et al., 1980). This trend appears in puberty particularly in females (von

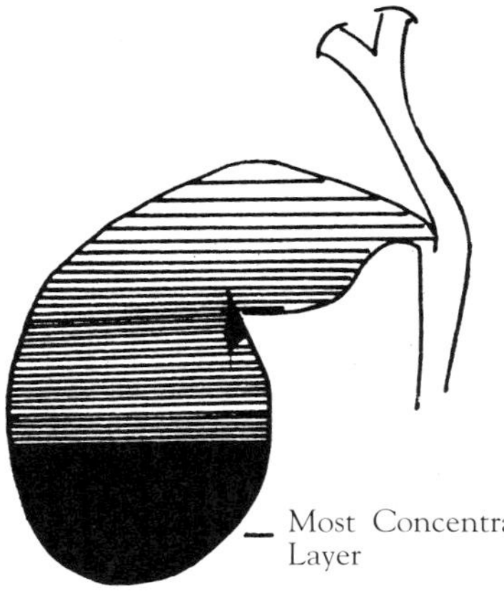


**Figure 18**

Stratification of Bile in Gallbladder: Schematic Representation

Bergmann et al., 1986). However, the gallbladder content is by no means homogeneous. Stratificaton of bile in the gallbladder, as exemplified by the occasional finding of floating stones, the so-called Åkerlund phenomenon (Åkerlund, 1933), has long been known (Figure 18) (Tera, 1960; Nakayama and Van der Linden, 1975). Incomplete emptying of the gallbladder and subsequent filling with fresh hepatic bile are responsible for layering of bile with different composition inside the gallbladder, but the possible role of such layering in gallstone formation is not well understood. Alteration of gallbladder motility resulting in bile stasis favors gallstone formation. Disordered gallbladder motility promotes nucleation, permitting continued growth of the crystals. In experimental animals, prevention of bile stasis by sphincterotomy abolishes gallstone formation in spite of the continued secretion of lithogenic bile and hypersecretion of mucin in the gallbladder (Hutton et al., 1981). Thus impaired gallbladder motility and bile stasis are important in gallstone formation.

The role of the gallbladder in gallstone formation may be divided conceptually into two parts. The first consists of modifying stored bile, favorable to gallstone formation, by absorption of water and electrolytes and secretion of various substances such as mucus, $H^+$ ion, and calcium. Nucleation of cholesterol monohydrate crystals takes place more rapidly in gallbladder bile than in hepatic bile. The second phase consists of providing a recess to allow sufficient time for cholesterol monohydrate crystals to form and grow via microliths to macroscopically recognizable gallstones by decreased contractility and motility of the gallbladder.

## Modification of bile in the gallbladder

A majority of hepatic bile, at least 80 %, enters the gallbladder during interdigestive periods (Lanzini et al., 1987; Lanzini and Northfield, 1990; Lanzini et al., 1987). After entering the gallbladder, bile is concentrated 5 to 10 times by the absorption of water and electrolytes. During overnight fasting, it is said to reach as much as 10 times the original concentration. In the gallbladder, the saturation index decreases and solubilization of cholesterol in bile becomes more stabilized (Nakayama and Van der Linden, 1975; Carey and Small, 1978). As early as 1932, experimental observation by Andrews et al. that the inflamed gallbladder wall increases permeability to bile salts led to the suggestion that this is the mechanism by which the bile salts : cholesterol ratio is decreased, leading to the precipitation of cholesterol from bile – a cardinal event in the formation of gallstones (Andrews et al., 1932). Diamond demonstrated that in the gallbladder of guinea pigs and rabbits, the gallbladder actively transports both Na and Cl, and water follows passively (Diamond, 1964). Using mice, Caldwell and Levitsky suggested that bile salt is absorbed but not cholesterol (Caldwell and Levitsky, 1967). A small amount of phospholipids is absorbed. A more recent study shows that gallbladder mucosa absorbs cholesterol from bile in animals (Neiderhiser et al., 1976) as well as in man (Svanvik et al., 1986), and more cholesterol is absorbed from bile with high cholesterol content. The lipid content of bile is an important determinant of alteration of ion transport across the gallbladder mucosa (Roslyn et al., 1989), i.e., lithogenic bile with a high cholesterol and phospholipids content and a high phopholipids : bile acid ratio significantly alters ionic transport. Absorption of water and sodium is dependent upon the intraluminal presence of lithogenic bile. In the early stage of experimental gallstone formation, gallbladder bile is more concentrated, which may partly be due to prolonged exposure to the gallbladder mucosa during bile stasis in the gallbladder (Roslyn et al., 1987a). Absorption in the gallbladder increases (Conter et al., 1986b), while $Na^+$ transport decreases (Moody et al., 1989b; Roslyn et al., 1989). Cytotoxicity of bile salt may be responsible for the change of transport, modified by the presence of phospholipids (Ammon, 1979; Roslyn et al., 1987a), and accentuated by the presence of supersaturated bile (Veraldi et al., 1991). In a later stage of experimental gallstone formation, transport is decreased, correlating well with the morphological changes (Nahrwold et al., 1976). In prairie dogs on a lithogenic diet, blood flow in gallbladder mucosa, as measured by hydrogen gas clearance, is increased significantly (Conter et al., 1992). In crossover studies, the addition of lithogenic gallbladder bile to control animals resulted in a significant increase in gallbladder mucosal blood flow. Addition of nonlithogenic gallbladder bile to the gallbladder of prairie dogs on a lithogenic diet resulted in a significant decrease in gallbladder mucosal blood flow. Similar results are observed with lithogenic and nonlithogenic hepatic bile. Thus, alterations in gallbladder mucosal blood flow are influenced by the presence or absence of lithogenic bile and may play a role in cholesterol gallstone formation. However, it may also be possible that the change in gallbladder mucosal blood flow is a nonspecific response to the cytotoxic property of supersaturated bile (Veraldi et al., 1991) resulting in the vasodilation from an inflammatory mediator such as prostaglandin or from hydrophobic bile acid (Bomzon et al., 1984). Ion transport in the gallbladder increases in the presence of lithogenic bile (Roslyn et al., 1989). Absorption in the gallbladder increases during the early stage of cholesterol stone formation when cholesterol monohydrate crystals are present in bile but before the macroscopic gallstone appears (Conter et al., 1986b; Roslyn et al 1987a).

## Role of intraluminal content

An increase in solute concentration resulting from enhanced water absorption may influence the concentration of pronucleating and antinucleating factors and thereby promote agglomeration of crystals, eventually leading to stone formation. Hence, in a sense, altered gallbladder absorption may itself be a prerequisite to cholesterol gallstone formation. Changes in gallbladder ion transport are determined in part by the interaction of a variety of intracellular stimuli, including cyclic adenosine monophosphate, neural and hormonal influences, and prostaglandins. It also occurs as a response of otherwise healthy mucosa to altered luminal content (i.e., lithogenic bile), not because of an irreversible alteration in the absorptive property of the tissue (Abdou et al 1985). Ammon (1979) first suggested that the phospholipids : bile acid ratio in bile may be a determinant of gallbladder absorption. Increase of bile salt relative to phospholipids in bile reduces gallbladder absorption, while absorption in the gallbladder increases as the phospholipids : bile salt ratio increases. Instillation of conjugated bile acid in dog gallbladder in concentrations well below the physiological level inhibits gallbladder absorption, but its effect is blocked by the addition of lecithin. Phospholipids reverse a bile salt-induced increase in transmural movement of dextran in rabbit gallbladder (Heuman et al., 1980). Recently, Roslyn et al. using prairie dog gallbladder in a Ussing-type chamber, determined the influence of bile salt and varying ratios of biliary bile salt and phospholipids on transepithelial potential difference Vms, resistance Rt, and short-circuit (Roslyn et al., 1989). They found direct evidence that the ratio of phospholipids to bile salt modulates ion transport across prairie dog gallbladder, which may be an important determinant of gallbladder absorption in health and disease. Thus luminal factors normally present in bile may help regulate the gallbladder's absorptive function. The mechanism underlying alteration of membrane permeability and ion transport by bile salt is said to consist of mucosal damage (Saunders et al., 1975; Gullikson et al., 1977), alteration of mucosal permeability (Heuman et al., 1980), or activation of adenylate cyclase (Binder et al., 1977) and alteration of the integrity of the intercellular tight junctional complex (Freel et al., 1983). On the other hand, the mechanism of phospholipids antagonizing the bile salt-induced effect on ion transport is suggested to be the increased concentration of phospholipids, which induces micellar "swelling" and facilitates incorporation of bile salt into these structures (Roslyn et al., 1989). Biliary lipids and bilirubin are concentrated by net absorption of water across the gallbladder epithelium (Wood and Svanvik, 1983). Absorption of electrolytes and water in the gallbladder increases bile acid concentration and enhances micellar solubilization of cholesterol (Carey and Small, 1978) but decreases the stability of phospholipids-cholesterol vesicles, predisposing to cholesterol precipitation and nucleation of cholesterol monohydrate crystals (Halpern et al., 1986b; Holzbach, 1986). During an overnight fast, dilute hepatic bile enters the gallbladder, where bile is concentrated, and results in the layer formation, i.e., stratification of bile in the gallbladder (Nakayama and Vander Linden, 1975), providing a microenvironment for gallstone formation.

### Role of inflammation

The concentrating activity of the gallbladder is subjected to physiological and pathophysiological variation. Mild inflammatory change and chronic cholecystitis are always found in the gallbladder wall upon histological examination of the specimen removed by cholecystectomy for cholesterol gallstones. Whether the inflammation observed is the cause or the effect of gallstones is not known. Svanvik et al. inserted human gallstones into cat gallbladder and found that slight to moderate inflammation was produced in the gallbladder; the concentrating activity of the gallbladder was not changed (Svanvik et al., 1981). However, inflammatory changes must affect mucosal transport in the gallbladder. Good correlation between the presence of gallstones and inflammation of the gallbladder on the one hand and an increase in goblet cells and mucus- secreting glands, on the other, is noted (Bouchier et al., 1965). Chronic cholecystitis reduces the concentrating activity of gallbladder mucosa and decreases absorption of water and electrolytes, secretion of $Na^+$, and active fluid secretion (Rådberg et al., 1988, Jacyna et al., 1988a). The ratio of biliary lipids in gallbladder bile to hepatic bile decreases with increasing histological abnormality of the gallbladder wall with a patent cystic duct (Rådberg et al., 1988). A similar relationship is found for bilirubin. The direction and rate of transport correlate with the degree of mural inflammation (Nahrwold et al., 1976; Jivegard et al., 1986). Inflammation of the gallbladder wall is associated with reduced absorption or even reversal of transport (Svanvik et al., 1981). In vitro, poor fluid absorption or even secretion into the lumen of the inflamed gallbladder occurs (Dumont et al., 1982). Slight absorption of biliary lipids and bilirubin may take place (Ostrow, 1967, 1969; Neiderhiser and Roth, 1972b; Neiderhiser et al., 1973). Further, Ostrow demonstrated that unconjugated bilirubin is absorbed much faster than conjugated bilirubin; passive non-ionic absortpion is suggested (Ostrow, 1967). Acute but not chronic inflammation of the gallbladder wall is associated with enhanced diffusion of bile acid from the gallbladder lumen. Differential absorption of organic components of gallbladder bile influences cholesterol solubility, particularly in the presence of mucosal injury (Ostrow, 1971). Conjugated bilirubin is only slowly transported across the normal gallbladder mucosa, and absorption of unconjugated bilirubin is unaffected by the presence of inflammation. Thus the ratio of bilirubin in gallbladder bile to hepatc bile is the accurate measure of concentrating activity on organic contents, since the secretion rate of bilirubin into bile is fairly constant (Riegel et al., 1932; Ostrow, 1967). Fluid secretion in the inflamed gallbladder is said to be mediated by prostaglandins (Svanvik et al., 1981; Jacyna et al., 1988a) and is reversed by nonsteroidal anti-inflammatory drugs (NSAID) which are known prostaglandin antagonists. It is known that in the inflamed gallbladder, secretion of cholesterol occurs from mucosa (Svanvik et al., 1986).

### Mucus secretion in the gallbladder

The gallbladder adds mucus to bile during its storage. The mechanism of secretion of mucin granules by gallbladder mucosa has been studied using quantitative electron microscopy (Wahlin et al., 1976). The increased levels of mucus and mucus degradation products are noted by Verschure (1956), using paper electrophoresis, and by Bouchier et al.

(1965) in gallbladder bile of gallstone patients by the analysis of hexosamine, a marker for mucin. Increased mucin glycoprotein content is also noted in the bile of gallstone patients by others (Lee et al., 1979; Sahlin et al., 1988; Mingrone et al., 1988), rising as much as 500% (Shiffman et al., 1993a). Gallbladder mucin increases either before or during the early phase of gallstone formation in man. This increase is not the result of gallstones within the gallbladder or cystic duct obstruction resulting in a secondary increase in mucin production. Excess mucin is preferentially located adjacent to gallbladder mucosa, forming a gel layer, and provides an environment for cholesterol monohydrate nucleation. Cholesterol monohydrate crystals are trapped in the mucin layer and aggregate. Mucin hypersecretion occurs shortly after the sustained increase in biliary cholesterol secretion and in the cholesterol saturation index induced in prairie dogs by feeding a 2% cholesterol-enriched diet followed by the appearance of cholesterol crystals in bile (Lee et al., 1981b). The early change in gallbladder mucus during the initial phase of gallstone formation was first documented in cholesterol-fed ground squirrels (Smith et al., 1987). Mucus granules are identified in the gallbladder epithelium of mice, preferentially in the cells of invaginations and crypts (Wahlin et al., 1976; Wahlin, 1977), and in ground squirrels (MacPherson et al., 1987; Pemsingh et al., 1987). Incorporation of [$^3$H]-galactose, a glycoprotein precursor, is noted in the membrane-bound granules localized in the supranuclear cytoplasmic regeon and later in apical cytoplasmic regions of epithelial cells as well as in the mucus present in the gallbladder lumen of mice (Wahlin, 1977). Golgi apparatus plays an important role in the synthesis of glycoprotein (Wahlin et al., 1974; Wahlin and Schiebler, 1975). In the course of gallstone formation in mice, a significant increase is noted in the volume density of Golgi complexes (Wahlin, 1977). Therefore, it seems apparent that glycoproteins formed in the cisternae of the Golgi complex migrate through the subapical and apical cytoplasm and are discharged into the gallbladder lumen. At the distal Golgi, secretory products can be segregated into distinct types of secretory vesicles that differ in their dependence on external stimuli for their release. In gallbladder mucosa, secretory granules are stored in the electron-dense secretory granules until exostosis is triggered by an extracellular signal such as hormone or neurotransmitter regulated exostosis (Wahlin et al., 1976; Axelsson et al., 1979). The mechanism of mucus secretion by the gallbladder epithelium may be nolocrine, merocrine, or apocrine secretion, but exostosis of granule content seems to be merocrine secretion in the ground squirrel, as in the mouse and guinea pig. MacPherson et al. found that in ground squirrel the cholesterol saturation index of bile rose within 12 hours on a lithogenic diet; there was a rapid rise of mucus by 18 hours and the appearance of cholesterol monohydrate crystals at 24 hours coinciding with a sharp decrease in the absolute concentration of bile acid and phospholipids and an increase in cholesterol (MacPherson et al., 1987). A significant increase in intracellular mucin granules is noted as early as 18 hours on a lithogenic diet. Mucus hypersecretion prior to cholesterol monohydrate crystal formation seems to be stimulated by lithogenic bile, since Lee et al. prevented the hypersecretion by prior ligation of the cystic duct (Lee et al., 1981b). However, in man, no evidence was obtained by electron microscopic morphometric study of the gallbladder epithelium to indicate that the degree of cholesterol saturation influences the mucin content in the gallbladder wall (Sahlin et al., 1990). A tendency toward an increased secretory granule volume was found in the gallbladder mucosa of gallstone patients compared with gallstone-free controls. Marked reduction in total lysosome area and in the volume density of lysosomes is found in gallstone patients, possibly relating to a decreased intracellular degradation of protein and/or mucin.

A thick sludge-like layer overlying the mucosal epithelium in the initial phase of gallstone formation is thought to consist of a mixture of acidic mucins. Hypersecretion of mucus and formation of this sludge like layer appear to be critical nucleating conditions in the formation of cholesterol gallstones (Pemsingh et al., 1987). Cholesterol monohydrate crystals occur in a mucus layer adherent to the gallbladder epithelium which provides a favorable environment for the nucleation process (Smith et al., 1987). In fact, Hulten observed this in resected human gallbladder specimen (Hultén, 1968a, 1968b, 1970). Hultén (1968a) found using a plastic cast, that gallbladder mucosa has well-developed niches in the whole gallbladder wall lined with epithelium, which greatly augment the mucosal surface in where water and electrolytes are absorbed and mucus is secreted. Hence, Hultén named them absorptive niches (Hultén 1968b). The diameters of the niches are pinheads in size and 1 to 2 mm in depth. The niches are blister-shaped structures which are more or less lobulated, ramify into diminishing cavities, and end in small, cup-shaped terminations. They are so tightly packed that the flat surface between them becomes negligible. They are neither Luschka's crypts nor Rokitansky-Aschoff sinuses. Changes in bile in these niches may lead to precipitation of cholesterol monohydrate crystals. Hultén (1968a) found particles of yellow cholesterol and sometimes also of black pigment enclosed in the lobulated plastic bubbles on the cast. Water absorption and pH changes toward acidity are more pronounced in niches transforming mucus into gel, in which precipitates become enveloped. The musculature of the gallbladder consists of a lattice of longitudinal and circular fibers. The former lie next to the mucosa and the latter next to the serosa. Since the gallbladder has no submucosa, its musculature lies directly against the mucosa. Gallbladder musculature compresses the mucosa, but because of the absence of submucosa, the mucosa cannot settle in folds. Thus the mucosal membrane is compressed and the contents of niches are pressed into the gallbladder lumen, cleansing the niches of their content. After a long interval, when the gallbladder contracts, it presses out a mucous clot of gel-like consistency loaded with precipitation products. Such clots were described by Naunyn (1892). He assumed that such a sedimentary, amorphous mass originated from a diseased mucous membrane due to a stone-forming "catarrh" caused by an infection from coli bacteria or irritation by stagnated bile—so-called inflammation theory of gallstone formation.

Gallbladder bile is mucous. The thickest and toughest mucus lines the mucosal surface of the gallbladder (Hultén, 1968b). The mucus becomes more viscous and more tenacious the longer the absorption of water and a shift in pH level continue. Precipitates in the niches may exert local irritation, which may stimulate mucus production. Caselli et al. found a layer of visible mucus suspended only above the metaplastic areas of the gallbladder mucosa. They suggested that such fully metaplastic zones may functionally represent "nucleating areas" and that the areas of the gallbladder lumen near mucus metaplasia might be the places where nucleation begins (Caselli et al., 1990). Gallinger et al. (1985) found that mucin from the bile of both gallstone patients and controls shortens nucleation time in a dose-dependent manner but they did not find any quantitative or qualitative differences in mucin (Harvey et al., 1986; Whiting and Watts, 1984). Mucin and nonmucin glycoproteins promote nucleation when added to in vitro (Gallinger et al., 1987).

### Role of prostaglandin

Mucus secretion by the gallbladder is said to be stimulated by prostaglandin and inhibited by blockers of prostanoid synthesis (LaMont et al., 1984; LaMorte et al., 1986; Wahlin et al., 1988). Factors affecting prostaglandin synthesis, such as diet, hormones, and inflammation, alter gallbladder mucin secretion and increase the risk of develpong gallstones. In addition, prostaglandin reduces sodium and water absorption by the gallbladder mucosa, mainly by inhibiting the active component of the transfer system (Leyssac et al., 1974) and initiating secretion of fluid and electrolytes in the gallbladder lumen, rendering bile less concentrated (Heintze et al., 1976). Prostaglandins are easily formed by various tissues, including the gallbladder (Leyssac et al., 1974), in response to chemical and mechanical injuries and are considered important mediators of the inflammatory response. Cholesterol given to experimental animals is found to increase the synthesis of prostaglandin by the gallbladder mucosa, i.e., $PGF_{2\alpha}$, $PGE_2$, and thromboxane, paralleling (LaMorte et al., 1985a, 1986) the hypersecretion of mucus into bile (Lee et al., 198lb). Indomethacin, a potent cyclooxygenase inhibitor, almost completely blocks in vitro prostaglandin biosynthesis (Leyssac et al., 1974), causes mucosal injury (Erickson et al., 1987), reverses the direction of net $Na^+$ flux in the secreting gallbladder, and causes absorption of $Na^+$ (Jacyna et al., 1988b). Prostaglandin release is enhanced by luminal lysophosphatidyl choline, gallbladder distension, and experimental cholecystitis (Neiderhiser et al., 1983; Thornell et al., 1986). When the gallbladder is perfused in vivo in the cat and overflow of prostaglandins from the gallbladder epithelium is used as an index of the balance between local prostaglandin formation and degradation in vivo, prostaglandin $E_2$ output is markedly raised during lysophosphatidyl choline perfusion; this response is inhibited by indomethacin administration. Prostaglandin E inhibits fluid absorption and induces fluid secretion in the gallbladder both in vitro (Leyssac et al., 1974) and in vivo (Thornell et al., 1981). Fatty acid, i.e., arachidonic acid, a precursor of prostaglandin synthesis, when added to an explant of prairie dog gallbladder in organ culture causes a two- to fivefold release of mucin (Lee et al., 1981a; LaMont et al., 1983b). Prostaglandins and their precursor, arachidonic acid, stimulate mucin secretion from gallbladder mucosa in man (Van Berge Henegouwen et al., 1987). However, exogenous prostaglandin fails to stimulate mucin secretion of gallbladder explants (O'Leary et al., 1991b). Carey et al. proposed that PC rich in arachidonic acid secreted from the liver could stimulate mucin secretion from the gallbladder mucosa of those who develop gallstones (Carey and Cahalane, 1988a). However, no relationship between gallbladder mucin and change in bile constituents could be elicited. Hence, an increase in gallbladder mucin during gallstone formation resulting from rapid weight loss in man does not seem to be the result of alterations in biliary arachidonic acid or bile salt composition in the hydrophobicity index of bile acids (Shiffman et al., 1993a). The amount of free fatty acid is significantly higher in bile with cholesterol gallstones (Mingrone et al., 1988). During gallstone formation in the prairie dog, PC in bile and gallbladder mucosa is enriched by arachidonic acid (Booker et al., 1989a), and there is an associated increase of prostaglandin synthesis in the gallbladder (LaMorte et al., 1986). Prostaglandin antagonists, such as NSAIDs – e.g. aspirin – prevent gallstone formation in animals in spite of the presence of supersaturated bile (Lee et al., 1981a, LaMont et al., 1983b). These earlier results have been refuted (Myers et al., 1989; Borch et al., 1994). However, more recently, in a careful, well-controlled study, Cohen et al. in Mosbach's laboratory showed that administration of aspirin does not alter the incidence of gallstones in the two established animal models, i.e., the prairie dog and hamster (Cohen et al., 1991). Feeding of aspirin plus cholesterol to hamsters even caused an increase in the incidence of cholesterol stones. Li et al. (1994) also found aspirin to have no effect on gallstone formation in the prairie dog, nor does it prevent a decrease in contractility despite a profound decrease in endogenous gallbladder prostanoid synthesis. In man, aspirin inhibits cholesterol precipitation and crystal formation (Broomfield et al., 1988). It also prevents gallstone recurrence in a population at high risk of cholelithiasis, i.e., after the complete dissolution of gallstones by oral administration of ursodeoxycholic acid (Hood et al., 1988). A retrospective study showed that regular users of NSAIDs had a significantly lower gallstone recurrence rate than nonusers. A prospective study of patients undergoing rapid weight reduction was inconclusive regarding the effectiveness of aspirin (Broomfield et al., 1988). The underlying mechanism is far from clear, but one of the most plausible mechanisms of action of NSAIDs in preventing gallstone recurrence is inhibition of mucoglycoprotein secretion by the gallbladder. Prostaglandins effect on motility and fluid absorption in the human gallbladder is mediated through intramural nerves present in the gallbladder wall (Lundgren et al., 1989). An other possible mediator is hydrophobic bile acid. O'Leary et al. showed that chenodeoxycholic and deoxycholic acids stimulate gallbladder mucin secretion in vitro (O'Leary et al., 1991a; O'Leary, 1994). This finding is in agreement with observations that the bile of gallstone patients contains more hydrophobic bile acid (Heuman et al., 1980; Marcus and Heaton, 1988) and that a shift from cholic acid to deoxycholic acid occur in the bile of prairie dogs on a cholesterol-supplemented lithogenic diet before the actual formation of gallstones (Brenneman et al., 1972). However, others could not find significant changes in the bile acid composition or the hydrophobicity index of bile acid with gallstone formation after gastric bypass (Shiffman et al., 1993a) or dietary-induced weight reduction (Broomfield et al., 1988, Marks et al., 1991).

Thus several studies suggested that gallbladder mucin hypersecretion is mediated by the increase in gallbladder prostaglandin synthesis (Booker et al., 1989). However, a recent study by O'Leary et al using the organ culture technique showed that prostaglandins do not regulate gallbladder mucin secretion in the prairie dog and that the increased prostaglandin synthesis in the gallbladder is not likely to be responsible for mediating gallbladder mucin hypersecretion during gallstone formation (O'Leary et al., 1991a).

Indomethacin inhibited the synthesis of prostaglandin almost completely but had no effect on mucin secretion by the gallbladder. The calcium ionophore A23187 significantly stimulates prostaglandin synthesis but does not stimulate mucin secretion. Exogenous prostaglandin does not stimulate mucin secretion of gallbladder explants. Furthermore, long term indomethacin treatment of prairie dogs on a lithogenic diet failed to inhibit gallbladder mucin hypersecretion or cholesterol monohydrate crystal formation. Gallbladder mucin secretion increases rapidly within days after the initiation of a cholesterol-supplemented diet, while increased prostaglandin synthesis becomes evident only after 2 or more weeks of cholesterol feeding (LaMorte et al., 1986). The increased prostaglandin synthesis rises to a plateau and remains elevated for 4 to 6 weeks (LaMorte et al., 1986), while the stimulus for mucin secretion increases sharply and then abates after 1 week (Lee et al., 1981a). The concentration of indomethacin required to inhibit gallbladder mucin secretion during organ culture is substantially higher than that required to inhibit prostaglandin synthesis (LaMont et al., 1983b). Thus increased mucin production may represent the mucosal response to the cytotoxic effect of lithogenic bile, perhaps mediated by cyclic nucleotide and/or inositol phosphate, as well as prostaglandins (Veraldi et al., 1991), and is enhanced by free $Ca^{2+}$ (Van der Meer et al., 1991). Biliary calcium ions also stimulate mucous glycoprotein secretion by the gallbladder mucosa, which is blocked by calcium antagonists (Malet et al., 1986a).

## Formation of sludge

Sludge is defined as gelation of gallbladder mucin with entrapment of particulate matter nucleated from bile (Carey and Cahalane, 1988a; Lee, 1990) and is sediments composed of cholesterol monohydrate crystals, cholesterol liquid crystals, and precipitates containing calcium salts of bilirubin, calcium carbonate, calcium phosphate, or with infection calcium salt of fatty acid anions embedded in a matrix of mucus gel strands (Lee and Nicholls, 1986; Shaffer, 1992). Bilirubin in sludge is composed mainly of unconjugated bilirubin (83.6%), monoglucuronide (16.3%), and a trace of diglucuronide. The importance of mucin in the formation of sludge as the first step in gallstone formation has been emphasized (Lee and Nicholls, 1986; Lee et al., 1988; Malet et al., 1986b, Carey and Cahalane, 1988a). Smith and LaMont found that the brown-black material composing the matrix of cholesterol stones has a mucin-bilirubin complex similar to that identified in biliary sludge (Smith and LaMont, 1985). This mucin gel matrix seems to play a pivotal role in the formation of gallstones, providing a nucleating matrix; enhances the adherence of cholesterol monohydrate crystals to grow into gallstones; and binds unconjugated bilirubin, providing an environment favorable for the polymerization of bilirubin. A striking increase of mucus glycoprotein in gallbladder bile of the sludge-forming group compared with the gallstone and control groups is noted. These differences are not noted in hepatic bile, suggesting that the differences occur in the gallbladder. Mucus hypersecretion and glandular metaplasia are noted in the gallbladder epithelium harboring sludge. These changes in the gallbladder lead to the increased mucus content of gallbladder bile, which, in turn, induces nucleation of cholesterol monohydrate crystals. Whether or not sludge should be regarded as an embryonic or harbinger stage of gallstone formation is controversial. Progression of biliary sludge to gallstones in man has been observed by several investigators (Messing et al., 1983; Lee and Nicholls, 1986; Lee et al., 1988; Maringhini et al., 1987; Janowitz et al., 1994). Lee et al. (Lee and Nicholls, 1986; Lee et al., 1988) and Carey and Cahalane (1988a) suggested that sludge might be regarded as the embryonic stage of gallstone disease. The frequency of the sludge-stone sequence is probably greater than that detected by ultrasonography (Shaffer, 1992). Prolonged fasting also induces sludge formation. In a prospective study of 38 patients after gastrointestinal tract surgery, Bolondi et al. (1985) using sequential ultrasonographic examination found that 10 days of fasting produced 12-sludge positive patients, (i.e., a prevalence of 33 %), 3 of whom developed gallstones after 1 to 2 years of follow-up. The effect of fasting on biliary composition is described in hepatic bile (Metzger et al., 1973) and in gallbladder bile (Bloch et al., 1980). Gallbladder bile is significantly supersaturated, with a cholesterol saturation index of 135 %, after 15 hours of fasting, but this index falls to 113 %, after 20 hours. Sludge may disappear with the resumption of oral intake and the return of normal gallbladder contractility (Messing et al., 1984; Bolondi et al., 1985). The ease with which these precipitates form during stasis of gallbladder bile suggests a role for this process in the formation of gallstones. However, Andersen et al. maintain, after longitudinal study of patients by ultrasonography, that if biliary sludge exists as a common condition it must be very short-lived, detectable only in monitored longitudinal studies, and it seems unlikely that sludge is a natural stage in the evolution of gallstones (Andersen and Højgaard, 1991). Sludge produces low-amplitude echoes without acoustic shadowing on the ultrasonogram, which change to gallstone echoes with the appearance of acoustic shadowing. At the end of the third trimester, 40 % of normal pregnant women are said to have biliary sludge in their gallbladder (Maringhini et al., 1987) which often disappears spontaneously after delivery (Maringhini et al., 1993). The prevalence of sludge in the immediate postpartum period in Italian females is reported to be 26.2 % compared to 0.5 % in controls (Maringhini et al., 1987). Sludge forming in pregnant women is said to be predominantly cholesterol monohydrate crystals. On the other hand, Jørgensen examined random population samples of 3,608 healthy subjects with ultrasonography and found sludge in only 5 persons, whereas 207 persons were found to have gallstones (Jørgensen, 1987). Slowed and incomplete emptying of the gallbladder, inadequate stimulation of gallbladder contraction, and biliary sludge formation are often associated with prolonged fasting or lack of stimulation to release CCK, such as after an abdominal operation (Bolondi et al., 1985) or total parenteral nutrition (Messing et al., 1983). Gallbladder sludge was detected by ultrasound scanning in 286 of 17,021 cases (1.68 %) and disappeared within a relatively short time (2.0+3.5 month) in 71.4 % (Janowitz et al., 1994). Lee et al reported that biliary sludge seems to disappear in 20 % of patients and to reappear in more than half, while 10 % go on to produce gallstones (Lee et al., 1988). Sludge formation in gallbladder is frequently observed by ultrasonography after bone marrow transplantation but the underlying mechanism is uncertain (Teefey et al., 1994).

## Gallbladder contractility and motility

Gallbladder emptying affects bile acid pool size and the composition of bile (Duane and Hanson, 1978). After cholecystectomy, the bile acids to be stored in the gallbladder, about 50–60 % of the total bile acid pool, enter the enterohepatic circulation. Biliary secretion of bile acid increases and cholesterol solubilization in bile improves (Shaffer and Small, 1977). Subsequently, the bile acid pool decreases but is compensated for by the increased frequency of the enterohepatic circulation. The gallbladder is no longer available to provide for the cholesterol monohydrate crystals growing into gallstones. Hence, there is no recurrence. When the gallbladder contracts, evacuation of the content is usually not complete, leaving 1/4–1/3 of the gallbladder bile in situ (Lawson et al 1983), where growth of cholesterol monohydrate crystals, microliths, and gallstones may continue (LaMorte et al., 1979). Weak contraction at long intervals causes stagnation of bile in the niches, leading to the accumulation of precipitates and the formation of tenacious mucus (Hultén, 1968b). Thus disordered gallbladder motility is associated with an increased risk of gallstones (Holzbach, 1983b; Everson, 1991). Gallbladder hypomotility can be clearly identified in animal models of cholesterol gallstones occurring early, even before the appearance of cholesterol monohydrate crystals in bile (Fridhandler et al., 1983). Periodic emptying of the gallbladder is demonstrated to prevent gallstone formation in the prairie dog (Roslyn et al., 1979, 1981a). Marked reduction in the incidence of gallstones in cholesterol-fed prairie dogs receiving a daily stimulus of noncholesterol, lipid-protein emulsion containing vegetable oil, peanut oil, and milk solids was observed in spite of the marked rise in the saturation index of bile. In these animals, good mixing of gallbladder content was elicited by a significantly higher gallbladder bile : hepatic bile ratio of bile acid specific activity compared to that of controls. Thus decreased exposure time of gallbladder mucosa to cholesterol-saturated bile and periodic flushing of cholesterol agglomerations from the gallbladder may be the mechanism by which stone formation is prevented. Therefore, gallbladder stasis which occurs in the presence of lithogenic bile has an essential role in the formation of gallstones. Sphincterotomy prevents gallstone formation in prairie dogs by alleviating gallbladder bile stasis with a reduction of gallbladder storage time below that require for crystal growth and agglomeration (Hutton et al., 1981). The increase in cystic duct resistance (Pitt et al., 1981) and a defect in gallbladder contractility occur very early in the course of gallstone formation in prairie dogs and ground squirrels even before bile becomes saturated with cholesterol and precipitation of cholesterol monohydrate crystals (Doty et al., 1983; Fridhandler et al., 1983). Physiological gallbladder contraction is mediated by gastrointestinal hormones such as CCK and motilin – the former being the major hormone initiating postprandial gallbladder contraction (Ivy and Oldberg, 1928). The mean peak of CCK is achieved after 8 minutes of infusion, and maximum gallbladder contraction occurs at 10 minutes (Lilja et al., 1982). The gallbladder is refilled within 40 minutes of the cessation of CCK infusion. Endogenous hypercholecystokinemia was found to reduce gallstone incidence in hamster model (Borsh et al., 1994). Motilin is probably important in the control of gallbladder motility. Intravenous motilin administration causes gallbladder contraction in vivo in several animal species (Takahashi et al., 1982). Loss of contractility of gallbladder muscle is observed not only in response to CCK octapeptide (humoral mediator) but also in response to an entirely different agonist, acetylcholine (neural mediator), and persists even after bypassing of all receptors using direct depolarization of muscle cells by means of a high external $K^+$ concentration, with no significant shift of normal dose-response curves. The progressive defect in smooth muscle contractility is not associated with any loss of sensitivity to these stimuli and appears to be localized specifically to the gallbladder muscle. Wahlin (1977) asserts that such a defect in two animal models of cholelithiasis indicates that biliary stasis is an important factor in the early stage of cholesterol gallstone formation.

In man, change of gallbladder emptying in the presence of gallstones has been variously reported to be increased (Maugdal et al., 1980; Northfield et al., 1980) or decreased (Shaffer et al., 1980; Fisher et al., 1982; Daignaut et al., 1988) or unchanged (Van Berge Henegouwen et al., 1978; Mok et al., 1980). Hypermotility of the gallbladder is observed when gallstones are present (Northfield et al., 1980), which seems to be due to the hyperreactivity to CCK. However, others failed to substantiate this findings (Fisher et al., 1982). Impaired gallbladder motility is encountered in about one-half of gallstone patients (Catnach et al., 1992). Impaired gallbladder emptying is seen even in the presence of lithogenic bile but without gallstones (Brugge et al., 1986). Hypomotility is not found in gallbladder with black pigment stones (Behar et al., 1989). A more recent study using ultrasonography demonstrated greater fasting and postprandial gallbladder volume but not reduced gallbladder contractility in gallstone patients (Festi et al., 1990). Abnormal gallbladder emptying is independent of stone size and number and seems to be intrinsic to the gallbladder (Pomeranz and Shaffer, 1985). This intrinsic smooth muscle defect is also demonstrated in human gallbladders harboring gallstones (Behar et al., 1989). Such defective gallbladder function persists in gallstone patients even after complete gallstone dissolution with oral bile acid therapy (Festi et al., 1990) or fragmentation and complete dissolution of gallstones (Spengler et al., 1989), suggesting that the defect is independent of the presence of gallstones. Although Sylwestrowicz et al. found that gallbladder emptying improves after gallstone dissolution (Sylwestrowicz and Shaffer, 1988), placement of inert prosthetic gallstones in the form of small glass beads in guinea pig gallbladder resulted in no change in the gross and microscopic appearance of the gallbladder (Pomeranz et al., 1986). Only moderately inhibited gallbladder contraction was observed. Therefore, abnormal gallbladder motility seems to be a major component of the pathophysiological process in gallstone disease rather than a late consequence of the presence of gallstones in the gallbladder. Thus, defective gallbladder contactility is implicated as one of the factors responsible for the gallstone formation by causing stasis of bile.

The female preponderance of gallstone disease has been well documented, with a male : female ratio of 1.0 : 1.5 to 2.0 in premenopausal women. Therefore, the female sex hormone may influence contractility of the gallbladder and thus formation of gallstones. Gerdes and Boyden (1938) used cholecystography to study postprandial evacuation of the gallbladder in women during pregnancy and after delivery. From the fourth month on delayed evacuation of the gallbladder was noted. After delivery, the evacuation rate soon returned to normal, coinciding with the increase in progesterone level (Short and Eton, 1959). Nilsson and Statin (1967), using oral cholecystography with CCK stimulation, examined women at estrogen and progesterone peaks during the menstration cycle (Short and Eton, 1959) and found that emptying of the gallbladder is impaired during the progesterone peak. Progesterone has an inhibitory effect on gallbladder emptying analogous to the well-known effect of progesterone on uterine muscle. Keane et al. (1986) demonstrated reduced spontaneous contraction and decreased magnitude of maximum contraction in human gallbladder specimens exposed to progesterone. The presence of progesterone receptor in the gallbladder wall was demonstrated in more than half of the human gallbladder specimens examined (Daignault et al., 1988). The presence of progesterone receptor can be correlated with impaired gallbladder emptying.

During late pregnancy, the conditions for gallstone formation are set by the emergence of supersaturated bile in the sluggish and enlarged gallbladder, with incomplete emptying (Everson et al., 1982). Progestin seems to be responsible for the impaired contractility of the gallbladder during pregnancy (Keane et al., 1986). Biliary sludge may appear because of gallbladder hypomotility (Maringhini et al., 1987). In the immediate postpartum period, sludge was noted by ultrasound examinations in 26% of the cases, most of which disappeared 1 year later. Fasting volume, residual volume after meals, and volume remaining in the gallbladder throughout the day increased two times during late pregnancy (Everson, 1991; Everson et al., 1982). Gallbladder enlargement and incomplete emptying are likely to be significant. Bile retention in the gallbladder is greatest in the second and third trimesters, a time when gallbladder bile is most lithogenic (Kern et al., 1981). Gallbladder bile retention could contribute to the pathogenesis of cholesterol gallstones by allowing more time for nucleation and precipitation of cholesterol crystals. The use of contraceptive steroids is associated with an increased incidence of gallstones (Boston Collaborative Drug Surveillance Program, 1974; Braverman et al., 1980; Everson et al., 1982; Shaffer et al., 1984). However, contraceptive steroids induce only minor changes in gallbladder motility (Braverman et al., 1980).

Retrospective studies show that the incidence of gallstones increases after vagotomy (Clave and Gaspar, 1969; Sapala et al., 1979). As much as 41% of patients who underwent selective vagotomy acquired gallstones after 3 to 5 years during follow-up (Csendes et al., 1978). Abnormal emptying of the gallbladder is found to be partly responsible for gallstone formation in man (Duane and Hanson, 1978). However, a later study showed that while the gallbladder enlarges, responsiveness of the gallbladder to CCK increases, improving emptying (Masclee et al., 1990). In the biliopancreatic bypass procedure for weight loss, in which the proximal half of the small intestine is anastomosed to the distal 50 cm of terminal ileum after dividing the small intestine in the middle, gallstones are reported to appear in 30% of patients (Scopinaro et al., 1981). Foods ingested completely bypass the upper small intestine. As a result, gallbladder emptying is impaired because of lack of stimulus.

Thompson et al differentiated two groups of gallstone patients in terms of gallbladder contractility (Thompson et al., 1982), i.e., contractors and noncontractors, based on the noted change in gallbladder volume examined by real-time ultrasonography before and after the ingestion of a fatty meal (Everson et al., 1980). Further, they found that contractile gallbladders with gallstones are more sensitive to challenge by endogenous CCK than those of normal volunteers. The gallbladder response of noncontractors appears to have decreased sensitivity. A high correlation is demonstrable between gallbladder kinetics and changes in plasma CCK concentration in man (Lilja et al., 1982). Zhu et al. confirmed their previous in vivo findings utilizing gallbladder muscle strips examined for the responsiveness to a graded dosage of CCK-8 (Zhu et al., 1985). Thickening and fibrosis of gallbladder tissue may have caused the decreased contractility of the gallbladder. Gallbladder contractility in vitro was compared in patients with cholesterol stones and black pigment stones (Behar et al., 1989). Muscle strips exposed to bile with excess cholesterol have reduced contractility, as revealed by marked reduction in the force of spontaneous phasic contractions and in response to CCK-8, acetylcholine, and potassium chloride compared to those with black pigment stones. Impaired gallbladder contractility precedes gallstone formation and results from muscle dysfunction (Behar et al., 1989). Smooth muscle cells isolated from human gallbladder with cholesterol stones contract less than those with black pigment stones in response to CCK, acetylcholine, and potassium chloride (Yu et al., 1993). $Ca^{2+}$ influx through voltage-operated $Ca^{2+}$ channels appears to be abnormal in smooth muscle cells from human gallbladder with cholesterol stones.

# Risk factors

## Age

Advanced age is a risk factor for gallstone formation. The incidence of gallstones increases with age (Zahor et al., 1974; Lindström, 1977). Gallstones in infants and children are rare (Klingensmith et al., 1988). They are uncommon under the age of 20 years, but do occur in Mexican-Americans (Andrassy et al., 1976; Odom et al., 1976). During routine obstetric ultrasound examinations, Klingensmith et al. reported the presence of multiple gallstones in fetal gallbladder, which resolved spontaneously 6 weeks after the birth together with the two previous descriptions on the presence of fetal gallstones. Cholelithiasis does occur in children and even in infants (Brill et al., 1982). Heubi et al. (1983) studied 17 infants and children aged 4 months to 9 years and compared them with 20 healthy adults aged 21 to 35 years. They found that the cholesterol molar fraction in bile was much greater in the adult subjects than in the infants and children, as was cholesterol saturation. The proportionately larger bile acid pool in children (adjusted to body size) was thought to be responsible. In the first weeks of life, the total and primary bile acid pools expand and are maintained during childhood at sizes exceeding those of adults. The absence of inhibition of bile acid synthesis by sex hormones may explain the proportionately larger pools in infancy and childhood, but the precise reason is unknown. Cholelithiasis in children is historically associated with adolescent pregnancy and hemolytic anemia, but this situation is now changing (Bailey et al., 1989). In addition to infants and children more frequently associated with cholelithiasis are those with prolonged fasting, diuretic therapy, and ileal abnormality. Children have primarily reduced biliary cholesterol: bile acid secretion ratios; therefore, even lower cholesterol saturation in bile is expected. Based on 6,050 cases with various childhood cancers, the cumulative risk of developing gallstones is calculated to be 0.42 % at 10 years and 1.03 % at 18 years; these rates are considerably higher than those for the general population (Mahmoud et al., 1991). Known risk factors for gallstones in childhood and young adults (Newman, 1973; Silverman and Roy, 1983; Friesen and Roberts, 1989) are hemolytic anemia, total parenteral nutrition, obesity, a family history of gallstones, previous abdominal operation and infection, cystic fibrosis, hepatobiliary disease, pregnancy, use of oral contraceptives, bronchopulmonary dysplasia, and malabsorption syndromes. Infants and children from a population at moderate risk for gallstone formation in adulthood begin life with relatively low biliary cholesterol saturation. A significant correlation is found between age and cholesterol secretion (Einarsson et al., 1985). A negative correlation exists between age and bile acid synthesis in patients with gallstones and those without gallstones but with supersaturated bile. Saturation indices and biliary cholesterol secretion most likely increase after puberty, especially in women (von Bergmann et al., 1986). The male: female ratio of gallstone prevalence is lowest in the younger age group but narrows to roughly 1 : 2 after age fifty (Diehl, 1991). In Pima Indians, abnormal biliary lipid composition may be present even in prepubertal age (Bennion et al., 1979).

Valdivieso et al found higher cholesterol saturation levels in older Chilean women (Valdivieso et al., 1978). In a more extensive study, the lipid composition of stimulated duodenal bile was compared in healthy subjects of various ages without gallstones, obesity, and hyperlipidemia, thus excluding possible disturbances secondary to the presence or absence of gallstones (Einarsson et al., 1985). Older persons have a considerably larger pool of circulating deoxycholic acid (Van der Werf et al., 1982), more saturated bile (Valdivieso et al., 1978; Einarsson et al., 1985), and a higher prevalence of gallstones (Marcus and Heaton, 1988). The increased deoxycholic acid pool in older age groups may simply be due to the slowing of colonic transit with age (Marcus and Heaton, 1988). A high concentration of deoxycholic acid in the circulating bile acid pool promotes secretion of biliary cholesterol and supersaturation of bile. In model bile, taurodeoxycholic acid is shown to shorten nucleation time compared with taurochenodeoxycholic acid (Van Berge Henegouwen et al., 1987). A positive correlation was found between the age-related increase in gallstone formation, on the one hand, and hepatic cholesterol secretion rate and biliary cholesterol saturation, on the other. Age is negatively correlated with bile acid synthesis and the size of the cholic acid pool. Using [$7\alpha$-$^3$H] cholesterol and tritium release assay, cholesterol $7\alpha$-hydroxylation, the rate-limiting step in the synthesis of bile acid from choelsterol, was found to be significantly reduced in the older age group, especially in females (Bertolottie et al., 1993); these changes probably occur on a transcriptional level (Jelinek et al., 1990; Pandak et al., 1991). Therefore, cholesterol saturation of bile increases with age as a consequence of enhanced hepatic secretion of cholesterol and decreased bile acid synthesis.

The relation between aging and gallstone formation in hamsters and guinea pigs has been studied. Hikasa and his colleagues found that young hamsters fed a lithogenic diet formed cholesterol stones exclusively, while older hamsters formed not only cholesterol stones in 60 % but also black pigment stones in 20 % of the animals tested (Hikasa et al., 1980). Older guinea pigs are more prone to form gallstones when fed a lithogenic diet (Poston et al., 1990). This enhanced susceptibility is suggested to be due to a reduced response of the gallbladder to CCK, since gallstone formation can be prevented by the administration of pharmacological doses of CCK. However, the effect of aging on gallbladder function in man remains controversial. In older men, the fasting gallbladder volume is said to be larger but the rate of emptying and fractional emptying are not changed (Boyden and Grantham, 1936). However, a later study using ultrasonography failed to find differences between fasting gallbladder volume and rate of emptying between older and younger age groups but older people appear to show earlier initiation of contraction (Khail et al., 1985).

## Fasting

Fasting exerts a profound effect on the cholesterol saturation of bile and the subsequent formation of gallstones (Danzinger et al., 1971; Holzbach et al., 1973; Metzger et al., 1973; Williams et al., 1977b, Bloch et al., 1980). On the other hand, using ultrasonography Jørgensen and Jørgensen found no relation in a Danish population between the prevalence of gallstones and the number of meals or snacks taken (Jørgensen and Jørgensen, 1989). In rhesus monkeys with intact enterohepatic circulation of bile acid, Redinger et al. found that fasting decreases the bile acid pool and greatly increases the relative amount of cholesterol in bile but does not produce supersaturated bile (Redinger et al., 1971). In man, cholesterol saturation in both hepatic and gallbladder bile occurs with increasing duration of fasting. Danzinger et al. noted a high incidence of supersaturated bile after 10 hours of fasting in young female siblings with gallstones (Danzinger et al., 1972a). Hepatic bile contains a greater proportion of cholesterol after an overnight fast than in a fed state (Shaffer et al., 1972; Metzger et al., 1973; Northfield and Hofmann, 1973, 1975). Williams et al. (1977b) studied the composition of gallbladder bile in man after random fasting for 9, 12, and 16 hours and found that the molar percentage of cholesterol in bile increased during fasting in both sexes but was significant only in women. Bile became more lithogenic with longer fasting, but mean values for both sexes became lithogenic only after a 16-hour fast. Using Hegardt and Dam's criteria (Hegardt and Dam, 1971) (Figure 14), an increased proportion of bile from both sexes was found to move into the metastable-labile and supersaturated zones on fasting, again with significant changes in women. The cholesterol saturation index is significantly greater after 15 hours than after 10 hours at fasting and maximum cholesterol saturation seems to occur between 10 and 20 hours (Bloch et al., 1980). Prolonged fasting for 4 to 6 days reduces the proportion of cholesterol in gallbladder bile (Duane et al., 1976). Therefore, there is an initial rise in cholesterol saturation of hepatic and gallbladder bile with an overnight fast but a fall during prolonged fasting (Northfield and Hofmann, 1975; Bloch et al., 1980). Because of interruption of the enterohepatic circulation of bile acid which is sequestered in less frequently contracting gallbladder, the bile acid secretion rate falls, especially with the reduced bile acid pool (Vlahcevic et al., 1970b). But because of the apparent uncoupling of cholesterol and bile acid secretion, cholesterol secretion continues somewhat independently of bile acid secretion leading to increased cholesterol saturation of bile (Metzger et al., 1973). This effect is more pronounced in American Indians, who have a reduced bile acid pool (Vlahcevic et al., 1972) and increased cholesterol secretion. Increased saturation of bile tends to occur in women, which may be responsible for their higher prevalence of gallstones (Williams et al., 1977b). Furthermore, Capron et al. (1981) found that the duration of overnight fast is greater in young women with gallstones in a well-matched prospective case-control study; no difference was found in older women. Fasting resulted in markedly decreased HMG-CoA reductase activity in rats. When expressed activity is taken as a percentage of total activity, fed animals use only about 10% of their available activity (Kelley and Story, 1985). The change in HMG-CoA reductase activity seems to be influenced by the kind of diet consumed before fast. The majority of the rise in HMG-CoA reductase, a rate-limiting enzyme of cholesterol synthesis, and cholestrol synthesis during the circadian rhythm seem to be due to food intake (Edwards et al., 1972). Indeed, the activity of HMG-CoA reductase seems to reach a nadir after 14 hours of fasting (Dugan et al., 1972; Edwards et al., 1972; Gregory et al., 1972) coinciding with the rise in cholesterol saturation of bile. In fasting subjects, there is a lack of dietary cholesterol, which may decrease hepatic secretion of cholesterol. During fasting the gallbladder empties (Van Berge Henegouwen et al., 1978), and then the content is replaced by more lithogenic hepatic bile. When mixing in the lumen is not complete, the region of lithogenic bile becomes a locus for crystal formation and growth (Metzger et al., 1973). Starvation decreases enterohepatic circulation of bile acid from 12 to 6 times per day, as well as the size of bile acid pool (Redinger et al., 1971).

## Diet

The role of diet in the pathogenesis of cholesterol gallstones has long been a matter of great interest, as exemplified by the aphorism "female, fair, fat, forty and fecund", (5f), attributed to Professor Deaver of the University of Pennsylvania at the beginning of the twentieth century. The prevalence of gallstones varies over time, and seems to be less frequent during the years of famine and the years immediately following it than in times of plenty (Martensson, 1937). Martensson quotes that the prevalence of gallstones decreased, especially in females in Rostock, Germany, during and right after World War I (i.e., from 1914–1922) as judged from the autopsy material. A marked increase in the prevalence of cholesterol gallstones in Japan is thought to be due to the changing diet with a higher fat intake in the years after World War II (Nakayama and Miyake Jr, 1970). Such change in diet may act via a change in HMG-CoA reductase activity, a rate-limiting enzyme in cholesterol synthesis (Kelley and Story, 1985). A higher prevalence of gallstones is found in overweight persons (Friedman et al., 1966; Scragg et al., 1984b; Pixley and Mann, 1988; Barbara et al., 1987; Rome Group for Epidemiology and Prevention of Cholelithiasis 1988b). Obesity and gallstone formation seem to be consistently associated in young women in cross-sectional and retrospective studies (Horn, 1956; Newman and Northup, 1959) and in women below 50 in case-control studies (Smith and Gee, 1979; Honoré 1980a). However, Sarles et al. did not find such an association with body weight, work habit and physical exercise (Sarles et al., 1969). A case-control study of diet, alcohol, and relative weight, involving 267 patients with newly diagnosed gallstones and 241 matched controls from the community and 359 patients in hospitals, was conducted by Scragg et al. (1984b). They found that the increased intake of simple sugars is associated with an increased risk of gallstones, and increased intake of fat and energy increases this risk in young subjects. Obesty is also associated with an increased risk only in young women. Intake of alcohol is inversely related to the risk. Maclure and his collaborators (1989, 1990) conducted an extensive prospective study of symptomatic gallstones based on a survey of 88,837 women—registered nurses, aged 34 to 59 years—by semiquantitative food frequency questionnaire followed for 4 years. A Quetelet index (QI) of relative weight (weight in kilograms/square meter in height) was used. Approximately linear relationship between relative weight and increased risk of the symptom-associated gallstones was observed, which may have been indiscernible in the previous studies because of their relatively small sample size. Overweight persons with QI > 32 kg/m$^2$ had a relative risk of 6.0, while slightly overweight persons of QI 24–24.9 kg/m$^2$ had a relative risk of 1.7. Weight gain was found to be associated with an increased risk of gallstones. Energy intake seems to be directly associated with the risk. Among 59,306 women with QI <25 kg/m$^2$, higher intake of energy of > 8,200 J/day is associated with an increased prevalence of symptomatic gallstones, with a relative risk of 2.1 compared with the lower energy intake of <4,730 J/day. Alcohol intake of >5g/day decreased the prevalence of gallstones and was inversely associated with the risk. An increased risk with age was evident only among the nonobese women. The prevalence of gallstones in vegetarians seems to be lower. Pixley et al. studied 130 vegetarian women and 632 controls, and found that the prevalence of gallstones in vegetarian women was 12% while in nonvegetarian women 25% (Pixley et al., 1985). Prevalence increases with age and body mass index. A lower than expected prevalence of gallstones is explained only in part by slimness. The 2,5-fold increase in the risk of developing gallstones in nonvegetarians compared with vegetarians was reduced to 1,9 when these two potentially confounding factors were controlled for. Vegetarians tend to consume less saturated fat, in addition to eating no meat and have a higher intake of fiber than nonvegetarians. An inverse relation was found with vegetable fat, vegetable protein, and total dietary fiber. Intake of legumes (i.e., beans, peas, and lentils) seems to be inversely associated with the risk of gallstone formation (Nervi et al., 1989). Self-reporting bias can be excluded because the data on weight and food intake were collected before the onset of gallstone symptoms. A lower deoxycholic acid pool is reported in vegetarians (Ahlberg et al., 1980). No association was found with energy-adjusted intakes of cholesterol, total fat, animal fat, total protein, total carbohydrate, and sucrose. The effect of obesity may have masked all association with the intake of nutrients. In overweight persons, hypersecretion of biliary cholesterol is frequent (Bennion and Grundy, 1975; Shaffer and Small, 1977), while secretion of bile acid and phospholipids does not change accordingly, thus resulting in the rise of cholesterol saturation index of bile.

Nutrients said to increase the risk of gallstone formation are total calories (Sarles et al., 1969, 1970, 1971; Scragg et al., 1984b), total fat (Borgman, 1965), animal fat (Osuga and Portman, 1971), vegetable fat (St Clair et al., 1980; Duffy et al., 1985; Lee et al., 1987b), total carbohydrate (Thornton et al., 1983), sucrose (Scragg et al., 1984a), total protein (Borgman, 1965; Sarles et al., 1971; Duffy et al., 1985), and animal protein (Kritchevsky and Klurfeld, 1983; Mahfouz-Cercone et al., 1984, Jaskiewicz et al., 1987). However, Masai of East Africa rarely develop gallstones despite a diet rich in animal fat (Biss et al., 1971). An Australian dietary survey did not show any difference in caloric intake, but the patients with gallstones ate less fat (Wheeler et al., 1970). Sarles et al. studied the diet of gallstone patients of similar age and, later, 101 female gallstone patients with age-matched controls, and found a statistically increased intake of total calories irrespective of dietary composition (Sarles et al., 1969). The number of meals and intervals between the meals were not different. Cholesterol concentration of hepatic bile over 3–37 days is significantly correlated with total calorie intake. A high calorie, high-protein diet has been shown to increase significantly the number of bile samples which fall outside of the metastable-labile zone of the triangular phase diagram of bile (Sarles et al., 1971). Only one-third of the cholesterol in the intestinal lumen comes from exogenous sources, i.e., diet. Dietary cholesterol is less efficiently absorbed when it must first be transferred to gut lumen in a micellar phase from an oily phase or from a phospholipids/cholesterol lamellar phase (tissue membrane) before it can be absorbed. On the other hand, Wilson et al. maintains that the time needed to absorb cholesterol in meal is long enough for mixing of endo- and exogenous cholesterol to be complete. Therefore, absorption from both sources is equal (Wilson and Rudel, 1994). Once absorbed, cholesterol from endogenous and exogenous sources is presumed to be indistinguishable and should have similar potential for affecting cholesterol homeostasis. Ingestion of large amounts of exogenous cholesterol by human subjects for short periods of time or lesser amounts of cholesterol for longer periods of time has been shown to lead to increased secretion of cholesterol in bile (DenBesten et al., 1973). On the other hand, Duane et al. found that increased consumption of cholesterol in man does not significantly alter the cholesterol saturation index, suggesting that dietary cholesterol may not be a major factor in cholesterol gallstone formation (Duane, 1994). A high-cholesterol diet increases the fractional turnover and synthesis rate of cholic acid, but not of chenodeoxycholic acid, without altering the pool size of either bile acid. In African green monkeys dietary cholesterol increases hepatic free and esterified cholesterol content and down-regulate cholesterol $7\alpha$-hydroxylase by transcriptional regulation (Rudel et al., 1994). In a series of investigations on biliary tract physiology using rhesus monkeys with intact enterohepatic circulation of bile acids (Dowling et al., 1970), Small and his co-workers fed animals for 2 to 3 weeks to obtain a steady state, with each animal acting as its own control. Feeding of safflower oil rich in saturated fatty acid, given as 20 % isocaloric substitution of normal monkey chow, doubles the bile acid pool size, but enterohepatic circulation remains unchanged. Secretion of bile acids and phospholipids increases, and lithogenicity of bile decreases (Redinger et al., 1971). Triolein, tricaprylin, a no-fat diet, and fasting affect the secretion and relative composition of bile but none of these produce supersaturated bile in rhesus monkeys with 5 % diversion of biliary constituents. Since the red blood cell fatty acid pattern is demonstrated to be an objective index of fatty acid composition of the habitual diet over a long period, Arca et al. (1987) did a cross-sectional study on the epidemiology of gallstone disease using ultrasonography. They found no difference in erythrocyte fatty acid composition between women with or without gallstones, and a raised erythrocyte linoleic acid : saturated fatty acid ratio was associated with the risk of gallstones only in women with very low serum triglycerides. In contrast to the previous studies by Bennion and Grundy (1978), Sturdevant et al. (1973), Miettinen et al. (1976), Sarles et al. (1978), Malhotra (1968), Scragg et al. (1984b), they concluded that dietary fatty acids do not play a major role in the pathogenesis of gallstone disease. A cholesterol-rich diet supplemented with fish (menhaden) oil demonstrated decreased appearance of cholesterol crystals in a prairie dog model (Booker et al., 1990) and a decreased incidence of gallstones in African green monkeys (Scobey et al., 1988). Fish oil rich in $\omega$-3 fatty acid has been shown to block cholesterol nucleation and subsequent gallstone formation (Magnuson et al., 1989a; Tierney et al., 1993), but whether it involves changes in cholesterol saturation of bile is uncertain. A recent study by Smit et al. showed that fish oil feeding in rats has a pronounced effect on biliary cholesterol secretion, but bile acid and phospholipids secretion increases much smaller extent (Smit et al., 1994). As a result the biliary cholesterol : bile acid ratio increases markedly. Fish oil feeding is thought to increase the disposition of cholesterol into bile by potentiating bile acid-dependent cholesterol secretion, presumably by facilitating the recruitment of bile-destined cholesterol.

In experimental animals, the effect of fat on gallstone formation has been studied with conflicting results, probably because of the species difference and specific lithogenic regimen used. In hamster, dietary palmitic acid (16 : 0) is highly lithogenic. In Syrian Golden Hamsters fed a low fat-diet supplemented with cholesterol, a palmitic acid-rich diet produced cholesterol stones and was associated with mucin accumulation in gallbladder bile. This effect was absent, with a decreased incidence of cholesterol stones, when, the hamsters were fed an oleic acid (18 : 1) rich diet (Jonnalagadda et al., 1993, 1995). However, a high intake of palmitic acid-rich fat decreased the incidence of cholesterol stones with a concomitant increase in the incidence of black pigment stones. Unsaturated fat, especially at levels over 10 % favors the development of amorphous pigmented stones but the total incidence of gallstones decreases (Christensen et al., 1964). Feeding of a lithogenic diet is associated with mucin accumulation in the gallbladder and with enhanced mucous secretion and cell proliferation (Sakata et al., 1993). Increased goblet cells secreting large amounts of sialomucin can be demonstrated in the epithelia. Dietary fat high in linoleic acid lowers the incidence of gallstones in SASCO hamsters by maintaining cholesterol in liquid crystalline vesicles by changing the composition of phospholipids even when bile is supersaturated (Ayyad et al., 1993). In prairie dogs, on the other hand, a diet rich in fat, especially polyunsaturated fat, increases the lithogenicity of bile and accelerates cholesterol stone formation. A diet with 40% corn oil rich in polyunsaturated fat increases the proportion of lecithins containing linoleic acid instead of the usual palmitoleic, oleic, and arachidonic acids (LaMorte et al., 1993).

## Obesity

Obesity has long been thought to be associated with gallstones, as exemplified by the aphorism, previously noted, attributed to Deaver (Rains, 1964) and later confirmed by several workers (Mentzer et al., 1926; Gross, 1929; Van der Linden, 1961; Friedman et al., 1966; Wheeler et al., 1970; Sturdevant et al., 1973; Honoré et al., 1980a; Diehl et al., 1980; Layde et al., 1982; Scragg et al., 1984b; Hanis et al., 1985). In the Framingham study (Friedman et al., 1966), the risk increases twofold in those whose weight is 20% above the median. Recently, Jørgensen (1989a), using ultrasonography on random samples of 5,581 men and women in a Danish population, found a positive association between gallstone and body mass index in women but not in men. Body mass index may not be as good an indicator of obesity in men as in women, since the index could be the same for those who are fat and those who are heavily muscled. The relation to the ratios of waist to hip girth (Hartz et al., 1984) and to subscapular to triceps skinfold thickness (Haffner et al., 1989) has been confirmed. Heavy body build with a tendency toward obesity in Pima Indians may be one factor contributing to the high prevalence of gallstones (Hesse, 1959). However, others failed to substantiate this finding (Comess et al., 1967). Gallstone diseases occur three times more frequently in patients with morbid obesity (Mabee et al., 1976). The relative risk rises sharply at the highest level of obesity (Layde et al., 1982; Petitti et al., 1988; Moran et al., 1993). Childhood obesity is associated with fatty liver but not with gallstones (Tominaga et al., 1993). Two strains of hereditarily obese mice were not found to be susceptible to gallstone formation on the Tepperman diet (Tepperman et al., 1964).

Overweight individuals with higher energy intake eating more dietary fat and cholesterol have elevated serum levels of LDL and VLDL. Obese persons have overproduction of total body cholesterol (Nestel and Monger, 1967; Nestel et al., 1969, 1973; Miettinen, 1971) and increased secretion of cholesterol (Bennion and Grundy, 1975, Mabee et al., 1976; Shaffer and Small, 1977). Parallel changes in cholesterol synthesis and secretion, which are both abnormally high, occur in obese subjects (Bennion and Grundy, 1975; Key et al., 1980). A gradation of secretory defects may exist between the massively obese and the nonobese. At one extreme lie the grossly obese subjects, whose main problem is excessive cholesterol secretion (Bennion and Grundy, 1975). Next come obese Caucasoid women with gallstones, with raised cholesterol secretion and marginally decreased bile acid output (Grundy et al., 1972), followed by obese American Indian women with combined defects, i.e., increased cholesterol secretion and reduced bile acid pool and secretion. Finally, at the other extreme, are nonobese Caucasoid women with only decreased secretion of cholesterol solubilizers, i.e., bile acid and phospholipids. There is likely to be a continuum of disturbed secretion between these extremes. Hepatic content of cholesterol ester is higher in obese subjects but ACAT activity is not increased (Sahlin et al., 1994). The cholesterol saturation index of bile in obese persons with gallstones is reported to be significantly higher than in those without gallstones (Reuben and Dowling, 1978) but some have failed to confirm this (Sahlin et al., 1994). Cholesterol secretion is related to total body weight (Grundy et al., 1974). Mean hourly hepatic cholesterol secretion in bile of obese subjects is three times greater than that of normal controls and twice that of subjects with gallstones (Mabee et al., 1976). Despite increased synthesis and normal or increased bile acid pool size with normal enterohepatic cycles (7.9 cycles per day) and increased secretion rates of bile acid and phospholipids, it is insufficient to compensate for increased cholesterol secretion, leading to the formation of supersaturated bile (Bennion and Grundy, 1975; Mabee et al., 1976). Thus formation of supersaturated bile in obese subjects seems to be attributable to a single defect in lipid metabolism, namely, excessive output of cholesterol in the presence of normal bile acid flux. The condition of supersaturation in obese subjects is not transient or related to fasting but persistent, and therefore is more predisposed to cholesterol crystallization and gallstone growth. In contrast, normal subjects may transiently secrete supersaturated bile (Nakayama and Van der Linden, 1970) or may even have microcrystalline cholesterol in bile (Juniper and Burson, 1957), but subsequent secretion of unsaturated bile rapidly reverses this cholelithogenic state (Mabee et al., 1976). A study of the effect of obesity on gallbladder function shows that fasting gallbladder volume and fractional emptying are similar in obese and nonobese subects, indicating that obesity per se does not alter gallbladder motor function (Vezina et al., 1990).

Weight reduction resulted in a significant reduction of cholesterol output but not of bile acid and phospholipids (Bennion and Grundy, 1975). Weight loss in obese persons is associated with a gradual decrease in the cholesterol saturation of bile, but its normalization is a slow process (Reuben and Dowling, 1978). The individual response is variable and unrelated to the magnitude or rate of weight loss. However, weight reduction is recommended in obese persons, since the saturation index of bile usually falls during weight loss. After weight loss and during maintenance of stable weight at a new lower level, biliary secretion of cholesterol falls (Bennion and Grundy, 1975), which, in turn, is due to decreased cholesterol synthesis (Miettinen, 1971). However, rapid dietary weight reduction may be associated with an increased risk of gallstones, with as many as 25 % of patients developing gallstones within 8 weeks (Liddle et al., 1989), and 26 % after 3 weeks (Broomfield et al., 1988), and 10.9 % after 16 weeks (Yang et al., '1992), possibly due to the decrease in bile acid synthesis and the bile acid pool, mobilization of cholesterol from adipose tissue stores, increased glycoprotein in bile (Broomfield et al., 1988), and decreased motility of the gallbladder (Nestel et al., 1973; Bennion and Grundy, 1975; Broomfield et al., 1988). As much as 36 % of the patients with morbid obesity develop gallstones, and an additional 13 % develop sludge within 6 months of a weight loss procedure (Mok et al., 1979). Half of the gallstones that form disappear rapidly once loss of weight ceases (Marks et al., 1994). Increased cholesterol concentration of gallbladder bile and increased cholesterol saturation index occur during rapid weight loss (Shiffman et al., 1992a). Risk of gallstone formation is said to increase exponentially as the rate of active weight loss increases. It is suggested that rates of weight loss should not exceed an average of 1.5 kg per week (Weinsier et al., 1995). Ursodeoxycholic acid prevents lithogenic changes in bile and the formation of gallstones (Broomfield et al., 1988; Everhart et al., 1993; Worobetz et al., 1993, Sugerman et al., 1995). Aspirin, a prostaglandin inhibitor, decreased the biliary glycoprotein concentration in bile and prevented a rise in the cholesterol saturation index of bile, thus preventing the formation of cholesterol monohydrate crystals and gallstones in obese individuals undergoing rapid weight loss. Hood et al. also succeeded in preventing the recurrence of gallstones by feeding NSAIDs such as aspirin, indomethacin, piroxicam, mefenamic acid, ibuprofen, naproxen, and fluorbioprofen after dissolution of gallstones by oral cholelitholytic agents (Hood et al., 1988). Gallbladder mucin increases as much as 18-fold and free $Ca^{2+}$ and total calcium increase 40 %. Jejunoileal bypass and gastric bypass for morbid obesity increase the incidence of gallstones in the first 2 years (Dietel and Petrov, 1987; Schmidt et al., 1988). No significant differences were found in either initial body weight or weight loss detected between those who formed gallstones or those who did not during the period of rapid weight loss, regardless of whether the weight loss was induced surgically or by dietary means (Broomfield et al., 1988; Liddle et al., 1989; Shiffman et al., 1991). Hence, it was suggested that the weight loss simply potentiates other risk factors. After the completion of weight loss, biliary cholesterol secretion and the cholesterol saturation index decline (Bennion and Grundy, 1975). Broomfield et al. found that saturation of bile with cholesterol and increased arachidonic acid, prostaglandin $E_2$, and glycoprotein occur 1 month after dieting begins and before the actual formation of gallstones (Broomfield et al., 1988). Recently, Marks and his colleagues in Schoenfield's laboratory studied obese patients on a very low calorie diet who are considered liable to form gallstones (Marks et al., 1991, 1992). Nucleation time decreased before the appearance of cholesterol crystals. Elevation of the biliary cholesterol saturation index, with no change in total lipid concentration and a significant increase of arachidonate, occurred, followed by an increase of prostaglandin $E_2$ and then of glycoprotein. Marks et al. suggested that the sequence of events occurring here is as follows. Biliary arachidonate, through synthesis of prostaglandin $E_2$, induces synthesis of glycoprotein, thus promoting cholesterol nucleation. This is in agreement with the prevailing hypothesis that synthesis and secretion of glycoprotein, a potent cholesterol nucleation promotor, is stimulated by the increase in biliary arachidonate through its conversion to prostaglandins (LaMorte et al., 1986; Mingrone et al., 1988). Undoubtedly obesity is one of the major mechanisms underlying cholesterol stone formation. However, nonobese women are also susceptible. Heaton and his colleagues found whole gut transit time is significantly longer and stool output is also lower in women with gallstones (Heaton et al., 1993).

## Sex difference and pregnancy

Growing evidence suggests that pregnancy, contraceptive steroid use, postmenopausal estrogen substitution, and estrogen therapy increase the risk of gallstones. Von Recklinghausen (1880–1887) is credited with observing that 90% of women with gallstones have been gravid at least once (Gerdes and Boyden, 1938). Subsequently, in 1890, Courvoisier noted that three times as many women have gallstones as men (Gerdes and Boyden, 1938).

**Gallstone prevalence in females**

The prevalence of cholesterol gallstones has long been known to be higher in females; the male: female ratio is usually 1.0 : 1.5–2.0 (Friedman et al., 1966; Nilsson, 1966). The highest male to female ratios, 1 : 7, was observed in Southwest American Indians (Hesse, 1959). The prevalence is the same in both sexes until puberty but increases slowly at first. In girls it increases more rapidly after 13 to 14 years of age, when most radical hormonal changes take place. A cross-sectional study by Jørgensen et al. (1988a) on women revealed that gallstones are significantly associated with young age at menarche, abortion, and multiple childbirth. In women the prevalence continues to rise until menopause (Nilsson, 1966). In sexually mature and postpubertal subjects, significantly higher cholesterol and low bile acid concentrations in bile are noted; phospholipid level remain the same as those before puberty (Heubi et al., 1992). The female : male ratio is highest in the younger age groups (Diehl et al., 1991). The difference between men and women in the prevalence of gallstones gradually diminishes. In the very old population, gallstone disease is as frequent in men as in women in agreement with earlier reports (Horn, 1956; Edlund and Olsson, 1956). The female preponderance of gallstones is also noted in nonhuman primates, i.e., all nine cases of previously reported, naturally occurring cholesterol gallstones are female (Kessler, 1982). Studies on nonobese prepubertal and postpubertal males and females indicated that hormonal changes at puberty may have great influence on biliary composition (von Bergmann et al 1986). Females have a marked increase in the cholesterol saturation index of bile, from 83% to 138% after puberty, in contrast to males, whose saturation indices do not change significantly. Schroeder also implicated pregnancy as a contributing factor in gallstone disease in 1892 (quoted by Thistle et al., 1971), which was later confirmed by several population studies (Friedman et al., 1966; Coronary Drug Project Research Group, 1977; Barbara et al., 1987; Rome Group for Epidemiology and Prevention of Cholelithiasis, 1988b; Murray et al., 1994). An increased risk of gallstones is noted with increasing parity (Friedman et al., 1966; Bernstein et al., 1973; Layde et al., 1982; Diehl et al., 1985); this tendency is more apparent in younger women (Bernstein et al., 1973). In a control study, Scragg et al. (1984c) showed an increased risk of gallstones after age 29 in women who had been pregnant and demonstrated that it is related to the number of pregnancies. In Chippewa Indians, Thistle et al. showed that pregnancy is associated with a higher prevalence of symptomatic gallbladder disease in American Indian women, especially in those less than 30 years old (Thistle et al., 1971). However, Robertson et al. showed that parity is not greater among those with gallbladder disease than among the general population at risk (Robertson and Dochat, 1944). Van der Linden et al. also contested the etiological relationship between parity and gallbladder disease (Van der Linden, 1961). Therefore, the role of pregnancy in the pathogenesis of cholesterol gallstones has been a subject of considerable interest but is far from settled. Several excellent reviews on the subject are available (Robertson and Dochat, 1944; Rådberg 1989).

### Change of bile composition

The reason for the increased risk of gallstones should be sought in the change of bile favorable to gallstone formation. In 1936, Potter analyzed 58 thick, and tarry gallbladder bile samples which were withdrawn during Caesarean section in 390 cases, and showed raised cholesterol and bile salt concentrations (Potter, 1936). In 1981 Kern and his colleagues, studied, using $^{13}C$-labeled bile acid, biliary lipid, and bile acid composition, bile secretion and kinetics at different stages of pregnancy and ovulation in young, nonobese, healthy women (Kern et al., 1981). They found that the phase of the ovulatory cycle, i.e., the follicular phase with the estrogen effect predominanting and the luteal phase with the progesterone effect predominating, had no effect. No relation could be elicited between cholesterol saturation and serum concentration of progesterone, luteinizing hormone, or estradiol in nonpregnant women. But in the last two trimesters of pregnancy, the mean secretion rate of biliary lipids is not altered. The rate of secretion of cholesterol relative to bile acids and phospholipids increases compared to the first trimester of pregnancy or in the nonpregnant women. As a result, the saturation index of fasting hepatic and gallbladder bile increases during the second and third trimesters of pregnancy, suggesting that pregnancy does indeed increase the risk of gallstones. According to Valdivieso et al. bile becomes unsaturated within a few weeks of delivery (Valdivieso et al., 1993). However, the change in cholesterol saturation in bile is not observed in the baboon (McSherry et al., 1977; Morrisey et al., 1977), rhesus monkey (Martin et al., 1972), or guinea pig (Holzbach et al., 1971). Weight gain during pregnancy may increase hepatic cholesterol secretion and increases the cholesterol saturation index of bile. There is a progressive decrease in the percentage of chenodeoxycholic acid and a similar increase in the percentage of cholic acid. The fractional turnover rate of both primary bile acids becomes slower during pregnancy. The pool size of each major bile acid is expanded in the first trimester. The chenodeoxycholic acid and deoxycholic acid pools, but not the cholic acid pool, subsequently decrease. The fractional turnover rate of both primary bile acids is slower during pregnancy. These changes are induced by one or both of the following: (1) changed liver function or (2) change in the biliary-intestinal part of enterohepatic circulation. The synthesis rate of chenodeoxycholic acid, but not of cholic acid, decreases linearly during the first 20 weeks of pregnancy. The rate of enterohepatic cycling of the bile acid pool is reduced throughout pregnancy. Marked alterations in bile acid kinetics occur which appear secondary to altered gallbladder function. The gallbladder stasis demonstrated in pregnant women (Nilsson et al., 1967; Braverman et al., 1980) causes accumulation of bile acid in the gallbladder lumen, altering the state of enterohepatic circulation of bile acid.

### Change of gallbladder function

Soon after the introduction of cholecystography by Graham and Cole in 1924, D'Amato et al. and Clauser et al. found that the gallbladder visualizes more slowly and remains visible longer during pregnancy (Kalk and Schöndube, 1926; Gerdes and Boyden, 1938).

In 1936 Potter observed the gallbladder to be distended in 75 % of 390 women undergoing Caesarean section (Potter, 1936). Gerdes and Boyden examined 21 pregnant women, 5 of whom were also studied postpartum (Gerdes and Boyden, 1938). Three of the five cases had a gallbladder more distended during pregnancy than afterward. Four of the five women had improved visualization 6 to 8 weeks after parturition, showing gestational alterations in the concentrating ability of the gallbladder. The rate of emptying of the gallbladder before and after parturition markedly increased 6 to 8 weeks postpartum. The rate of emptying is not altered in the first trimester but is markedly retarded during the first part of a phase of contraction in the second and third trimesters. Retardation seems to be due primarily to an initial delay in emptying. Mechanical pressure does not seem to be the primary factor in gallbladder stasis, but position and pressure may be contributing factors. They concluded that stasis of bile in the gallbladder sets the stage for the sequence of events which result in the greater prevalence of gallstones among women who bear children. Ultrasonography, which is convenient, accurate, reproducible, and believed to be without hazards, is applied to determine gallbladder volume using a sum-of-cylinder method, assuming a circular shape of transverse projection of the gallbladder. Braverman et al. studied 11 control women, 33 pregnant women, and 17 on contraceptive steroids (Braverman et al., 1980). Gallbladder volume increased to twice the normal amount, and reduced emptying of the gallbladder was noted in the second and third trimesters. Gallbladder volume was not affected by contraceptive steroids. Everson et al., also found that gallbladder volume, residual volume after contraction, and average hourly volume estimated by ultrasonography increase during pregnancy but return to normal in the postpartum period (Everson et al., 1982; Rådberg et al., 1989). Contraction of the gallbladder in pregnant women (contracted to 40 % of the fasting volume) did not differ significantly from controls, as did CCK levels (Rådberg et al., 1989). Therefore, increased fasting gallbladder volume is not due to different CCK levels but rather to some other factor, such as progesterone, which is elevated in pregnancy and known to relax smooth muscle (Bruce and Behsudi, 1979). Estrogen, although elevated during pregnancy, has no effect on gallbladder motility. However, absorption of water from the gallbladder depends on the sodium pump in the gallbladder mucosa, believed to be sodium-potassium ATPase, which is decreased by estrogen present in high concentrations in late pregnancy. The rate of emptying is slower in pregnancy.

Next, consider the effect of changed gallbladder physiology on bile acid kinetics. The volume of the fasting gallbladder and the residual volume after physiologically stimulated contraction are directly correlated with bile acid pool size. The volume of bile in the gallbladder after an overnight fast is the net result of the amount of bile secreted, its distribution between the gallbladder and the intestinal tract, and, the concentrating function of the gallbladder. Delayed gastrointestinal transit from mouth to cecum in the third trimester of pregnancy (Wald et al., 1982) may be partly responsible for the reduced bile acid pool size. The residual volume of the gallbladder after the contraction is also directly related to total bile acid synthesis. Increased retention of bile in the gallbladder may contribute to the increased risk of gallstones in pregnant women by allowing more time for nucleation and precipitation of cholesterol initiating the growth of gallstones. The continued sequence is not interrupted when gallbladder emptying is delayed and incomplete. No index of bile saturation can be correlated significantly with serum levels of progesterone, luteinizing hormone, or estradiol (Kern et al., 1981). However, in certain laboratory animals, the gallbladder is enlarged and empties poorly during pregnancy. These changes can be reproduced in guinea pigs by administration of ovarian hormones (Smith et al., 1941). To determine the cause of the enlarged gallbladder observed during pregnancy, the absorptive capacity of gallbladder mucosa, concentrating function of the gallbladder and hepatic bile flow were measured in the cat (Rådberg and Svanvik, 1986). It was found that the rate of absorption in the gallbladder of pregnant animals doubled. Outflow of hepatic bile increased in pregnancy. However, pregnant baboons appear to lack or at least have a diminished capacity to concentrate preferentially bile salts in the gallbladder (McSherry et al., 1971). Thus, the ovulatory cycle has no effect on gallbladder function, but pregnancy induces major changes such as retention of bile in the gallbladder (Kern et al., 1981; Everson et al., 1982). Increased biliary sludge is noted during pregnancy and immediately postpartum but frequently disappears spontaneously (Maringhini et al., 1988).

### Oral contraceptives

Hormonal changes during pregnancy must influence biliary physiology. Administration of the female sex hormone increases supersaturation of bile (Pertsemlidis et al., 1974). In the same vein, the prevalence of gallstones increases in women on oral contraceptive steroids (Boston Collaborative Drug Surveillance Program, 1973). In a cross-sectional study using ultrasonography, the users of oral contraceptive steroids (both combined estrogen/progestin and pure progestin preparations) had an increased incidence of gallstones (Jørgensen, 1989b). A two fold increase in the risk of gallstones in noncontraceptive estrogen users was found (Petitti et al., 1988). However, chance may have played a role in these findings, which differed from those of Kakar et al. (1988), in which an excess risk of only 20% was found in users. Estrogen-progestin intake increases cholesterol saturation of bile accompanied by a decrease in bile acid concentration (Pertsemlidis et al., 1974). Bennion and her coworkers (1976, 1980) found that the cholesterol saturation index increases in women during oral contraceptive steroid use but decreases thereafter. They found a significant rise in biliary cholesterol secretion but no change in secretion of bile acids and phospholipids in bile. As a result, the molar percentage of cholesterol was increased in both gallbladder and hepatic bile. There was no change in bile acid pool size and bile acid composition. The authors concluded that oral contraceptive steroids increase biliary cholesterol secretion, raise the level of cholesterol saturation of bile, and predispose to cholesterol precipitation and gallstone formation. This situation is analogous to that observed in obesity. However, a review of the evidence does not support the causative role of hormone replacement therapy (Bateson 1988). In male patients with prostate carcinoma randomly allocated to estrogen therapy and orchidectomy, Henriksson et al., (1989) found, after 1 year of estrogen treatment, a significantly higher incidence (up to 18%) of new gallstone formation and progressive gallstone disease during ultrasonographic follow-up. Appearance of more new gallstones or increased size or number of gallstones were observed compared to the orchidectomy group. Pharmacological doses of estrogen increased the relative concentration of biliary cholesterol, and the cholesterol saturation index of bile, which agrees well with the findings of previous studies (Pertsemlidis et al., 1974; Bennion et al., 1976; Anderson et al., 1980). Estrogen affects the metabolism of cholesterol (Kern and Everson, 1987) and bile acid (Everson et al., 1988, 1991) in man and animals. Ethinyl estradiol increases receptor-mediated uptake of LDL by hepatocytes (Windler et al., 1980). In their comprehensive study on the effect of estrogen on hepatobiliary function, Everson et al. found that premarin, exogenous estrogen, used extensively by postmenopausal women, increases biliary cholesterol secretion by enhancing hepatic lipoprotein uptake and inhibiting bile acid synthesis, thus diverting excessive cholesterol (Everson et al., 1991). Estrogen may selectively inhibit chenodeoxycholic acid synthesis and stimulate cholic acid synthesis (Everson et al., 1988, 1991). As a result, the cholesterol saturation index is increased. A majority of studies have found that estrogens, given alone or in combination with progestin, stimulate biliary secretion of cholesterol and phospholipids but not of bile acid (Henriksson et al., 1989) and increase lithogenicity of bile. The exception is the studies by Down et al. (1983) and Everson (1991). Kern et al., after giving low estrogen in combination with progestin, suggested that contraceptive steroids affect biliary cholesterol by increasing cholesterol entering the common metabolic pool and/or by inhibiting hepatic ACAT activity, a known effect of progesterone, so that an increase in free cholesterol entering the pool leads to an increase in output (Kern and Everson, 1987). Henriksson et al. suggest that increased inflow of lipoprotein cholesterol is a major determinant of the increased concentration of cholesterol in bile (Henriksson et al., 1989). Stimulated LDL cholesterol uptake would, in turn, have to be explained by increased cholesterol production, either in extrahepatic organs or in the liver, based on their observation that the change in serum LDL cholesterol is inversely related to that in biliary cholesterol. The liver is the key organ in the regulation of LDL. Catabolism of LDL is highly dependent on the expression of specific LDL receptors in the liver. This receptor capacity and the catabolism of LDL are increased in estrogen therapy (Eriksson et al., 1989). Increased biliary cholesterol secretion is related to the dose and potency of estrogen used. Thus changes in biliary cholesterol seem to be related to the induced changes in serum lipoprotein metabolism. Premarin also lowers chenodeoxycholic acid synthesis and the bile acid pool altering biliary bile acid composition, stimulates cholesterol esterification, and enhances the clearance of chylomicron remnants. The increased incidence of gallstones associated with contraceptive steroid use does not seem to involve abnormal gallbladder kinetics (Braverman et al., 1980). However, the presence of estrogen and progesterone receptors in the gallbladder wall was recently identified, pointing to a possible relation between sex hormone, gallbladder and gallstone formation (Singletary et al., 1986). Lower levels of gallbladder filling and diminished emptying are noted in women taking medroxyprogesterone (Shaffer et al., 1984). Administration of progesterone, but not estrogen, reduces the amplitude of spontaneous gallbladder contraction (Keane et al., 1986), suggesting that progestin, not estrogen, is responsible for the impaired contractility of the gallbladder characteristic of pregnancy. The blood progesterone level increases from the 11th to the 35th week of pregnancy (Short and Eton, 1959). After the delivery, blood progesterone level falls rapidly. Thereafter, the level rises more rapidly and remains high during labor. There seem to be species differences in response to estrogen. Ethinylestradiol decreases the synthesis and biliary secretion of cholesterol (Davis and Kern, 1976) and decreases the biliary cholesterol concentration (Morrisey et al., 1977) in baboons. Estrogen, although used in high doses, decreases the synthesis and secretion of bile acid in rhesus monkeys (Lynn et al., 1973), rats (Kern et al., 1977), and hamsters (Coyne et al., 1978). Estriol, a significant estrogen in human pregnancy, produces profound changes in bile salt-dependent as well as bile salt-independent flow in baboons with intact enterohepatic circulation, as studied by using a stream splitter for bile (Lynn et al., 1973). The cholesterol saturation index of bile increased due to the marked reduction in the relative amount of bile acid and the moderate increase of cholesterol and phospholipids. The effect is dose related. Addition of norethiosterone to estrogen reduced the cholesterol concentration in the bile of baboons (Morrisey et al., 1977), but progetin had no effect. The cat behaves like man rather than like the baboon or rat (Hirst et al., 1979). Treatment with estrogen-progestin for 18 days did not alter cholesterol in bile but did reduce the proportion of bile acids and phospholipids, increasing the cholesterol saturation index of bile in the cat. These changes reverted rapidly on cessation of the treatment. Female mice tend to develop stones earlier (Tepperman, 1965). They have significantly higher rates of bile production than males. Estrogen increases the rate of bile flow in the male while androgen decreases the rate in the female, suggesting that the well-known relationship between pregnancy and gallstones may be due in part to high levels of bile flow induced by the hyperestrogenization of pregnancy.

A sex difference in the incidence of gallstones in man is evident even in nonpregnant women, suggesting that factors in addition to pregnancy are operative (Horn, 1956). The bile acid pool in women is smaller than that in men, increasing the risk of gallstones in women (Bennion et al., 1978). Premenopausal women have bile that is more supersaturated with cholesterol and a smaller bile acid pool (Bennion et al., 1978, 1979). One of the dominant risk factors is female sex hormones, as suggested by the preponderance of gallstones in females (Robertson, 1945; Zahor et al., 1974). The lithogenic effect of exogenous female sex hormones is mediated, in part by an increase in biliary cholesterol saturation (Pertsemlidis et al., 1974; Tritapepe et al., 1972; Bennion et al., 1976). Einarsson et al. failed to demonstrate any difference between the sexes in biliary lipid metabolism in terms of hepatic secretion rate of cholesterol, bile acid synthesis, and bile acid pool size (Einarsson et al., 1985). Glycodeoxycholic acid decreased mRNA levels of HMG-CoA reductase and cholesterol $7\alpha$-hydroxylase in males but not in females (Xu et al., 1993). Bile acid synthesis is sustained in females because of continued synthesis of cholesterol, providing substrate for cholesterol $7\alpha$-hydroxylase and a stimulus for enzyme formation. Since deoxycholic acid levels increase with age (Van der Werf et al., 1981), and since hepatic deoxycholic acid flux does not suppress HMG-CoA reductase in females, more cholesterol is produced in older females. This, according to Xu et al, may partly explain the female preponderance of gallstones (Xu et al., 1993). Major factors in the more frequent development of gallstones in women may be sought in late pregnancy, such as an increase in biliary cholesterol saturation and altered motility of the gallbladder.

## Genetic and ethnic influences

### Population studies

The underlying reason(s) for the extremely high incidence of cholelithiasis in American Indians have been a subject of great interest. As many as 70% of young American Indian women have cholelithiasis (Sievers and Marquis, 1962). The prevalence pattern of cholelithiasis parallels the degree of Amerindian admixture, strongly implicating a genetic mechanism (Hanis et al., 1985). African-Americans have a lower prevalence of gallstones (Newman and Northup, 1959). In 1988 Lowenfels suggested an interesting hypothesis to explain the high prevalence of gallstones in northern Europeans and Amerindians (Lowenfels, 1988). According to the result of the recent analysis of mitochondrial DNA, Homo sapiens sapiens, modern human beings, evolved first in sub-Saharan Africa about 200,000 years ago, driven out of Africa via the Great Rift Valley by the change in the earth's climatic conditions to populate the other continents 90,000 years ago (Fagan, 1990). They expanded to northern Europe as the glaciers of the last so-called Würm glaciation receded, and via, the then existing Beringia land bridge, entered the Americas quite late in the last ice age of 15,000 years ago. In this cold climate, their survival depended on hunting and gathering strategies, with unpredictable periods of nutritional and caloric insufficiency. Those capable of storing excess calories as fat had pronounced survival advantages. Thus, over time, repeated exposure to the adverse conditions and cold climate of the last glacial period with marginal food supplies could have produced a genetic drift with eventual development of the so-called thrifty genes. The survivors, such as northern Europeans, northern Siberian populations such as the Yakut and Chukchi, Inuit (Eskimo), and Amerindians would still carry the same trait. The high prevalence of gallstones in Amerindians is well known (Hesse, 1959). Glenn also mentions the frequent gallbladder cases among Alaskan Eskimos (Yamase and McNamara, 1972). The low metabolic rates found in some Pima Indians (Ravussin et al., 1988) would have had considerable survival advantage. The lowest-risk populations for gallstones are restricted to Africa, India, and Southeast Asia, where prior exposure to cold temperatures would have been impossible. However, attractive as the above hypothesis seems, genetic difference alone is not sufficient to explain the difference in the prevalence of gallstones in the world population. Yamase et al. compared the incidence of gallbladder disease among eight ethnic groups residing in Hawaii, i.e., Caucasoid, Chinese, Filipino, Hawaiian, Japanese, Korean, Portuguese and Puerto Rican (Yamase and McNamara, 1972). Based on the hospital records with a diagnosis of gallbladder disease on discharge at the Queen's Medical Center in Honolulu, the highest incidence was found among Chinese descendants. However, no difference in age distribution was observed. The authors concluded that the incidence of gallbladder disease is determined primarily by environmental factors rather than ethnic differences.

## Genetic disposition

Gallstone disease was once suggested to be inherited as a Mendelian trait (Jackson and Gay, 1959). Cholelithiasis seems to appear in definite clusters in some families, reflecting both genetic and environmental factors. For instance, Rinaldo et al. described a family in which 8 of 11 members of the two generations studied had gallstones or symptoms suggestive of gallstones (Rinaldo and Baltz, 1957). First-degree relatives have a double risk of gallstones (Gilat et al., 1983; Jørgensen, 1988b; Pixley et al., 1985). The prevalence of gallstones is higher in siblings of patients with the disease than in their spouses, who supposedly share similar environmental factors including diet, suggesting that a genetic factor plays a role in the development of gallstone disease (Van der Linden and Lindelöf, 1965; Van der Linden and Westlin, 1966). Sisters of young women with gallstones develop bile saturated with cholesterol at an earlier age, suggesting a polygenic predisposition to gallstones (Danzinger et al., 1972a). Parents of patients younger than 20 years of age suffering from cholelithiasis developed the disease more frequently than parents of young controls in the general population and than sex- and age-matched controls without gallstones (Van der Linden and Simonson, 1973). A significant increase in the family prevalence of gallstones was noted among 1,616 symptom-free individuals by ultrasound examinations in six out of nine age groups compared with a stone-free group (Nürnberg et al., 1989). On the other hand, concordance of cholelithiasis in twins has been reported (Tesler, 1946). However, a prospective study of Danish twins showed considerable discordance for gallstone disease in monozygotic twins over 40 years old (Harvald and Hauge, 1956). A genetic predisposition toward developing gallstones associated with the ABO blood group has been sought, but no strong and concordant correlations were found (Kjølbye and Nielsen, 1959; Hauch and Moore, 1963; Bodvall and Overgaard, 1966; Wheeler et al., 1970). An increased frequency of HLA-Aw19 is found in 33 % of patients with cholelithiasis compared to 22 % of controls (Papasteriades et al., 1990). The frequency of Aw19 is even higher (44 %) in patients with a family history of the disease. The study suggests that there is a genetic predisposition toward cholelithiasis, with expression through the HLA system. Genetic determinants of cholesterol gallstones in mice have been sought (Fujihira et al., 1978; Alexander and Portman, 1987) using Tepperman's model (Tepperman et al., 1964). Two strains, $C_{57}$BL/6 and Nc, out of eight inbred strains were highly susceptible to gallstone formation (Fujihira et al., 1978). Later Alexander and Portman found that male black mice ($C_{57}$BL/6) produced gallstones with a 50 % incidence after 2 weeks on the diet, while in male agouti (CBA/J) mice and females of both strains no gallstone formation was observed (Alexander and Portman, 1987). All mice given a lithogenic diet had bile supersaturated with cholesterol after an overnight fast, but only one half of black male mice formed gallstones and all agouti males were free from gallstones. A dramatic difference was found in the increased fasting gallbladder volume between black mice and agouti mice within 3 days after the change from a stock to a lithogenic diet. Strain differences in gallbladder volume may be due to differences in gallbladder size or function (Barnett and Hilbun, 1966; Parkin et al., 1973) or to differences in the function of the choledochoduodenal junction (Cox et al., 1985). Resistance to cholesterol gallstone formation in certain groups of mice may be explained by the high activity in the liver converting free cholesterol, derived mainly from plasma lipoproteins, to bile acids, which are secreted into bile, and to esterified cholesterol, which is stored in the liver. Different strains of hamsters also vary considerably in cholesterol stone formation associated with difference in biliary cholesterol, bile acid and plasma lipoprotein profiles (Trautwein et al., 1993). A difference in susceptibility to gallstone formation is also observed in squirrel monkeys (Saimiri sciureus) (Portman et al., 1980). About half of Brazilian squirrel monkeys of both sexes on a lithogenic diet for over 6 months produced cholesterol gallstones. A definite sex difference exists in Bolivian squirrel monkeys; males are completely resistant, in contrast to females, with high susceptibility. The gallbladder bile of nearly all monkeys studied was supersaturated with cholesterol. The bile of Bolivian monkeys had a much greater concentration of total lipids, i.e., cholesterol, bile acids, and phospholipids. Male Bolivian monkeys had the highest percentage of chenodeoxycholic acid, the lowest percentage of deoxycholic acid and larger cholic acid and chenodeoxycholic acid pool sizes. The cholesterol saturation index of all Bolivian squirrel monkeys with gallstones was greater than that of all Brazilian monkeys free of gallsotnes. Male Bolivian monkeys had lower levels of plasma HDL, especially of $HDL_2$. The occurrence of low plasma $HDL_2$ levels in a population resistant to gallstone formation is consistent with the suggested role of that fraction in the net transport of cholesterol to bile and HDL as the preferred precursor of biliary cholesterol in squirrel monkeys. However, these findings do not necessarily mean that genetic factors are more important than environmental facotrs in the development of gallstone disease (Van der Linden and Westlin, 1966). For instance, familial aggregation of diabetes mellitus and gallstone disease suggests shared genes, environment or both in their separate etiologies (Hanis et al., 1985). Genetic influence, if it exists, may be independent of other risk factors for gallstone formation. Although the above discussion suggests the presence of a genetic disposition toward cholelithiasis, one is advised not to overlook the etiological role played by other factors such as diet, as exemplified by an emigration study in which genes do not change but environmental factors do (Loefler, 1988).

## Socioeconomic Status

Whether or not socioeconomic status affects the prevalence of gallstones is controversial. After adjusting the potential confounding factors, Diehl et al. found that women of lower socioeconomic status are at greater risk of developing gallstone disease (Diehl et al., 1985), in agreement with the findings of Layde et al. (1982). Using ultrasound survey, Jørgensen found that the crude incidence was lowest in women of the highest social class and rose with decreasing social class (Jørgensen 1988b). So far, no significant difference in gallstone risk in relation to socioeconomic status has been reported among men (Diehl et al., 1985, Jørgensen, 1988b).

## Diseases

### Diabetes

The association of gallstones and diabetes mellitus has attracted attention because of the unfavorable outcome of cholecystectomy in diabetics (Turrill et al., 1960, Mundth, 1962). There has been much controversy over whether gallstones are in fact associated with diabetes mellitus. Some studies found such an association; others failed to do so. An increased incidence of gallstones with diabetes mellitus has been well documented (Gross, 1929; Newman and Northup, 1959). The prevalence of gallstones is positively associated with diabetes mellitus and increasing age. Lieber reported that, based on 34,666 autopsies of patients over 20 years of age, the prevalence of gallstones in diabetics was found to be 30.2 % as against 11.6 % of controls (Lieber, 1952). He also noted an appreciable increase in gallstone prevalence after the third decade. Kravetz (1964) found that 20 % of cholecystectomized consecutive Southwest American Indians had diabetes mellitus. Diehl et al. reporting in 1980 their cross-sectional study on Mexican-Americans, found that diabetics had a higher prevalence of gallbladder disease, mostly cholelithiasis, than nondiabetics (Diehl et al., 1980). When taken with age-specific data, diabetes is found to contribute to gallstone prevalence even after age, ethnic group, and adiposity have been considered (Diehl el al., 1980). This is in agreement with Hanis et al. (1985), who found a significant association between gallbladder disease and diabetes mellitus beyond that which could be explained by body mass alone. Gallbladder disease and diabetes mellitus dominate the health status of the Amerindian population, and those having the highest rates of diabetes mellitus consistently show a high rate of gallbladder disease. The prevalence pattern parallels the degree of Amerindian admixture, which strongly implicates a genetic mechanism. Increased plasma insulin values were found to be associated with an increased risk of gallstones in young subjects in a case-control study (Scragg et al., 1984a). A recent ultrasonographic study using uni- and multivariate analyses failed to reveal a significantly increased gallstone prevalence in diabetics (Jørgensen, 1989a). Other studies confirm no increase of gallstone prevalence in diabetics. Feldman and Feldman (1954) found no such association in the Framingham study. There was no significant correlation between cholelithiasis and diabetes mellitus, which may be due to the presence of too few diabetics in the study population (Friedman et al., 1966). Zahor et al. found no correlation between cholelithiasis and diabetes mellitus in their autopsy studies in Prague and Malmö (Zahor et al., 1974). Honoré et al also failed to find a statistically significant association between diabetes mellitus and symptomatic cholesterol stones in a large series of 775 patients treated surgically (Honoré 1980b). Diehl and Elford studying the population in England and Wales using multiple-cause mortality tables found no evidence to support the contention that diabetics are at increased risk of death from gallstone-related diseases (Diehl and Elford, 1981). In large cross-sectional surveys in Italy, no relation was found between the prevalence of gallstones and diabetes mellitus (Barbara et al., 1987; Rome Group for Epidemiology and Prevention of Cholelithiasis, 1988a). In Japan, gallstones are found to be associated with glucose intolerance but not directly with diabetes mellitus (Kono et al., 1988). Thus even the existence of an increased prevalence of gallstones in diabetics is not clear.

Whether cholelithiasis and diabetes mellitus are causally related in some stepwise fashion, or whether they represent different manifestations of a common underlying etiology, or, whether the observed association is mediated by other factors remains to be determined. Two concepts have been advanced on the relation between cholelithiasis and diabetes mellitus. The first concept is that cholelithiasis precedes and initiates diabetes mellitus by causing pancreatitis, pancreatic scarring, and islet cell damage (Twiss and Carter, 1964). Robertson found, after reviewing extensive literatures that almost all authors thought diabetes mellitus follows gallstone formation (Robertson 1945). In Pima Indians, diabetes mellitus occurs many years after the onset of gallbladder disease (Lam, 1954). The other concept is that diabetes mellitus precedes cholelithiasis and that gallstone formation reflects the generalized derangement of metabolism of the diabetic patients (Goldstein and Schein, 1964; Norton et al., 1968). Norton et al. found that serum insulin levels in a fasting patient were high normal or above the usually accepted normal range in 13 randomly selected cases from among 240 postcholecystectomy patients (Norton et al., 1968). They thought that the increased prevalence of diabetes mellitus seems to be another expression of altered lipid and cholesterol metabolism resulting in gallstone formation and concomitant diabetes mellitus and related to adult-onset diabetes mellitus, in which fasting serum insulin levels are normal or elevated (Yalow and Berson, 1960). Bennion and Grundy have studied cholesterol metabolism in Pima Indians with adult-onset diabetes mellitus who have a high prevalence of diabetes mellitus and gallstones (Bennion and Grundy, 1977). Generalized increase in hepatic lipid production, greater excretion of cholesterol and bile acid, and elevation of plasma cholesterol and triglycerides were present. Increased bile acid production and expansion of the bile acid pool of all four bile acid species during diabetic hyperglycemia which gives no biochemical basis for the increase in gallstone incidence resulted in decreased cholesterol saturation in bile. This trend seems to be reversed by insulin treatment and is therefore conducive to cholesterol precipitation and gallstone formation, although Tanno et al. (1988) could not confirm it. Gallbladder bile is significantly more saturated with cholesterol during insulin treatment than during uncontrolled hyperglycemia (Bennion and Grundy, 1977). Bennion et al. hypothesized that the reported association of gallstones and diabetes mellitus may be due to a causative factor shared by both conditions, such as obesity. Obesity and hyperlipidemia are commonly associated with diabetes mellitus, and the often cited association between diabetes mellitus and gallstones may actually be a result of diabetics being obese and having type IV hyperlipidemia. Bile composition has been studied in diabetics and healthy controls matched for age, sex, and body mass index (Harber and Heaton, 1979). Cholesterol saturation and molar percentages of bile acids, phospholipids, and cholesterol are not significantly different. Bile is mostly supersaturated in both groups. Adult-onset diabetics who are almost always obese have increased biliary secretion of cholesterol and more saturated bile than slimmer juvenile-onset diabetics. Cholesterol supersaturation of gallbladder bile is not a feature of juvenile diabetics, as is suspected by the similar prevalence of cholelithiasis in controls (de Leon et al., 1978). Therefore, it is possible that the increased prevalence of gallstones in diabetics may be due not so much to diabetes itself as to the frequently associated obesity. Obesity is a strong risk factor for both cholesterol gallstones and adult-onset diabetes mellitus. In fact, one-third of adult-onset diabetics have raised triglyceride levels, but their bile is no more saturated than that of their obesity-matched controls. Gallstones may not be caused by diabetes mellitus but rather may share a major etiological factor with it.

Gallbladder dysfunction in diabetics was shown long ago by cholecystography (Tedstrom et al., 1926) and more recently by real-time ultrasonography (Onodera et al., 1983; Braverman, 1986). A large, poorly contracting, poorly filling gallbladder is frequently found in diabetics, regardless of the presence or absence of symptoms of gallbladder disease. These signs are especially frequent in diabetic patients who have autonomic neuropathy, with impaired gallbladder emptying and a reduced peak ejection rate, and occur less frequently in nondiabetics (Stone et al., 1988). This suggests the occurrence of a "diabetic neurogenic gallbladder" syndrome exemplified by large size, poor contraction, and/or poor visualization of the gallbladder and lack of symptoms of gallbladder disease (Gitelson et al., 1963; Grodzki et al., 1968). The gallbladder is frequently enlarged, resembling cholecystomegaly induced by vagotomy (Bloom and Stachenfeld, 1969; Clarke et al., 1979), and the fasting gallbladder volume is considerably larger in diabetics (Braverman, 1986). Contraction of the gallbladder in diabetics is poor (Onodera et al., 1983; Braverman, 1986; Stone et al., 1988) especially with autonomic neuropathy (Onodera et al., 1983). The rate of gallbladder emptying is significantly slower. Gallbladder hypotony is more frequently found in diabetics (Grodzki et al., 1968). However, diabetic cholecystoparesis is not entirely related to autonomic neuropathy, since it is not corrected by the administration of metoclopramide, a known cholinergic stimulant. It may be related to defective endogenous cholecystokinin release or to decreased responsiveness of the gallbladder wall. Bile is less concentrated in female diabetics than in controls (Harber and Heaton, 1979) which is consistent with impaired gallbladder emptying. Thus, whether a causal relationship between diabetes mellitus and gallstone exists remains controversial.

### Hyperlipidemia

Hypertriglyceridemia is associated with supersaturated bile and an increased prevalence of cholesterol gallstones (Ahlberg et al., 1979b, 1980). Others could not confirm that observation (Scragg et al., 1984a, Diehl et al., 1987). The relation between hypertriglyceridemia and gallstones disappears when the body mass index and other variables are controlled for by multivariate analysis (Kono et al., 1988; Jørgensen, 1989c). Primary hyperlipoproteinemia is often accompanied by abnormalities in cholesterol and bile acid metabolism (Hellström and Einarsson, 1977). Diabetics tend to be obese and to have triglyceridemia. Both of these disorders are associated with an increased risk of gallstones and cholesterol saturation of bile (Mentzer, 1926; Einarsson et al., 1975). Thijs et al. (1990) in a case-control study, found the highest risk for gallstones in low HDL levels and high triglyceride levels, while others found a greater risk in low serum HDL-cholesterol

(Pettiti et al., 1981; Scragg et al., 1984a; Diehl et al., 1987; Jørgensen, 1989c). Only a weak association with total cholesterol level is present (Scragg et al., 1984a, Rome Group for Epidemiology and Prevention of Cholelithiasis, 1988b). An association between HDL cholesterol and biliary cholesterol saturation (Thornton et al., 1981), and between reduced HDL cholesterol concentration and gallbladder disease, mostly cholelithiasis, in female twins pairs (Pettiti et al., 1981) has been reported, but the contention could not be confirmed (Henriksson et al., 1989). Einarsson et al. found that the prevalence of gallbladder disease (cholelithiasis, cholecystitis, and cholecystectomy) in consecutively admitted hyperlipoproteinemia patients is increased in type IV but not in type IIa hyperlipidemia (Einarsson et al., 1975), and the peak prevalence occurs in a somewhat younger age group (40 to 49 years). Total synthesis of cholesterol and bile acid is normal in type IIa and type IIb but abnormally high in type IV hyperlipoproteinemia (Einarsson et al., 1974; Angelin et al., 1976; Ahlberg et al., 1979a). The ratio between the synthesis of two primary bile acids, i.e., cholic acid and chenodeoxycholic acid, is decreased in the former and increased in the latter. High HMG-CoA reductase may explain the increased synthesis of cholesterol in type IV hyperlipoproteinemia. The most supersaturated bile is found in prebeta-hyperlipoproteinemia (Cahlin et al., 1973a), in which total biliary bile acid and lecithin concentrations are decreased significantly. Precursor incorporation into lecithin is significantly decreased in prebeta-hyperlipoproteinema (Cahlin et al., 1973b).

**Coronary heart disease**

A relationship between gallstone disease and coronary heart disease, including myocardial infarction, sudden death, coronary insufficiency, and angina pectoris, has been suspected ever since cholesterol was found to be a common constituent of both atheroma and cholesterol gallstones (Schoenheimer and Breusch, 1933). Epidemiological studies on the subject have so far been inconclusive (Friedman et al., 1966; Paul et al., 1983). Longitudinal surveillance of health conducted on a population aged 28 to 62 at the baseline in 1948 to 1950, examined biennially in the town of Framingham, Massachusetts – the Framingham Study – presented a good opportunity to investigate such a correlation. However, due to the limited number of gallstone disease cases available and the relatively short period of follow-up of 10 years, the study has been inconclusive (Friedman et al., 1966). Later, using 5,209 cases, members of the original cohort of the Framingham Study, and a longitudinal cohort study approach, followed for 26 years, during which nearly all members passed through the peak ages of risk for both diseases, Bortnichak et al. studied the relationship of diagnosed cholesterol cholelithiasis to subsequent incident coronary heart disease (Bortnichak et al., 1985). Univariate examination, with no correction for time ordering of the conditions or for shared risk factors, indicated a significant but modest positive correlation in men but not in women. This finding is supported by logistic multiple regression analysis allowing for the effects of time ordering and for eight standard coronary risk factors. Framingham men with cholecystectomy had nearly twice the risk of subsequently developing coronary heart disease for the first time. Male gallstone patients are at increased risk for subsequent coronary heart disease. Indeed gallstone disease and coronary heart disease may have shared factors, most notably age, obesity, blood lipid levels, and possibly diet. However, it should be noted in this connection that American Indians have a very high prevalence of gallstone disease but a low incidence of atherosclerotic disease (Gilbert, 1955; Hesse, 1959).

### Cystic fibrosis

As more and more cystic fibrosis patients have survived in recent years, it has become apparent that the incidence of cholelithiasis in adult cystic fibrosis is far greater (autopsy incidence of 27.5 %) than in the general population of 8–17 % (Vawter and Schwachman, 1979; Scott and Block, 1989). However, the mechanism underlying the formation of gallstones in cystic fibrosis is not well understood. Malabsorption of bile acid in pancreatic insufficiency, resulting in the production of supersaturated bile (Weber et al., 1973; Goodchild et al., 1975; Roy et al., 1977), the presence of abundant mucoproteins (Esterly and Oppenheimer, 1962; Bennion et al., 1978), frequently associated ductal anomalies, anomalous emptying of gallbladder promoting bile stasis, and growth of gallstones (Esterly and Oppenheimer, 1962; Vawter and Schwachman, 1979) have been suspected as contributing to gallstone formation.

### Distal ileopathy, ileal resection and colectomy

Cholelithiasis may be considered a late complication of disorders of the terminal ileum (Heaton and Read, 1969). The prevalence of gallstones in terminal ileopathy is variously reported to be 24–34 % (Heaton and Read, 1969; Cohen et al., 1971; Dowling et al., 1972; Hill et al., 1975; Whorewell et al., 1984) and is about three to four times higher than the expected prevalence in the general population. A rise in prevalence is noted with the increased duration of ileal disorders (Heaton and Read, 1969). The greatly increased prevalence of gallstones in younger patients under 40 years of age is noteworthy (Hill et al., 1975; Pellerin et al., 1975). The prevalence does not seem to rise with the passage of time (Hill et al., 1975). Andersson et al. found that the overall prevalence of gallstones in patients with Crohn's disease treated surgically was 17 %, i.e., with minor resection (less than 100 cm) was 9 %, while with major resection (over 100 cm) it was 35 % (Andersson et al., 1987). They estimated that the probability of developing gallstones after 20 years is about 50 %. With minor small bowel resection, the liver can compensate for bile acid loss by increasing its synthesis, but with more extensive resection the liver can no longer compensate for the fecal loss of bile acid, resulting in decreased bile acid concentration in the duodenum (Hardison et al., 1967; Percy-Robb et al., 1971). This is in agreement with the recent finding that a significant correlation is found between the length of ileum resected, on the one hand, and activities of HMG-CoA reductase and cholesterol 7$\alpha$-hydroxylase in the liver, on the other (Åkerlund et al., 1991). This increase is reflected by the increased serum level of both lathosterol (a marker for cholesterol synthesis) and 7$\alpha$-hydroxycholesterol (a marker for bile acid synthesis). Resection of 20 to 40 cm of the ileum stimulated enzyme activities two to three times, while resection of 80 to 150 cm stimulated enzyme activities four times. Malabsorption of bile acid leads to parallel stimulation of LDL receptor expansion, cholesterol synthesis, and degradation in the liver. An unusually large proportion (57.1 %) of gallstones encountered in terminal ileopathy was radiopaque – three times the figure of controls (Heaton and Read, 1969); however, this increase was not noted by others (Hill et al., 1975).

Development of gallstones in distal ileopathy is considered to be due to the loss of distal ileal function by diseases involving the distal ileum, such as Crohn's disease or resection of the distal ileum. The site and state of absorption of bile acid were determined in dogs by analyzing the bile acid composition of portal venous blood from the respective branches coming from the different parts of the intestinal tract. The technique was gas chromatography-mass spectrometry-selected ion monitoring, using deuterated bile acid as the internal standard (Fujii et al., 1988). The major site of absorption of conjugated bile acid was established to be the distal small intestine, in agreement with earlier studies (Dietchy, 1968). As much as 74 % of bile acid was absorbed at the distal small intestine during enterohepatic circulation. Exclusion of the terminal ileum results in impaired bile acid and cholesterol absorption (Färkkilä et al., 1988). Absorption of cholesterol is more sensitive to reduction in an absorption area than is bile acid absorption. Thus diseases involving the terminal ileum or ileal resection induce bile acid malabsorption, stimulating de novo bile acid synthesis in the liver, enhance conversion of cholesterol to bile acid, and reduce inflow of cholesterol to liver. As a result, the demand for cholesterol in liver increases. Malabsorption of bile acid leads to a two to three fold increase of rate-limiting enzymes in cholesterol synthesis, HMG-CoA reductase activity, and bile acid synthesis, cholesterol $7\alpha$-hydroxylase activity, as well as hepatic LDL receptor expression, with a significant reduction in LDL cholesterol (Åkerlund et al., 1991). When the demand is no longer compensated for by a stimulated cholesterol synthesis and enhanced receptor-mediated uptake of LDL cholesterol (Havel, 1988) to maintain the bile acid pool size, the result is a decreased bile acid pool and reduced bile acid secretion from the liver, with subsequent production of lithogenic bile and an increased cholesterol saturation index, predisposing to gallstone formation (Hardison et al., 1967; Garbutt et al., 1969; Heaton and Read, 1969; Dowling et al., 1972; Marks et al., 1977). However, no such increase was noted in prairie dogs (Pitt et al., 1984) or rhesus monkeys (Dowling et al., 1970, 1971), and neither in human infants nor in children (Heubi et al., 1983). In a follow-up study, Heubi et al. found a significantly higher cholesterol saturation index in young adults when compared with themselves before puberty, which may predispose them to gallstone formation in adulthood (Heubi et al., 1992). The bile salt pool appears to be better preserved in childhood. Hence, bile salt secretion is maintained and the cholesterol saturation index is kept down. After puberty, bile salt secretion declines but cholesterol secretion is maintained. Consequently the cholesterol saturation index rises. Recent study by Makino et al. showed that after total or subtotal colectomy risk of developing cholesterol stones increases as judged from the rise of molar percentage of cholesterol and decrease of bile acid in bile (Makino et al., 1994). Distinct species difference exist as ileal resection in prairie dogs induces pigment stones (Pitt et al., 1984).

## Primary Immunoglobulin Deficiency

Immunoglobulin deficiency has been found to be associated with cholelithiasis based on cholecystographic findings (Diaz-Buxo et al., 1975; Danon et al., 1983). Putative action of immunoglobulin has been advanced as nucleators (Holzbach et al., 1984) and antinucleators (Gallinger et al., 1987). However, when ultrasonography was used to include truly asymptomatic gallstones, no increased prevalence was noted (DeSantis et al., 1990). This discrepancy may be due to selection bias, as the previous studies may have included older and more seriously ill patients (Dias-Buxo et al., 1975).

## Dublin-Johnson syndrome

In Dubin-Johnson syndrome with specific defects in the transport of certain organic anions, such as bilirubin glucuronide, from hepatocyte to bile, two cases associated with gallstones are reported. In one case reported by Skornick et al., gallstones analyzed chemically were found to have very high cholesterol content, and the bile had a high cholesterol saturation index (Skornick et al., 1983). A defect in bilirubin and bile acid transport may be responsible for the higher lithogenicity of the bile.

## Spinal cord injury

A high incidence of gallstones has been noted after spinal cord injury, i.e., the incidence at autopsy increased from 11% to 29% (Apstein and Dalecki-Chipperfield, 1987). When the incidence of past cholecystectomy is added, the incidence of gallstones after spinal cord injury rises as much as 49%. The underlying mechanism is not clear.

## Cholecystectomy

The removal by cholecystectomy of the gallbladder, the site of formation of cholesterol gallstones, completely cures the disease. After removal of the gallbladder, the bile acid pool falls slightly but lack of trapping in the gallbladder results in a greater fraction of the bile acid pool cycling in the enterohepatic circulation per hour and, subsequently, more bile salt made available for solubilization of cholesterol (Shaffer and Small, 1977). More rapid cycling produces an increase in bile acid and phospholipid secretion; cholesterol secretion does not rise consistently. The net result is a lowering of cholesterol saturation of bile following cholecystectomy. Therefore, further gallstone formation is unlikely. In nonobese subjects, bile acid and phospholipid secretion increases and there is a definite improvement in bile compostion. In obese subjects, the effect is similar but less marked. The appearance of keto bile acid in bile has been noted after cholecystectomy (Hepner et al., 1974), but its significance in relation to gallstone formation is unknown.

## Vagotomy

The anterior vagal nerve sends the hepatic branch, while the posterior vagal nerve sends the celiac branch. During total vagotomy, both hepatic and celiac branches are divided together with the main gastric branches, while in selective vagotomy hepatic vagi are preserved. Johnson and Boyden (1952) were the first to warn of an increased gallstone incidence after total vagotomy; this was later corroborated by Rudick and Hutchison, (1965). The increased incidence of gallstones after total vagotomy was reported to be 16–24 % or four to six times (Nobles, 1966; Clave and Gaspar, 1969; Tompkins et al., 1972; Sapala et al., 1979) of the 4.5 % control rate in the 10-year Framingham Study (Friedman et al., 1966). Johnson and Boyden suspected that the gradual development of dilatation and noncontractility of the gallbladder was responsible and demonstrated that the fasting volume of the gallbladder is doubled within a year after vagotomy (Johnson and Boyden, 1952). Gallbladder tonus is maintained by hepatic vagi, and electric stimulation of hepatic vagi elicits gallbladder contraction (Stavney et al., 1963). Gallbladder contraction is wholly under the control of CCK. Increased sensitivity of the gallbladder to CCK is noted after vagotomy (Malagelada et al., 1974). Selective vagotomy preserves gallbladder tonus (Rudick and Hutchison, 1965). Stasis of bile in the gallbladder and delayed emptying occur in spite of decreased outlet resistance at the cholecystocholedochal junction (Schein and Gliedman, 1970). Ihasz and Griffith compared the incidence of gallstones after total vagotomy and selective vagotomy in which hepatic and celiac vagi are preserved (Ihasz and Griffith, 1981). A marked increase in the occurrence of gallstones was noted in markedly dilated noncontracting gallbladder i.e., in 9 of 46 cases of the former while in slightly hypotonic gallbladders, only 1 of 45 cases of the latter. Whether or not the lithogenicity of bile increases after vagotomy remains controvertial. The cholesterol saturation index decreases after truncal vagotomy (Stempel and Duane, 1978; Shaffer, 1982). A concomitant increase in the cholesterol saturation index of bile is shown in dogs (Sheen , 1971). This does not hold true after selective proximal vagotomy (Fujino, 1974). Bile acid malabsorption seems to play a significant role in the pathogenesis of gallstones after vagotomy but decreased bile acid synthesis is suggested to be important (Thompson et al., 1994).

### Gastric resection

In total gastrectomy, vagal nerves are divided at their main trunks; in subtotal gastrectomy, hepatic branches are usually spared and the celiac branch is transected. Majoor and Suren are credited with being the first to note the occurrence of gallstones after subtotal gastrectomy (Majoor and Suren, 1947). They reported an incidence of 3.4 %. An increased incidence of gallstones after truncal vagotomy and partial gastrectomy has been reported by several investigators (Tompkins et al., 1972; Sapala et al., 1979; Ihasz and Griffith, 1981; Horwitz and Kirson, 1965; Lorusso et al., 1988). Sapala et al. (1979) found that truncal vagotomy with subtotal gastrectomy is associated with a far greater incidence of postgastrectomy cholelithiasis than subtotal gastrectomy alone. They concluded that truncal vagotomy, not subtotal gastrectomy, is responsible for the increased incidence of gallstones, as the incidence of gallstones after subtotal gastrectomy alone is no different from that found in the Framingham Study (Friedman et al., 1966). Cattey et al. followed 14 patients who had a normal gallbladder and underwent total gastrectomy for Zollinger-Ellison syndrome, with a mean follow-up period of 6.3 years (Cattey and Wilson, 1989). Later, 10 of the 14 patients, or 71 % developed gallstones. They predicted that by 13 years after total gastrectomy, more than 90 % of patients at risk will have developed cholelithiasis.

Hada and his colleagues followed for 6 years 158 patients who underwent gastrectomy for gastric carcinoma, in which wide dissection of surrounding tissues is usually carried out around the esophagical hiatus (Hada et al., 1993). The incidence of gallstones is influenced by the extent of gastric resection (i.e., higher for total than subtotal gastrectomy) and the mode of reconstruction (i.e., higher for the procedure bypassing than passing the duodenum). The reasons given for the increased prevalence of gallstones after gastrectomy are altered motility of the gallbladder (Johnson and Boyden, 1952; Inoue et al., 1992), denervation of the gallbladder (Tinker and Cox, 1969), gallbladder stasis (Clave and Gaspar, 1969), and increased cholesterol saturation index of bile (Cowie and Clark, 1972).

### Gastric Bypass Surgery

A high incidence of gallstones during weight loss after gastric bypass surgery for morbid obesity has been documented (Wattchaw et al., 1983). Following gastric bypass surgery, as many as 35 % of patients develop gallstones (Shiffman et al., 1991, 1993b). Glycoprotein increases in conjunction with the formation of gallstones during rapid weight loss after bariatric surgery (Broomfield et al., 1988). The change in gastrointestinal hormones after gastric bypass may induce a defect in gallbladder motility (Kellum et al., 1990) which permits mucin accumulation within the gallbladder. The temporary reduction in gallbladder emptying observed coincides with the formation of gallstones (Shiffman et al., 1991) in the early postoperative period after gastric bypass. Postoperative changes noticed following gastric bypass may be explained by the change in gallbladder emptying and stasis in the gallbladder.

## Drugs

### Smoking

There has been controversy whether or not there is a higher risk of gallstones associated with smoking. No relation was found between the prevalence of gallstones and smoking in some studies (Diehl et al., 1987; Kono et al., 1988). Others found that smokers tend to have gallstone disease (Layed et al., 1982; Rome Group for Epidemiology and Prevention of Cholelithiasis, 1988b; Jørgensen, 1989a). A marginal tendency was reported by Freedman et al. (1986). During the Royal College of General Practitioners (RCGP) Oral Contraceptive Study on a cohort of 46,000, smokers were more likely to develop symptomatic cholelithiasis than nonsmokers (relative risk, 1.19), and there was a significant correlation with the number of cigarettes smoked daily (Murray et al., 1994). Women who smoked at the beginning of the study had a 50 % higher crude incidence of gallstones than nonsmokers (Layed et al., 1982). The relative risk was 1.6, but there was no dose-response relationship. Since the risk of gallstones was not related to how heavily the women smoked, it may indicate a threshold effect of smoking. Jørgensen (1989a) found that smoking had a significant association with gallstones among men when eight parameters were included in the multivariate analysis, but found no substantial dose-response effect. A positive trend was seen among women. In twin women smokers, Petitti et al. found a relative risk of 1.8 for gallbladder disease history after controlling for confound factors such as age, body mass index, alcohol and estrogen use, and various lipoproteins (Petitti et al., 1981). Pastides and his colleagues conducted a case-control study on 84 patients with gallbladder disease and 171 controls for smoking, among other characteristics such as demography, reproduction, and diet (Pastides et al., 1990). They found that gallstone patients were less frequent smokers. Smoking was found to increase degradation of exogenous estrogens resulting in correspondingly lower plasma level to the extent and since gallstone formation is estrogen related, a negative association between tobacco smoking and cholelithiasis should be expected. In postmenopausal women, Jensen et al. (1985) found that smoking increases the degradation of exogenous estrogens, resulting in correspondingly lower plasma estrogen levels. The lower concentrations of HDL cholesterol and higher triglyceride levels found in smokers than in nonsmokers (Freedman et al., 1986) are compatible with a lower incidence of gallstones in the former. However, Pastides's work has been criticized (Lowenfels, 1991), since the controls were taken from a large trauma center where smoking is a known risk factor for various types of injury and increases the risk of motor vehicle accidents and traffic violations by 50% even after adjusting for alcohol consumption. Therefore, it appears more likely that the apparently protective effect of smoking on gallstones noted by Pastides and his colleagues may largely be attributable to excess smoking in their controls. The risk of gallstone disease in relation to smoking seems to be small, if any.

### Alcohol consumption

The relation between alcohol consumption and the prevalence of gallstones is controversial. Several studies showed no relationship (Rome Group for Epidemiology and Prevention of Cholelithiasis, 1988b; Kono et al., 1988). On the other hand, in the Framingham Study, a low risk of gallstone disease among those with high alcohol consumption was reported (Friedman et al., 1966). In a case-control study, an inverse relationship between alcohol use and the risk of gallstones was found. A protective effect of alcohol was noted only with a modest intake of alcohol (Scragg et al., 1984c). Lowering of cholesterol saturation induced by alcohol is found in animals (Schwesinger et al., 1988).

### Blood cholesterol-lowering drugs

A serum cholesterol-lowering diet with large amounts of polyunsaturated fatty acids increases the prevalence of cholelithiasis (Sturdevant et al., 1973). Specific inhibitors of HMG-CoA reductase such as simvastatin, pravastatin, and lovastatin seem to have a beneficial effect on cholesterol saturation (Duane et al., 1988a; Hoogerbrugge van der Linden et al., 1990; Reinhér et al., 1990b; Mitchell et al., 1991a; Smit et al., 1992; Logan and Duane, 1990; Bateson, 1990). Clofibrate, a lipid-lowering drug, enhances cholesterol saturation of bile by increasing biliary secretion of cholesterol (Coronary Drug Project Research Group, 1977; Einarsson and Angelin, 1986). In fact clofibrate administration is associated with a twofold increase in the prevalence of gallstones (Coronary Drug Project Research Group, 1977). Administration of gemfibrozil, a fibric acid derivative and structually different, with biological actions distinct from those of clofibrate, which reduces levels of total and LDL-cholesterol and triglycerides but raises HDL cholesterol, is not associated with an increased incidence of diagnosed gallstones (Coronary Drug Project Research Group, 1977; Frick et al., 1987). Another dietary fiber, psyllium (psyllium hydrophilic mucilloid), lowers LDL-cholesterol primarily via stimulation of bile acid synthesis (Everson et al., 1992).

### Bile acid sequestrants

Bile acid sequestrants such as cholestyramine did not significantly increase the incidence of diagnosed gallstones (Coronary Drug Project Research Group, 1977; Frick et al., 1987).

### Nicotinic acid

Administration of nicotinic acid is not associated with an increased incidence of diagnosed gallstones (Coronary Drug Project Research Group, 1977; Frick et al., 1987).

### Female sex hormones

Treatment with estrogen and clofibrate increases the incidence of gallstones, as judged by the life table analysis (Coronary Drug Study Research Group, 1977). In women on estrogen therapy, the relative risk of symptomatic gallstone disease increased to 2.0 (Petitti et al., 1981, 1988) and 3.7 (Honoré, 1980c). Postmenopausal women undergoing cholecystectomy were 2.5 times more likely to have used estrogen (Boston Collaborative Drug Surveillance Program, 1974). The incidence of gallstones increases in estrogen-treated men (Henricksson et al., 1989). However, others found no significant relationship (Kakar et al., 1988; Jørgensen 1988a). Using liver biopsy specimens, estrogen at pharmacological doses was found to stimulate hepatic LDL receptor expression and the rate-limiting enzyme step in cholesterol biosynthesis, HMG-CoA reductase activity, in man (Angelin et al., 1992). The former is responsible for the enhanced clearance of LDL from the circulation (Ericksson et al., 1989). More than half of the receptor-mediated elimination of plasma LDL occurs in the liver (Havel and Hamilton, 1988). In estrogen-treated men, a decrease in the concentrations of total and free cholesterol in liver microsomes was observed despite increased activity of both pathways for cholesterol delivery to and within hepatocytes, i.e., the LDL receptor and HMG-CoA reductase (Angelin et al., 1992). The most plausible explanation for the effect of estrogen administration is that the effects of estrogen treatment are exerted on biliary canalicular membranes and/or on the intracellular distribution of cholesterol avaiblable for subsequent biliary excretion. Thus, membrane cholesterol is lost because of the increased secretion of free cholesterol into bile (Henricksson et al., 1989). The close correlation between the increase in biliary cholesterol output and the decrease in plasma LDL cholesterol levels (Henricksson et al., 1989) tend to support the above concept.

The use of oral contraceptives seems to increase the risk of gallstones to some extent. A case-control study found the risk to increase twofold (Boston Collaborative Drug Surveillance Program, 1973). Using ultrasonography, Jørgensen showed increased risk in a Danish population (Jørgensen, 1988a). Current users of oral contraceptive were found to have a moderately increased risk of symptomatic gallbladder disease (relative risk, 1.15), unlike former users (relative risk, 1.05) (Murray et al., 1994). Others found little increase in risk (Petitti et al., 1981; Layde et al., 1982; Royal College of General Practitioners Oral Contraceptive Study, 1982) or none (Barbara et al., 1987; Rome Group for Epidemiology and Prevention of Cholelithiasis, 1988b). The above result may be due to the difference in estrogen dose used, as Strom et al. found a dose-response relationship (Strom et al., 1986). The risk seems to be increased more in younger age groups (Scragg et al., 1984c; Strom et al., 1986).

## Other drugs

By giving aspirin, the occurrence of gallstones during severe weight loss in man can be prevented (Broomfield et al., 1988). Administration of ceftriaxone and glaphenine has been found to induce gallstones in man. The presence of unconjugated glaphenic acid, its central location, and the presence of large quantity of glaphenine and its derivatives (amounting to 30–80 % of the dry weight of gallstones induced), as revealed by Fourier transform infrared (FTIR) spectrometry, indicates the important role played by glaphenine (Moesch et al., 1993).

Treatment with the long-acting somatostatin analog, octreotide, which inhibits growth hormone and insulin-like growth factor (IGF) release effective on acromegaly, seems to be associated with a high risk of cholelithiasis (Daughaday, 1990; Ho et al., 1990; Hussaini et al., 1994). The gallstones that occurred were radiolucent cholesterol stones (Hussaini et al., 1994). Marked inhibition of gallbladder contractions after a test meal by both somatostatin and octreotide seems to be caused by suppression of CCK release by the intestine (Lembcke et al., 1987) and inhibition of gallbladder contraction in response to CCK (Fisher et al., 1987). Bile flow may also be inhibited (Marteau et al., 1989). Deoxycholic acid is increased, and the lithogenicity of bile is enhanced (Hussaini et al., 1994). The percentage of cholesterol in vesicles and vesicular cholesterol : phospholipids molar ratios are increased. As a result, the incidence of cholelithiasis became as high as 30–70 %. Thus, the pathogenesis of octreotide-induced gallbladder gallstones seems to be (1) gallbladder stasis; (2) prolongation of intestinal transit by inhibition of prokinetic hormone release, favoring the transformation of cholic acid to deoxycholic acid; (3) secretion of supersaturated bile with cholesterol transported by unstable vesicles with a higher cholesterol : phospholipids ratio (Hussaini et al., 1994). Thus acromegalic patients with octreotide-associated gallstones and gallstone-free acromegalic patients treated with octreotide have changes in bile composition similar to those in patients with conventional cholesterol stones.

d-Thyroxine was found to favor the formation of gallstones when given under a relatively short period (Bergman and Van der Linden 1964). In hypothyroid rats, bile acid synthesis, biliary secretion of cholesterol, and phospholipids diminish. A single injection of triiodothyronine increases cholesterol secretion 13-fold and phospholipids secretion 3-fold; an increase in bile acid synthesis occurs somewhat later (Gebhard and Prigge, 1992). Although the thyroid state greatly influences biliary lipid secretion, its clinical implication in gallstone pathogenesis is uncertain.

# Pigment Stones

## Black Pigment Stones (Black Stones)

Black (pigment) stones are multiple, dark brown to black, and lustrous (Maki et al., 1982). They are hard and brittle. Their outer surface is rugged; their cut surface is smooth, devoid of any crystal structure (Figure 1c). Black pigment stones are composed of unconjugated bilirubin, 5–15 % (Yamashita et al., 1988), and insoluble bilirubin polymers (Black et al., 1982; Ohkubo et al., 1984), with an admixture of calcium carbonate and phosphate (Wosiewitz and Schroebler, 1978). Black pigment stones containing and not containing carbonate seem to be present (Trotman et al., 1977). The mechanism of polymerization of bilirubin is not well understood. It may involve calcium acting as a bridge between bilirubin molecules (Soloway, personal communication). From 40 % to 50 % of black pigment stones are radiopaque (Maki et al., 1982). They occur in the gallbladder and occasionally migrate into the bile duct.

### Epidemiology

The proportion of black pigment stones in all gallstone cases differs according to the area. In Japan it is about 1–5 % (Miyake Jr et al., 1963; Kameda et al., 1981) and in the United States and Europe it is about 27 % (Trotman and Soloway, 1975). Postmortem studies showed that the prevalence of gallstones is approximately two times higher in cirrhotics than in noncirrhotics (Bouchier, 1969; Nicholas et al., 1972); these are mostly black pigment stones. An ultrasound survey showed an even higher prevalence of gallstones in cirrhotics (Acalovschi et al., 1988; Steinberg et al., 1988; Sheen and Liaw, 1989). The prevalence of gallstones is not increased in cirrhotics with age, and no sex difference is present (Bouchier, 1969). The prevalence of gallstones increases in liver cirrhosis, whether alcoholic or nonalcoholic (Summerskill et al., 1960; Davidson, 1962; Bouchier, 1969; Nicholas et al., 1972; Acalovschi et al., 1988; Steinberg et al., 1988). The frequency of gallstones in cirrhotics ranges from 25.6 % for prenecrotics to 35.8 % for alcoholics but no one form of cirrhosis has a greater prevalence of gallstones (Bouchier, 1969). Prevalence of gallstones increases from Child's A to Child's C, with a significant trend (Fornari et al., 1990). A case-control study showed an inverse relationship between alcohol intake and gallstone formation (Scragg et al., 1984b). In cirrhotic men, increased levels of estrogens and progesterone may cause impairment of gallbladder emptying similar to that observed in pregnant women (Fornari et al., 1990). Chronic mild hemolysis occurs in cirrhotics (Jandl, 1955; Cawein et al., 1960). Its relation to gallstone formation is discussed by Jones et al. (1955). Concentrations of total bilirubin and unconjugated bilirubin are not increased in cirrhotics (Soloway et al., 1977), but they are increased with hemolysis (Shull et al., 1977; Trotman et al., 1981; Keida et al., 1991). Conditions in cirrhotics favoring black pigment stone formation is discussed in detail by Ostrow (Ostrow 1984).

## Etiology

Spherocytosis (Bates and Brown, 1952) and sickle cell anemia are associated with an increased incidence of black pigment stones. The prevalence of gallstone disease in sickle cell anemia varies from 27% to 58% (Weens, 1945; Green et al., 1953; Jordan, 1957; Cameron et al., 1971; Karayalcin et al., 1979; Lachman et al., 1979; Sarnaik et al., 1980; Stephens and Scott, 1980; Rennels et al., 1984; Bond et al., 1987; Malone and Werlin, 1988). However, many do not develop gallstones. Therefore, mechanisms other than increased hemolysis must be considered. Fasting and residual volumes of the gallbladder after fasting are said to be twice those of controls (Everson et al., 1989). The rate of emptying and fractional emptying is similar. It was concluded that gallbladder enlargement, bile stasis, impaired emptying of sludge, and reduction of the bile acid pool may be important in the formation of black pigment stones, in addition to the overproduction of bilirubin. However, others found no change in the motility of gallbladder containing black pigment stones by comparing muscle strips from the gallbladder wall (Behar et al., 1989). Gallstones in sickle cell anemia have been reported not only in African blacks but also in Arabic populations (Perrine, 1973). In sickle cell anemia, whether homozygous or heterozygous, there is an increased prevalence of gallstones, i.e., hemoglobin SS, hemoglobin SC, hemoglobin S-beta-thalassemia (Rennels et al., 1984). Sludges also occur (Sarnaik et al., 1980; Senaati et al., 1993). The prevalence of gallstones in homozygous thalassemia, both major and intermedia, has been reported to be 52% based on ultrasonographic examination or plain abdominal X-ray (Goldfarb et al., 1990). There is a correlation between the presence of gallstones and increasing age. No difference in the severity of the disease between those with hemoglobin SC or hemoglobin S-beta-thalassemia, with or without gallstones, is present. The presence of gallstones is not related to sex, geographical origin, or hematological variables and is not associated with abnormal liver function (Bond et al., 1987). Gallstones and sludge in the gallbladder are detected by ultrasound examination in multiparas with hemoglobin SD disease (Spinapolice et al., 1982). Mean hemoglobin levels and reticulocyte counts, previously reported to be related to the development of gallstones (McCall et al., 1977), may not be accurate determinants of hemolytic rates. Intravascular hemolysis occurs in long-distance runners as a consequence of trauma to erythrocytes in the feet. This may be followed by the formation of black pigment stones because of the increased biliary excretion of bilirubin (Leslie et al., 1985). Any conditions associated with chronic hemolysis may lead to the formation of black pigment stones. Shift from bilirubin diglucuronide normally present in bile to monoglucuronide and further to unconjugated biliruhin (UCG) occurs in bile with black pigment stones (Ostrow 1984). Acid calcium salt $Ca(HUCB)_2$ forms readily at pH typical of bile (Ostrow 1984). As the ion product of Ca and monoacid species of UCB which is extremely insoluble in water lead to the precipitation of bilirubin. However, it should be noted that, more often than not, black pigment stone cases are associated with apparent hemolysis. Under these circumstances, a decrease in micelles and vesicles carrying unconjugated bilirubin and binding calcium increases unbound bilirubin and ionized calcium, thus promoting precipitation of unconjugated bilirubin.

Hypersecretion of mucin occurs in the gallbladder with black pigment stones (LaMont et al., 1983a, Malet et al., 1989). Formation of concretion is said to start within mucous gel accumulated in the crypts of gallbladder mucosa (Trotman et al., 1982). Supersaturation is facilitated by defective acidification by gallbladder (Moore 1990). Recently, calcium-regulatory protein has been isolated by sodium dodecyl sulfate-polyacrylamide gel electrophoresis from black pigment stones, inhibiting both the initiation and growth of calcium carbonate crystals (Okido et al., 1992). This acidic protein has an apparent molecular weight of around 5 kDa and has a very tight (possibly covalent) binding of a diazo-positive yellow pigment, presumably bilirubin. The protein is bound to the crystal and accompanied by transformation of the crystal habit from hexagonal to rectangular, but in general it is not recognizably crystalline (Okido et al., 1993). The protein seems to inhibit vaterite formation by interacting with the nascent crystals to modify their growth, as reflected by the change in the infrared spectrum. Anion polypeptide fraction (APF), the most abundant protein in human bile after albumin and immunoglobulin, may play a role in black pigment stone formation, possibly by its calcium and phospholipids binding property; previously it was known as calcium-binding protein (Lafont et al., 1993).

Significant bacterial infection is not associated with black pigment stones (Goodhart et al., 1978; Tabata and Nakayama, 1981). Pigment stones studied by Kaufman et al. containing no bacteria were black pigment stones (Kaufman et al., 1989). This finding is compatible with the previous bacteriological finding (Tabata and Nakayama, 1981) that the presence of bacteria in the bile of patients with black pigment stones does not necessarily mean bacterial involvement in the formation of black pigment stones. Although the incidence of bacteria increases when black pigment stones advance into the common bile duct (Tabata and Nakayama, 1981), bacteria do not seem to play an important role in the formation of black pigment stones.

Increased prevalence of gallstones in cases of total parenteral nutrition (TPN) with minimal or no oral feeding has been well documented (Whitington and Black; 1980; Roslyn et al., 1981b, 1983a, b, Doty et al., 1982, Messing et al., 1983; Pitt et al., 1983b; Roslyn et al., 1983b). Gallstones occur only in cases where sludge develops and incidence increases with the length of TPN. They are black pigment stones (Pitt et al., 1983a). Anderson (1972) were the first to suggest the cause-and-effect relationship between gallbladder disease and TPN, which was later corroborated by Petersen et al (Petersen and Sheldon, 1979). TPN favors the clinical expression of gallbladder disease, especially in high-risk patients such as those with ileal disease or resection. The occurrence of gallstones in children maintained on intravenous alimentation (Whitington and Black, 1980) and the appearance of sludge (Messing et al., 1981) have been noted. A prospective ultrasonography study of a large population of patients with TPN over 15 years disclosed that the incidence of gallstones was as high as 45 % which is significantly higher than predicted from the autopsy data (Pitt et al., 1983b). Patients with minimal or no oral intake during TPN administration have a nearly twofold increase in gallbladder diseases compared with those who have oral supplementation in addition to TPN. With ileal disease such as necrotizing enterocolitis, antenatal volvulus, lymphangioma of the mesentery and radiation injury to the ileum or ileal resection, bile acid malabsorption from terminal ileum further increases the risk of gallstone disease (Roslyn et al., 1983b; King et al., 1987). The mechanism underlying this increased incidence is not well understood. During TPN, intestinal hormone secretion is not activated, resulting in alteration of normal enterohepatic circulation of bile acids, change in bile composition, reduced daily contraction of the gallbladder, and bile stasis. These effects predispose to calculous and acalculous cholecystitis. Gimmon et al. found that the supersaturation of bile increases after the administration of TPN solution in rats, regardless of the route of administration i.e. parenteral or intragastric (Gimmon et al., 1982). However, in prairie dogs, Doty et al. (1982) found that supersaturation of bile decreases significantly after 10 days of TPN. Long term TPN seems to induce biliary sludge and may lead to eventual gallstone formation (Messing et al., 1983). Sludge formation is infrequent during the first 3 weeks of TPN but becomes constant after 6 weeks. No food intake and subsequent inactivity of the bowel may also have contributed to the formation of lithogenic bile (Messing et al., 1983). The increased prevalence of sludge and gallstones during TPN also seems to be due to stasis of bile in the gallbladder, as judged by ultrasonography, because of the absence of oral food intake and subsequently diminished gallbladder contraction (Cano et al., 1986). During TPN, bile stasis leads to sludge formation and eventual gallstone formation (Messing et al., 1983). Stasis in the gallbladder seems to be an important contributor to the development of gallstones effected by the loss of enteral stimulation by oral nutrient intake during TPN (Holzbach, 1983b). The sludge formed during TPN is said to be calcium bilirubinate granules. The main component of most gallstones induced by TPN seems to be calcium bilirubinate (Pitt et al., 1983a). TPN was found to induce lithogenic effect in hepatic bile by increasing concentration of bilirubin and calcium and decreasing hepatic bile flow in rats (Li and Stahlgren, 1995). Gallbladder stasis and altered bilirubin metabolism are thought to be important. During TPN, absence of neural and hormonal stimuli to the extrahepatic biliary tract in the form of food intake leads to decreased contraction of the gallbladder, with failure of the sphincter Oddi to relax, resulting in the preferential flow of bile and stasis in the gallbladder, favoring gallstone formation. A randomized double-blind controlled study indicated that administration of cholecystokinin octapeptide (CCK-OP) effectively prevents biliary sludge formation in persons receiving TPN by inducing significant periodic contractions of the gallbladder and prevents TPN-induced biliary stasis (Sitzman et at., 1990). Normalization of gallbladder motility and disappearance of sludge take place after the cessation of TPN (Messing et al., 1983).

On the other hand, after reviewing the references on various hepatobiliary disorders and TPN, Quigley et al. found that it is difficult to separate the effects of TPN on hepatobiliary function from many other hepatotoxic factors which may be operative (Quigley et al., 1993). They concluded that a loss of enteric stimulation, not TPN per se, may be the primary factor in the development of biliary sludge and gallstones. The apparent predirection of infants to TPN-related cholestasis may be based on the relative immaturity of the neonatal biliary excretory system. Although biliary sludge formation and gallstone incidence increase after prolonged TPN, Quigley et al. could not find bile to be supersaturated (Doty et al., 1984; Innis, 1985).

# Brown Pigment Stones (Calcium Bilirubinate Stones)

Brown pigment stones (or calcium bilirubinate stones or earthy stones) are brown, reddish-brown or dark brown, not lustrous, soft, and pliable. Their surface is usually slightly rough. They come in various shapes, from round to cylindrical, and are sometimes faceted when several stones are present in the bile duct in close proximity. In most instances, their cross section shows a layered structure with the spokes, like cholesterol crystals, radiating from the center of the stones (Figure 1d). The stones are composed of bilirubin, almost exclusively in free unconjugated form (20–40 %), cholesterol (5–20 %), fatty acid, mainly palmitic acid (5–20 %) and calcium (3–4 %) (Nakayama, 1968; Yamashita et al., 1988). Calcium combines with bilirubin in a ratio of 1 to 14.6 on a molecular weight basis. Hence brown pigment stones are usually not radiopaque (Maki et al., 1982) unless they have a calcium-rich shell. Unlike cholesterol stones, they contain large amounts of bilirubin in the form of calcium bilirubinate, which can be dissolved in appropriate solvents, indicating that free unconjugated bilirubin molecules are not cross-linked (Wosiewitz et al., 1983). Brown pigment stones contain a smaller amount of cholesterol, usually less than 20 % and calcium salt of fatty acids, mainly palmitic acid (Nakayama, 1968; Yamashita et al., 1988). They are present mainly in the extrahepatic bile duct and occasionally in the gallbladder and intrahepatic bile duct. The majority of common bile duct stones (59 %) found more than 21 months after cholecystectomy in the United States are said to be brown pigment stones and are thought to be formed de novo in situ (Malet et al., 1988). Their number ranges from 1 to a few 10s. In older patients, the proportion of brown pigment stones in the gallbladder, as well as in the extrahepatic bile ducts, is much greater than in younger ones. Intrahepatic calculi are mostly brown pigment stones, but a smaller proportion of cholesterol stones is also present (Mukaihara, 1981; Yamashita et al., 1988).

## Epidemiology

Brown pigment stones (or calcium bilirubinate stones) occur mainly in East Asia, including Japan, China, Korea, Taiwan, the Philippines, Indochina, Thailand, Malaysia, Singapore, and Indonesia (Nakayama, 1968). In the West, brown pigment stones are usually found as recurrent common bile duct stones formed de novo after cholecystectomy. The great majority of gallstones are brown pigment stones related to bile stasis and infection (Cetta, 1986). The proportion of brown pigment stones in a given population is always changing. In 1913, Miyake Sr noted the proportion of brown pigment stones (calcium bilirubinate stones) was much greater and constituted the major form of gallstone in Japan at that time (Miyake Sr, 1913). Since then, the proportion of brown pigment stones has been steadily declining (Miyake Jr and Johnston, 1968; Nakayama and Miyake Jr, 1970) and becoming 20–30 % of all gallstones in the 1980s (Tabata and Nakayama, 1981). At present, the proportion of brown pigment stones is about 10 % among gallbladder stones and 20 % among common duct stones in Japan; in the West, the proportions are 3 % and 20 % respectively (Kaufman et al., 1989). Brown pigment stones are more common in the West than has been previously stated (Stewart et al., 1987).

## Etiology

Biliary tract infection and stasis are thought to be important in the formation of brown pigment stones (calcium bilirubinate stones). In a prospective study, biliary infection precedes the formation of brown pigment stones rather than resulting from the stasis caused by the presence of gallstones (Cetta, 1986). Bacteria are almost always present with brown pigment gallstones, but the incidence is low with black pigment stones (Tabata and Nakayama, 1981; Cetta et al., 1984; Kaufman et al., 1989). Bacterial enzymes produced cleave the biliary constituents such as conjugated bilirubin to free unconjugated bilirubin, phosphatidyl choline (lecithin) to lysolecithin, and free fatty acid and conjugated bile acids to unconjugated bile acids. As a result, transformation of micelles and vesicles takes place. With the presence of ionized calcium, calcium bilirubinate and calcium salt of fatty acid are produced, which precipitate because of their poor aqueous solubility. The interior of gallstones is studied by scanning electron microscopy in the secondary electron image (SEI) and back-scattered electron imaging (BEI) modes (Kaufman et al., 1989). These studies found bacteria only within the calcium bilirubinate-protein matrix of brown pigment stones or in the pigmented portion of combination stones (Stewart et al., 1987), stressing that bacterial infection is important only in the formation of brown pigment stones. In fact, in two patients, Cetta et al. showed that bacterial infection precedes brown pigment stone formation (Cetta, 1986). Although, at initial common duct exploration, bacterial culture of bile was negative, it became positive and later formed brown pigment stones in the common bile duct. Thus, biliary infection seems to be a primary event and, in addition to bile stasis, seems to play a crucial role in the pathogenesis of brown pigment stones. Although bile acids present in normal bile are almost entirely in conjugated form (the free unconjugated form amounts to less than 0.1 % of the total) (Matoba et al., 1986), the presence of a large amount of free bile acids in brown pigment stones suggests that a considerable amount of free bile acid must have been present in bile both at the time when the brown pigment stones were being formed and during ensuing stone growth (Akiyoshi and Nakayama, 1990). A comparison of the free : conjugated bile acid ratios of paired biles and gallstones shows that they are consistently higher in the stones than in the corresponding biles, as conjugated bile acid is much more hydrophilic. Calcium salt of unconjugated bile acid has a high pK value and very low aqueous solubility (Jones et al., 1986), and hence is easily precipitated out and preferentially incorporated into stones. Un-ionized or partially ionized bile acids formed are (1) absorbed by the biliary tract by passive, nonionic diffusion (passive absorption), (2) precipitated as crystals, (3) form gels, and (4) become hydrophobically bound to biliary mucin. As a result, biliary bile acid concentration decreases. Furthermore, the simultaneous presence of bacterial phospholipase A leads to hydrolysis of biliary lecithin, with absorption of the lysolecithin formed and absorption/precipitation of the released fatty acid as calcium salt (Nakano et al., 1988b). This depletes the biliary phospholipid content and decreases the solubilization of cholesterol and bilirubin in bile. Since the infection by bacteria with $\beta$-glucuronidase activity is the key event in the formation of brown pigment stones, the predominant presence of free bile acid in the stones appears to indicate that bacterial species present at least at the beginning of stone formation may have possessed both hydrolases for bile acid and bilirubin conjugates. Such bacterial species can be found in some cases of brown pigment stones (Tabata and Nakayama, 1981; Akiyoshi and Nakayama, 1990). Recently, a close relation between biliary infection and the low level of secretory immunoglobulin A in bile has been emphasized in regard to the role played by the mucosal immune system in the biliary tract (Yio et al., 1992). It agglutinates bacteria, inhibits their motility, and prevents their adherence to mucous membranes (Xian et al., 1992). Its resistance to digestion by most proteolytic enzymes in the gastrointestinal tract (Bienenstock and Befus, 1983) may also contribute greatly to its role in mucosal immunity. The prevalence of cholelithiasis has been noted in patients with idiopathic late-onset immunoglobulin deficiency (Danon et al., 1983). Bile stasis favors continued bacterial presence and growth of calcium bilirubinate precipitates into brown pigment stones. Therefore, both stasis and infection seem to be necessary for brown pigment stone formation.

## Role of bilirubin

Bilirubin occurs in conjugated form as glucuronide, glucoside and xyloside and sulfate (Spivak and Carey, 1985; Keida, 1991). Its composition in human bile is bilirubin diglucuronide 50–60 %, monoglucuronide 20–30 %, monoglucuronide monoglucoside 10 %, diglucoside 5 %, monoxyloside 3 %, monoglucoside monoxyloside 1 %, monoxyloside 0.5 % and unconjugated bilirubin only 1 % (Keida et al., 1991). However, bilirubin found in brown pigment stones or calcium bilirubinate stones is almost exclusively in free unconjugated form (Yamashita et al., 1988) and is present as acid, neutral, and intermediate salts of calcium – the last having 1 1/2 molecules of bilirubin per calcium atom and containing both acid and neutral salts by X-ray diffraction study (Sutor et al., 1977a). Acid or intermediate salts, but no neutral salt, have been found in 14 out of 70 gallstones analyzed. Therefore, transformation of conjugated bilirubin to the free unconjugated form must have taken place in the course of stone formation, for which bacterial $\beta$-glucuronidase is mainly responsible (Maki, 1966; Tabata and Nakayama, 1981; Stewart et al., 1987; Cetta, 1986). Bilirubin diglucuronides are more readily deconjugated than bilirubin diglucoside and bilirubin monoglucoside monoxyloside (Keida et al., 1991). Therefore, glucuronides are more likely to be the main source of unconjugated bilirubin in the formation of both black and brown pigment stones (calcium bilirubinate stones). It has been well recognized that bacterial infection in bile almost always accompanies brown pigment stones (Tabata and Nakayama, 1981). Bilirubin is excreted in bile mainly as diglucuronide (BDG) and partly as monoglucuronide (BMG) (Ostrow and Murphy, 1970). Because of absence of the formation of intramolecular hydrogen bonds, bilirubin glucuronides are highly water soluble and enter into the duodenum via the biliary tract. However, under certain circumstances, they are transformed to unconjugated bilirubin (UCB), which is virtually insoluble in bile at physiological pH due to the formation of intramolecular hydrogen bonding (Figure 10) (Schmid, 1978; Yang et al., 1993). Because of the instability of UCB, its solubility is not well known. However, it seems to be influenced by pH and by the presence of ionized calcium, with which it forms insoluble salts. Solvent partition of UCB from chloroform to buffered aqueous sodium chloride indicated that aqueous solubility of bilirubin diacid ($H_2B^0$) is 66 nM and the two carboxylic pKa values of bilirubin are 8.1 and 8.4 (Hahm et al., 1992). UCB-$XI_\alpha$ exists as uncharged diacid ($H_2B$), two isomeric monoanions ($HB^-$) and dianions ($B^{2-}$). The proportion of each of the trinity of species, bound and unbound, in various body fluid have been reviewed (Ostrow et al., 1994). Dominant UCB is $H_2B$ and dominant UCB anion is $HB^-$ but not dianion ($B^{2-}$) at the physiological pH of bile. Maximum concentration of UCB in bile (35 $\mu$M) is several orders greater than its solubility in aqueous media at physiological pH (Spivak and Yuey, 1986). The solubility of UCB falls from di-anion to mono-anion and to fully protonated UCB, in this order (Brodersen, 1979). In model bile, UCB is almost exclusively bound to micelles, and its concentration is less than 1 % of total bilirubin (Ostrow et al., 1988). UCB is also bound to vesicles (Tipping et al., 1979) in the form of $H_2B^0$; with increasing pH, uptake of UCB by phospholipid vesicles decreases. Binding of UCB to micelles versus vesicles may be important in determining the precipitation of UCB leading to the formation of pigment gallstones (Donovan and Carey, 1991).

UCB combines with ionized calcium present in bile to form calcium bilirubinate, which precipitates because of its poor solubility in aqueous media, especially in the low concentrations of bile salt (Ostrow et al., 1988) usually encountered in bile with brown pigment stones (calcium bilirubinate stones) and leading to gallstone formation. Calcium salt of free UCB has varied stoichiometry because of the pH dependency of its ionic state. The predominant form is said to be the salt of the mono-anion, $Ca[HUCB]_2$, with a 1 : 2 stoichiometry (Womack et al., 1963). UCB in gallstones is found only as calcium salt and not as diacid ($H_2B^0$) (Ostrow, 1984), suggesting that bile is not supersaturated with UCB per se and/or that antinucleating factors for UCB are present in bile (Ostrow, 1990). Solubility products of calcium salts of bilirubin anions, and therefore the unbound concentrations of $Ca^{2+}$, $HB^-$ and $B^=$ must be determinants of the precipitation of bilirubin in bile. Ion products of these salts, and therefore their relative saturation in bile, increase with the increasing pH of bile. The activity of calcium in bile is controlled principally by the formation of soluble calcium complexes with bile salt (Rajagopalan and Lindenbaum, 1982) and other biliary constituents such as protein. The concentration of ionized calcium depends on the concentrations of bile salts and protein (Moore, 1984; Gleeson et al.,

1990). When the bile salt concentration in bile is high, free UCB is solubilized in biliary micelles, reducing the concentration of ionized calcium and thus hindering the formation of calcium bilirubinate and subsequent brown pigment stone formation.

## Role of *β*-glucuronidase

The endogenous β-glucuronidase level is low and is probably of hepatic or biliary tract origin (Ho et al., 1986). During stasis in the gallbladder UCB increases (Magnuson et al., 1990), not only by the postcanalicular action of endogenous β-glucuronidase but also, to a lesser degree, by nonenzymatic transformation (Oyabu et al., 1987; Spivak et al., 1987). Maki emphasized that β-glucuronidase in bile derived from Escherichia coli is responsible for its transformation during formation of brown pigment stones (Figure 19) (Maki, 1966). Until recently, very little attention was paid to the β-glucuronidase activity produced by other bacterial species. The presence of certain anaerobes in bile, such as Clostridium perfringens has been recognized. However, the advances made in anaerobic culture techniques and the use of selective media for anaerobes permitted the detection of additional species of anaerobes such as Bacteroides, Peptococcaceae, Eubacterium and Veillonella (Tabata and Nakayama, 1981). Although they are numerically inferior to the aerobes present in bile, they are potentially more important in biliary tract pathology due to their endotoxin production and their resistance to antibiotics. Tabata et al. found that, in addition to E. coli, Bacteroides fragilis and C. perfringens, Klebsiella produces β-glucuronidase activity (Tabata and Nakayama, 1981) (Table 9). In addition, some strains of Citrobacter freundii are found to produce β-glucuronidase (Skar et al., 1989a). Microcolonies of bacteria are detected by scanning electron microscopy throughout the interior of 78 % of pigment stones, both brown and black, but are absent in cholesterol stones (Stewart et al., 1987). According to Kaufman et al. bacteria may be seen only within the calcium bilirubinate-protein matrix, not in the calcium palmitate or cholesterol phases of brown pigment stones on scanning electron microscopy. In addition, bacteria was not demonstrated in cholesterol and black pigment stones (Kaufman et al., 1989). Measurement of bacterial adherence to the gallstone surface in vitro shows that biliary bacteria adhere to 90 % of

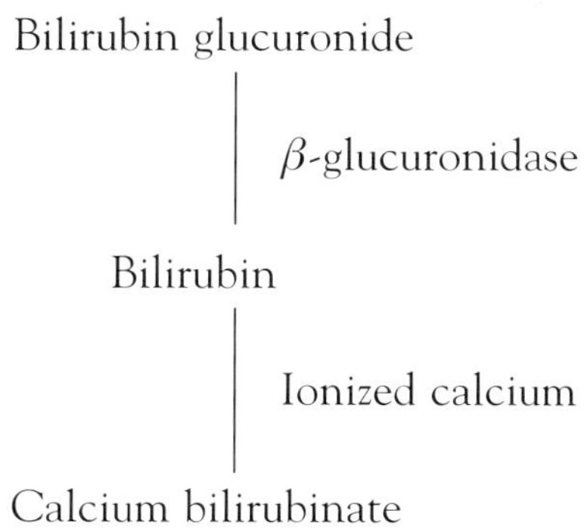


**Figure 19**

Cleaving of Bilirubin Glucuronide by β-Glucuronidase

brown pigment stones compared to only 8% of cholesterol stones (Stewart et al., 1987). The majority of bacteria isolated from brown pigment stones is found to produce glycocalyx, a charged glycoprotein (Costerton and Irvin, 1981) which may be responsible for precipitation and subsequent agglomeration of bilirubin pigment. D-Glucaric acid, a metabolite of D-glucuronic acid, is present in bile (Matsushiro et al., 1977); part of it is converted to D-glucaro-1,4-lactone, a potent inhibitor of $\beta$-glucuronidase. Oral administration of D-glucaro-1,4-lactone was found to reduce bacterial $\beta$-glucuronidase activity in bile in man (Matsushiro, 1965). However, recently, Ho and Ho, using an improved assay technique, showed that biliary $\beta$-glucuronidase activity is not affected by the D-glucaric acid present because (1) no negative correlation is present between D-glucaric acid content and $\beta$-glucuronidase activity in bile and (2) minimal conversion of D-glucaric acid to D-glucaro-1,4-lactone takes place at the usual pH of bile (Ho and Ho, 1990). Therefore, they concluded that biliary D-glucaric acid plays no role in the prevention of brown pigment stone formation.

**Structure of brown pigment stones**

The cross section of brown pigment stone shows an apparent layer formation with concentric pigment rings (Figure 1e), suggesting rhythmic growth and concomitant changes in bile composition (Malet et al., 1984). Bilirubin in brown pigment stones is almost exclusively in an unconjugated form. Therefore, for precipitation of UCB to occur, either an increase in concentration or a decrease in solubility is necessary. The concentration of

Table 9

**Bacteria with $\beta$-glucuronidase Activity isolated from Bile with Brown Pigment Stones**

| Bacteria | Number of strains | $\beta$-glucuronidase positive | |
|---|---|---|---|
| | | No. of Cases | % |
| Aerobes | | | |
| Escherichia coli | 29 | 29 | 100.0 |
| Klebsiella | 16 | 1 | 5.9 |
| Enterobacter | 17 | 0 | 0.0 |
| Streptococcus (D) | 13 | 0 | 0.0 |
| Citrobacter | 9 | 0 | 0.0 |
| Pseudomonas | 7 | 0 | 0.0 |
| Others | 8 | 1 | 12.5 |
| Anaerobes | | | |
| Bacteroides | 13 | 12 | 92.3 |
| Clostridium | 10 | 10 | 100.0 |
| Peptococcaceae | 2 | 0 | 0.0 |

Source: Tabata and Nakayama (1981).

UCB in bile from brown pigment stones is repeatedly shown to be similar to that of controls. The only difference found is a higher proportion of UCB to total bilirubin in bile with brown pigment stones than in controls (Masuda and Nakayama, 1979; Oyabu et al., 1987). Patients with brown pigment stones often suffer from repeated episodes of cholangitis inducing cyclic changes in the composition of bile, which may be responsible for the periodic precipitation of UCB on the stones. The proportion of UCB in bile with cholangitis is significantly higher than in that in bile without cholangitis (Nakano et al., 1988a), indicating that transformation of conjugated bilirubin is enhanced when bacterial infection is followed by cholangitis rather than by bacterial infection alone. When cholangitis is present, the proportion of UCB to total bilirubin in bile with $\beta$-glucuronidase-positive bacteria is significantly higher than that in bile without $\beta$-glucuronidase-positive bacteria. Furthermore, in cholangitis the pH of bile becomes lower toward the optimal pH of bacterial $\beta$-glucuronidase and promotes hydrolysis of conjugated bilirubin by $\beta$-glucuronidase. In control bile, the pH ranges from 7.4 to 8.5, but in brown pigment stones without cholangitis the mean pH value is 7.7; with cholangitis, it is still lower i. e. 7.4 (Nakano et al., 1988a). After the release of biliary obstruction and subsidence of cholangitis, total bilirubin concentration increases and the proportion of UCB to total bilirubin in bile decreases rapidly, indicating that cholangitis is an important factor in the increased proportion of UCB to total bilirubin in bile. The presence of cholangitis decreases bilirubin secretion and promotes hydrolysis of conjugated bilirubin secreted to UCB. Together with the lower concentration of bile acid, the lower pH of bile results in lower solubility of UCB promoting its precipitation. Thus occasional bouts of cholangitis may result in periodic deposition of UCB on brown pigment stones with layered structures by inducing cyclic changes of bile composition in situ during their growth.

### Solubilization of UCB

The solubilization of UCB in bile has attracted attention recently because it affects the formation and precipitation of calcium bilirubinate. UCB is solubilized in unilamellar and multilamellar vesicles and even by bile salt micelles (Mazer et al., 1980). The bile acid concentration in bile is significantly less in bile from patients with brown pigment stones than in those with cholesterol stones or in controls. This may partly be explained by the rapid absorption of bile salts from the biliary tract in the presence of inflammation (Ostrow, 1969) or depletion by bacterial digestion. Once the free bile acid is formed, passive absorption of bile acid takes place in the biliary tract, resulting in a decreased bile acid concentration in bile. The concentrating activity of the gallbladder with brown pigment stones is decreased, as evidenced by reduced visualization of the gallbladder by cholecystography. Prairie dogs fed on corn and alfalfa produce gallstones composed of cholesterol 45 %, bile pigment 30 % and calcium bilirubinate 25 % (Strichartz et al., 1989) – similar to the composition of human brown pigment stones. Decreased transepithelial potential difference and short-circuit current indicate the changes in gallbladder mucosal function. A decreased concentration of bile salts in bile diminishes micellar solubilization of bilirubin and cholesterol, thus favoring the formation of brown pigment stones. The glycoprotein matrix of brown pigment stones is probably derived from bacteria or inflamed gallbladder mucosa or both.

### Origin of free fatty acid

Brown pigment stones (calcium bilirubinate stones) contain considerable amounts of free fatty acid and phospholipids – mainly phosphatidyl choline (PC) (Nakayama, 1968; Robins et al., 1982). Molecular species of fatty acids in PC studied by HPLC showed great similarity to species of fatty acids present in gallstones, indicating that fatty acids in brown pigment stones are derived from PC in bile (Robins et al., 1982). Free fatty acids found in brown pigment stones are composed of various fatty acids but mainly palmitic acid (Nakayama, 1968, Sutor, 1970, Cetta, 1986), which constitutes one of the predominant fatty acids in biliary PC. A later study by Robins et al. showed that, in addition to 16:0, other fatty acids present in biliary PC are 16:1, 18:0, 18:1, 18:2, 20:4, 22:5, and 22:6 (Robins et al., 1982). Therefore, free fatty acid in brown pigment stones is most likely to be derived from biliary PC, main phospholipid in bile (Johnston et al., 1939; Nakayama and Blomstrand, 1961), since only a very small amount of free fatty acid is usually found in bile (Nakayama and Johnston, 1962). Free fatty acid and phospholipase activity in bile have been compared in cases with and without bacterial infection (Nakano et al., 1988b). The concentration of free fatty acids in bile of cases with bacterial infection is considerably higher, but no difference in fatty acid composition has been found. Biliary phospholipase activity, determined by incubating [$^{14}$C]-dipalmitoyl PC in bile, is higher when bacterial infection is present. A positive correlation is present between biliary phospholipase activity and the concentration of free fatty acid in bile. Bacterial species isolated, i.e., Serratia marcescens, Klebsiella pneumoniae, K. oxytoca, Enterobacter cloacae, Pseudomonas aeruginosa, Proteus vulgaris, B. fragilis, C. freundii, E. coli, C. perfringens and Enterococcus faecalis were found to have both phospholipase $A_1$ and $A_2$ activity. Two PCs predominant in human bile are 1-palmitoyl-2-oleoyl and 1-palmitoyl-2-linoleoyl PC (Ahlberg et al., 1981b). Since fatty acid present in brown pigment stones is mainly palmitic acid and must have been cleaved from the first position in the biliary PC molecule, bacterial phospholipase $A_1$ seems to play an important role in the formation of brown pigment stones. In the presence of bacterial infection, not only saturated but also unsaturated fatty acids may be released from biliary PC. Since saturated fatty acids, even when ionized, have lower aqueous solubility than unsaturated fatty acids (Hofmann and Mekhjian, 1973), this may lead to the preferential precipitation of saturated fatty acid, mainly palmitic acid. Cetta and De Nisi (1986) speculated that bacterial phospholipase C, with the presence of lipase, may be responsible for the release of free fatty acid from PC in bile. They found a high level of phospholipase C activity in the presence of recurrent common bile duct brown pigment stones, but with neither cholesterol stones nor black pigment stones (Cetta and De Nisi, 1986; Cetta and Lombardo; 1991) unlike Pattinson and Willis (1990). Some of the bacteria occurring in bile, such as C. perfringens and S. marcescens (Nakano et al., 1988b), show phospholipase C activity. Therefore, they may be partly responsible for the release of palmitic acid from biliary PC in conjunction with a lipase of either bacterial or pancreatic origin. Thus biliary PC is hydrolyzed by bacterial enzymes present in bile. Fatty acid, mainly palmitic acid, released in the presence of biliary concentrations of calcium binds with ionized calcium in bile, precipitates as water-insoluble calcium salt of fatty acid and participates in the formation of brown pigment stones.

### Location of anatomical variation

Recently, low and often left-sided entry of the cystic duct into the bile duct has been claimed to be associated with the presence of gallstones in the bile duct; the pathogenetic relevance of this condition is uncertain (Browman et al., 1988). The influence of juxtapapillary duodenal diverticula on the biliary tract and pancreas was first discussed by Lemmel (1934). The role of juxtapapillary duodenal diverticula has been considered in the formation of brown pigment stones (Løtveit et al., 1980; Osnes et al., 1981; Løtveit, 1982, Suzuki et al., 1984; Skar et al., 1989a; Sandstad et al., 1994). An increased incidence of common bile duct stones has been noted in patients with juxtapapillary duodenal diverticula (Skar et al., 1989b; Kennedy and Thompson, 1988; Hall et al., 1990). More frequent occurrence of gallstones after cholecystectomy is noted compared with patients without duodenal diverticula (Løtveit et al., 1982; Leinkram et al., 1980). Løtveit et al. studied gallstone patients without common bile duct stones, and either with or without juxtapapillary duodenal diverticula, and found that the incidence of bacteria is much higher in the bile of patients with diverticula (Løtveit et al., 1978). The presence of periampullary diverticula may inhibit ampullary function and predispose to ascending infection. In fact identical bacteria are found in diverticula and the biliary tract (Hall et al., 1990). Frequently, these stones are brown pigment stones or calcium bilirubinate stones; bile stasis and ascending infection are responsible. Subsequently, Skar et al. compared the bile of patients with and without duodenal diverticula treated with endoscopic papillotomy. They found an increased incidence of $\beta$-glucuronidase-producing bacteria and increased activity of bacterial $\beta$-glucuronidase (with an optimal pH of 7.0) in the bile of patients with duodenal diverticula (Skar et al., 1989a). Comparison of sphincter function by manometry in patients with and without juxtapapillary diverticulum showed papillary dysfunction or loss of papillary muscle tone (Kubota et al., 1989). This is claimed to be related to the increased incidence of common bile duct stones when a juxtapapillary duodenal diverticulum is present.

### Relation to sludge formation

Since the introduction of ultrasonography as a screening procedure for gallstone disease, fluid substance layers in the dependent portion of the gallbladder, producing low-amplitude echoes without the posterior acoustic shadowing characteristic of gallstones have been repeatedly recognized and named sludge (Conrad et al., 1979; Filly et al., 1980). Detection of sludge is equipment and operator dependent. Enhancement by using a high-frequency transducer of 5 to 7.5 mHz distinguishes small gallstones with poor shadows from sludge (Lee, 1990). Usually the presence of sludge cannot be established by either computed tomography, scintigraphy, or cholecystography. Its nature and its relation to the etiology of gallstones are hotly debated (Allen et al., 1981; Lee and Nicholls, 1986, Lee, 1990). Ma analyzed biliary sludge or mud in human bile with liver fluke infestation in Hong Kong, and found it to contain large amounts of bile pigment and lesser amounts of cholesterol, calcium, and sodium. He suspected that polyphenol oxidase from the parasite eggs plays an important role in the formation of sludge in the presence of E. coli (Ma, 1968). Calcium bilirubinate granules are consistently present in the sludge in human bile (Allen et al., 1981). Twelve percent of solid material is found to be UCB or its calcium salt. Biliary sludge is most often found after the prolonged stasis of gallbladder bile associated with other illnesses or mechanical obstruction of the common bile duct. Development of biliary sludge in the absence of anatomical obstruction in the common bile duct after reconstruction of the biliary tract following orthotopic liver transplantation has been a major complication (Starzl et al., 1977; McMaster et al., 1979).

Sludge is a suspension of pigment precipitates in bile and is at least in part calcium bilirubinate but not cholesterol crystals (Allen et al., 1981). Although calcium bilirubinate granules are consistently present in the sludge in human bile (Allen et al., 1981), as are cholesterol monohydrate crystals (Filly et al., 1980; Lee and Nicholls, 1986), other constituents of bilary sludge include crystals of calcium carbonate, calcium phosphate, or calcium salt of fatty acid. No difference in lipid composition and cholesterol saturation of bile, either hepatic or gallbladder, is found in sludge-forming patients from those with gallstones and controls (Leė and Nicholls, 1986). The relative proportion of UCB to total bilirubin in bile from patients with sludge (12.2 %) is much higher than from controls (4.6 %) ($p<0.025$), although the concentration of UCB in bile varies widely. This is in agreement with the previous finding of an increased proportion of UCB and monoconjugated bilirubin in bile in the presence of brown pigment stones (Masuda and Nakayama, 1979).

## Bile stasis

During stasis of gallbladder bile, bilirubin diglucuronide is hydrolyzed to bilirubin, which forms precipitates. In contrast to supernatant bile, bilirubin in sludge is almost entirely in the free unconjugated form, with small amounts of monoconjugated bilirubin (Allen et al., 1981). Enzymatic hydrolysis of bilirubin conjugates in the presence of low-grade biliary inflammation or infection (Nakano et al., 1988a) and/or nonenzymatic hydrolysis (Oyabu et al., 1987; Spivak et al., 1987) during bile stasis may be responsible. Ostrow et al. found that the solubility of bilirubin in bile decreases as pH and bile acid concentration in bile decrease (Ostrow et al., 1988). Bilirubin monoglucuronide or UCB forms insoluble salt with calcium ion present in bile or may undergo molecular restructuring to form insoluble bilirubin polymers. During prolonged bile stasis, bile becomes more concentrated and pH falls. Lower pH enhances the activity of $\beta$-glucuronidase activity in bile (Ho et al., 1979) and accelerates hydrolysis of bilirubin diglucuronide to free UCB. The bile acid concentration in bile of patients with brown pigment stones is decreased (Masuda and Nakayama, 1979), probably because of the presence of inflammation with resultant absorption of bile acid through the mucosa. Thus, lowering the pH and the bile acid concentration in bile decreases the solubility of bilirubin and its derivatives in bile and facilitates the formation of bilirubin precipitate, leading to the production of sludge or brown pigment stones. In addition, the bilirubin granules thus formed may serve as a nidus for the growth of cholesterol stones, as suggested by the presence of a pigmented center (Malet et al., 1986b). Thus, sludge formation may represent an important intermediate phase in the formation of various kinds of gallstones (Allen et al., 1981). The importance of mucin, a major component of mucus, in the formation of sludge must be emphasized. A marked increase of mucus in the gallbladder is the most striking feature in patients with sludge. Mucin binds to other macromolecules, such as protein and lipids, to form native mucus. Both small particles, either cholesterol or calcium bilirubinate, and mucus seem to be required for the characteristic low-amplitude echoes of sludge on ultrasound examination. Mucus provides a framework for the deposition of gallstone constituents by binding bilirubin, cholesterol, and calcium (Levy et al., 1984; Gallinger et al., 1985; Smith, 1987). The hydrophobic domain of mucin interacts with cholesterol and phospholipids to promote cholesterol nucleation by perturbing the stability of biliary vesicular lipids (Lee and Smith, 1989) and, ultimately, the formation of cholesterol crystals. Hypersecretion of mucus and other proteins, such as glycoprotein or glycolipids co-secreted, act as pronucleating agents and contribute to sludge formation, as observed in a dog model (Bernhoft et al., 1983). Inflammatory mediators, namely, prostaglandins or free oxygen radicals, may be important in the formation of sludge (Lee, 1990). Recently, Lee proposed an interesting hypothesis on the formation of sludge (Lee, 1990). A substantial change in bile composition triggers messengers present in intramembrane compartments such as cAMP inducing hypersecretion of mucus and cell proliferation. At the same time, it inhibits smooth muscle contraction and the apical sodium-hydrogen mechanism causing gallbladder stasis and non-acidification of gallbladder bile, leading to sludge formation.

# Fatty Acid Calcium Stones

In 1938, Nishimura described three cases of gallstones composed mainly of fatty acids (Nishimura, 1938, Nakayama 1968, Cowie et al., 1973). Free fatty acid, almost exclucively palmitic acid, is also present in considerable amounts in other types of gallstones, such as cholesterol stones and brown pigment stones (Sutor 1970; Yamashita et al., 1988). They have a dark brown to dark gray surface, are irregularly shaped, variable in size, and fragile. Their cross section is yellowish white, with a waxy luster, and shows multiple non-concentric layers (Figure 1e). They are present mostly in the common bile duct. Nakayama found that in addition to palmitic acid, other fatty acids, such as palmitoleic, stearic, linoleic, myristic, and pentadecanoic acids, are also present, in this order but in very small amounts (Nakayama, 1968). Later, Cowie et al. analyzed 31 gallstone specimens using the X-ray powder method and found two cases of common bile duct stones composed solely of calcium palmitate (Cowie et al., 1973). In human bile, palmitic acid together with oleic and linoleic acids comprise 80% of the fatty acid present, and fatty acid of biliary phosphatidyl choline, PC (lecithin) accounts for more than 90% of the fatty acid present in bile (Blomstrand and Ekdahl, 1960). The concentration of free fatty acid in bile is very low (Nakayama and Johnston, 1962), yet free fatty acid accounts for 1.5% in human cholesterol stones (Nakayama, 1968). Cowie et al. state that calcium palmitate is the fourth most abundant crystalline component of gallstones (Cowie et al., 1973). Among 331 cases of gallstones from eight countries, Sutor et al. found that calcium palmitate was present in 36% and accounted for 6% of all crystalline material (Sutor and Wooley 1971). Therefore, the concentration of free fatty acid or palmitic acid in bile must have been increased in some cases of cholelithiasis. Although the gallbladders containing fatty acid calcium stones appear remarkably normal, with no histological signs of inflammation, the common bile duct shows inflammation where fatty acid calcium stones are usually located. Phospholipase from bacteria is thought to be responsible for the release of fatty acid from biliary phospholipids (Nakano et al., 1988b), where over 90% of fatty acids in bile are located (Blomstrand and Ekdahl, 1960). Phospholipase A catalyzes the conversion of PC to lysolecithin and fatty acids. The resulting products, i.e., lysolecithin and free fatty acids, are as effective as lecithin, maintaining cholesterol solubilized in bile in conjunction with bile salts (Neiderhiser and Roth, 1970). Cholesterol is more or less kept in solution but is invariably present in fatty acid calcium stones in small amounts (Nakayama, 1968; Sanjo, 1970). Histochemical examination of fatty acid calcium stones shows a diffuse network of acid mucopolysaccharides containing sulfate radicals between the fatty acid calcium crystals (Sanjo, 1970). Therefore, it seems that, following infection of the biliary tract, fatty acids are released in bile from biliary PC, a major phospholipid in bile, bind with the calcium ions present, and are cemented together by acid mucopolysaccharide, thus forming fatty acid calcium stones.

# Inorganic Stones

Inorganic stones are composed of calcium carbonate and/or calcium phosphate in varying proportions. They come in different shapes, sizes, and colors (Figure 1f) and are present in the gallbladder (Phemister et al., 1931). Their color is white to whitish yellow, and they are sometimes covered with a brown pigment layer. By the X-ray powder diffraction method, calcium carbonate has been found to occur in three different forms, i.e., vaterite, calcite, and aragonite, in this order of frequency (Tamura, 1942; Bogren and Larsson, 1963; Sutor and Wooley, 1973; Aho et al., 1985). Milk of calcium contains calcium carbonate as calcite or aragonite (Phemister et al., 1939). Although Epprecht et al. suggest that vaterite is initially formed and then transformed to calcite or aragonite (Epprecht et al., 1953), the phase transition between three polymorphs of calcium carbonate, such as from solid aragonite to solid calcite, is an exceedingly slow process at room temperature. No transition was found by analyzing the same gallbladder stone specimen after storage in room air at room temperature for 20 years (Bogren, 1983). Therefore, the three polymorphs of calcium carbonate, i.e., vaterite, calcite, and aragonite, appear to precipitate in vivo mixed with each other in various proportions and/or with the other constituents. Practically no transition is likely to occur within the short time between surgery and analysis of gallstones.

In bile, much of the calcium present is bound to bile salts (Williamson and Percy-Robb, 1980; Moore et al., 1982; Moore, 1984). The recent introduction of the $Ca^{2+}$ electrode has permitted a fresh appraisal of the solubility of calcium carbonate and calcium equilibrium in bile (Moore and Verine 1985). Major determinants of calcium solubility in the proximal biliary tract are the secretion of calcium, bicarbonate, and calcium-binding bile salts (Williamson and Percy-Robb, 1979; Moore et al., 1982; Moore, 1984). In the gallbladder, solubility of calcium is further influenced by the mucosal absorptive function (Rege and Moore, 1986). Calcium in bile has two sources, i.e., hepatic bile and the gallbladder wall. Using the $Ca^{45}$, Tera found, that calcium ions pass fairly freely into gallbladder content directly from the blood via the gallbladder wall (Tera, 1961). Passage of calcium is dependent not only on active cellular secretion but also on diffusion of calcium ions. Calcium in bile exists in two forms, i.e. either bound, probably, to micelles, or in ultrafiltrable form or free calcium ions (Sutor and Wilkie, 1977a). Bile salts act as major buffers for free calcium ions in bile (Moore et al., 1982). Only 29 % of biliary calcium is said to be present in gallbladder bile as free $Ca^{2+}$ ion. Sutor et al. compared calcium values in bile from different types of gallstone formers and found that deposition of calcium carbonate in gallstones is not related to any calcium values in bile (Sutor and Wilkie, 1977a). Mean ionized and total calcium concentrations are similar in the bile of patients with calcified and noncalcified gallstones and in normal controls (Knyrim and Vakil, 1992). Calcium precipitation in bile is the cardinal event in the formation of inorganic stones. When the ion product; $[Ca^{2+}] \cdot [CO_3^{2-}]$ exceeds, the solubility product, ($K'_{sp}$), the bile becomes supersaturated (metastable) and calcium precipitation is thermodynamically possible (Rege and Moore, 1986). Hepatic bile is usually supersaturated with calcium carbonate, but gallbladder bile is not because of the marked decrease of $[CO_3^{2-}]$ upon concentration and acidification of bile in the gallbladder, for which secretion of hydrogen ion by the gallbladder is responsible (Shiffman et al., 1990). Hence, gallbladder functions, i.e., concentration and acidification of bile, play an important role in reducing the calcium carbonate lithogenicity of bile. Abnormal carbonate concentrations caused by defective acidification of bile appear to be the key factor in the precipitation of calcium carbonate (Knyrim and Vakil, 1992). Bile from normal controls completely inhibits precipitation of calcium carbonate from the supersaturated solution (Sciarretta et al., 1984; Knyrim and Vakil, 1992), while bile from calcified stones lacks antinucleating activity for calcium carbonate and decreases the size of spheres formed (Sutor and Wilkie, 1978; Knyrim and Vakil, 1992). Certain compounds or ions may have a profound effect on the growth rate of crystals and on their composition, which form a suitable stable complex with any of the ions or are absorbed onto certain crystal faces, causing habit modification and reducing or even preventing crystallization (Sutor and Percival, 1976, 1978). In case of bile, mixed micelles present are thought to be responsible. Aragonite is somewhat more soluble than calcite (Browman et al., 1937). The raised concentration of total $CO_2$, which is the sum of bicarbonate, carbonic acid, dissolved $CO_2$, and carbonate, is related to the presence of calcium carbonate in gallstones (Sutor and Wilkie, 1978). Precipitation occurs when such bile enters the gallbladder before the relationship between pH and total $CO_2$ has been attained. Human and canine gallbladder bile contains the substance which inhibits precipitation of calcium carbonate crystals (Dawes et al., 1991). Calcium precipitation is abolished completely by the addition of gallbladder bile from the controls and is ubiquitous in human gallbladder bile (Lipsett et al., 1993). Recently, calcium-binding protein was isolated from cholesterol stones (Shimizu et al., 1989) and from black pigment stones (Okido et al., 1992), which have common properties and immunological cross-reactivity with amphipathic anionic polypeptide (Domingo et al., 1992), suggesting that these proteins may be identical.

Calcium phosphate occurs in two polymorphic forms, i.e., apatite and whitlockite or hydroxyapatite, in this order of frequency (Sutor and Wooley, 1973). A significant increase in ultrafiltrable calcium in bile is related to the presence of calcium phosphate in gallstones (Sutor and Wilkie, 1977a). Bile prevents or inhibits precipitation of calcium phosphate and subsequent growth of the crystals (Sutor and Percival, 1976). When calcium ions and phosphate ions are mixed, an amorphous precipitate is formed which, over times changes into crystalline material with an apatite structure. Bile strongly inhibits the formation of the precipitate. Many molecules are capable of preventing hydroxyapatite formation by poisoning the growth of nascent crystals. This is done by forming a suitable complex with any of the ions which would normally precipitate out or be absorbed onto certain crystal faces, causing habit modification and alteration of the crystal growth (Sutor and Percival, 1976). The presence of an inhibitor in bile is responsible for the rare occurrence of calcium phosphate in gallstones. The inhibitor(s) are of hepatic origin, as they are present in common bile duct bile, and have a molecular weight of over 10,000. The bile salt-phospholipids micelles responsible are polyvalent anions, particularly containing sulfate or phosphate groups, having a strong affinity for bivalent or trivalent cations. Therefore, they bind calcium and inhibit crystal growth through adsorption on crystal faces. Recently, glycodeoxycholic acid and glycochenodeoxycholic acid, unlike other bile acids, have been found to prevent hydroxyapatite formation. They have higher affinity and a greater capacity to bind hydroxyapatite (Crowther and Okido, 1994). Glycocholic, taurocholic, taurodeoxycholic, and taurochenodeoxycholic acids specifically inhibit amorphous calcium phosphate formation, probably by lowering $Ca^{2+}$ activity.

# Porphyrin-containing gallstones

An association between erythropoietic protoporphyria (EPP), nonacute prophyria, and gallstones was noted in 1961 (Magnus et al., 1961). Partial enzyme defects in the heme biosynthesis pathway, with consequent overproduction of the heme precursor, protoporphyrinogen, and increased biliary concentration of protoporphyrin, may be related to the increased risk of gallstone disease (Herrick et al., 1990). Gallstones occurring in EPP had a higher protoporphyrin content (300 to 400 mg/g) than controls (Cripps and Scheuer, 1965; Feurle et al., 1980), which precipitates in bile because of its low solubility and serves as a nidus for stone formation. Gallstones with a high porphyrin content are reported in congenital erythropoietic porphyria (Günther's disease) associated with chronic hemolysis (Feurle et al., 1980). The incidence of gallstones in variegate porphyria is as high as it is in EPP (Herrick et al., 1990).

# Parasite stones

Biliary helminthiasis has been extensively reviewed by Ong, based on his vast experience at the University of Hong Kong (Ong, 1979). Of helminths, Ascaris lumbricoides and Clonorchis sinensis (liver fluke) (Teoh et al., 1963) have been found to be responsible for the formation of parasite stones by the deposition of calcium bilirubinate on the whole or a fragment of carcass of the parasites. In addition to the gallstones formed by the carcass of A. lumbricoides which inadvertently entered the biliary tract, eggs or cuticulae were frequently found in gallstones in Japan immediately after the Second World War, when the infestation of intestinal parasites was high (Miyake Jr, 1962). Maki emphasized the importance of such parasitic elements in gallstones, especially brown pigment stones, based on his finding that, upon close examination of gallstones, sometimes over 50% contained cuticulae and/or eggs of A. lumbricoides. Precipitation of biliary constituents can be induced by the incubation of parasite eggs or cuticulae (Maki, 1961). If the parasitic elements are responsible for the formation of gallstones, they should be present exactly in the centers of gallstones, but that does not necessarily occur (Miyake Jr, 1962). Since the postwar period, the infestation rate of intestinal parasites decreased dramatically in Japan. Today we seldom encounter these parasitic elements in gallstones, but brown pigment stones (calcium bilirubinate stones) still occur. However, in endemic areas such as Kashmir, India, where the infestation rate of intestinal helminths reaches 30%, bile duct stones with acalculous, intact gallbladders are frequent, and close inspection of soft pigment stones, i.e., brown pigment stones, invariably reveals worm segments or fragments (Khuroo and Zargar, 1985; Khuroo et al., 1989).

# Combination stones

When a layer consisting of bile pigment, cholesterol, and calcium carbonate is deposited on cholesterol stones, they are called combination stones or Kombinationsstein (Aschoff and Bacmeister, 1909) (Figure 1g). When the outlet from the gallbladder becomes incompletely blocked, calcium and bile pigment are deposited on the stones in increasing amounts, proceeding from the outlet, usually from the cystic duct to the gallbladder fundus, apparently as a result of increasing stagnation in the compartment formed by the stones (Phemister et al., 1939). Increasing pigmentation of the outer layer of the stones from the ampulla to the fundus can be noted. The radiopaque shadow also increases from the ampulla to the fundus. In some cases, there are stones with a calcium bilirubinate center surrounded by a cholesterol layer (Japanese Society of Gastroenterology, Committee for the Study of Cholelithiasis, 1986).

# Gallstone Formation in Animals

## Spontaneous gallstone formation

Spontaneous formation of gallstones is relatively rare but is known to occur in several animal species. From ancient times, gallstones in animals have been prized for their supposedly potent medicinal effect (Rains, 1964). In 1863, in his classic Treatise on gallstones, Thudichum reviewed the literatures on the subject up to that time (Thudichum, 1863). Gallstones occur spontaneously in cattle (Ford, 1955), pigs (Schoenheimer and Johnston, 1937; Danalis and Penny, 1967; Splitter, 1972), beavers (Fox, 1923), geese (Fox, 1923), sheep (Mentzer, 1934; Wood et al., 1974), goats (Rains, 1964), llamas (Rains, 1964), dogs (Cartmell et al., 1964; Binns, 1964; Nelson et al., 1968; Verine et al., 1969; Scott et al, 1973; Schall et al., 1973; Wales et al., 1982), cats (Naus and Jones, 1978; O'Brien and Mitchum, 1970), mongoose (Fox, 1923), polar bears (Fox, 1923), tigers (Thudichum, 1863), and monkeys (Fox, 1923) but also in animals without a gallbladder such as horses (Sastry, 1945; Kataruam and Verma, 1967; McDole, 1980; Traub et al., 1982) and elephants (Thenard, quoted by Thudichum, 1863; Rolleston and McNee, 1929; Decker and Krohn, 1973). The prevalence is recorded to be as follows; cattle 0.68 %, pig 0.24 %, horse 0.08 %, dog 0.04 % (Mårtensson, 1941) to 5.6 % (Wales et al., 1982) and sheep 1.75 % (Mentzer, 1934). Wales et al. (1982) found amorphous black pigment stones in 10 out of 180 dogs taken randomly from a local dog pound. No female preponderance is noted. The stones present are solitary to multiple (up to 50) and are greenish-brown to black, with a rubber-like to firm consistency. They are composed of bilirubin, insoluble bile pigment, and protein, with traces of bile acids and cholesterol similar to those produced experimentally in dogs (Englert et al., 1969). Naturally occurring gallstones in dogs are not likely to contain much cholesterol, as in man, since canine bile is much less saturated with cholesterol (Nakayama, 1967). Gallstones occur in as many as 50 % of fetal sheep (Wood et al., 1974). In nonhuman primates, spontaneous cholelithiasis is rare but does occur. For instance, no gallstones were found in 300 velvet monkeys (Circopithecus ethiops) (Lorentz, 1966), in 19 squirrel monkeys (Saimiri sciureus) (Osuga and Portman, 1971), in 17 rhesus monkeys (Macacus mulatta) (Dowling et al., 1971), in 1,512 nonhuman primate necropsies (McClure, 1974) and in 981 postmortem examinations of six species of monkeys (Kessler, 1982). A high bile salt:cholesterol ratio is noted in the bile of velvet monkey compared to that of man (Lorentz, 1966). However, naturally occurring gallstones were reported in the orangutan (Pongo pygmaeus) (Fox, 1930; Ruch, 1959), marmoset (Hamerton, 1932; Lapin and Yakovleva, 1963), baboon (Papio anubis and cynochealus) (Lapin and Yakovleva, 1963; Glenn and McSherry, 1970; McSherry et al., 1971, Lapin et al., 1979), owl monkey (Aotus trivirgatus) (Anver et al., 1972), rhesus monkey (Martin et al.,

1973; Kessler, 1982) and green monkey (Lapin, cited by Martin et al., 1973). A female preponderance has been noted (Glenn and McSherry, 1970; Anver et al., 1972; Martin et al., 1973; Lapin et al., 1979). The size of the gallstones ranged from 2–3 to 7 mm, and the number of gallstones from 1 to over 100. Gallstones occurring in animals contain less cholesterol and are composed mostly of bile pigment, calcium, and bile salt, such as in dogs (Wales et al., 1982). Gallstones in pigs consist mainly of lithocholate (Schoenheimer and Johnston, 1937) and $3\beta$, $6\alpha$-dihydroxy-$5\beta$-cholanoic acid (Haslewood, 1955), while those occurring in cattle are composed of large amounts of bile pigment, as well as deoxycholic acid, with lithocholic acid as a minor component (Fischer, 1911). Gallstones occurring in fetal sheep are composed of crystalline aggregates of calcium palmitate and amorphous bile pigment (Wood et al., 1974). Gallstones in nonhuman primates contain primarily cholesterol (Lapin and Yakovleva, 1963; Mc Sherry et al., 1971; Anver et al., 1972; Martin et al., 1973; Lapin et al., 1979), but calcium bilirubinate stones do occur (Kessler, 1982). Kessler found multiple gallstones in the distended, edematous gallbladder of an aged rhesus monkey born in India. They were irregularly rounded, brownish, and crumpy when sectioned, weighing 14 to 720 mg. Analysis by UV spectrophotometry revealed, that such gallstones are composed entirely of calcium bilirubinate.

## Experimental gallstone formation

Comparative study of experimental gallstone formation in different animal species is important, as it may give important information on the factors responsible for the formation of gallstones and may aid in selecting species suitable for further investigations. While human studies are criticized for missing the event or introducing extraneous events, animal studies, although permitting longitudinal sampling, may be examining a process that has little to do with human gallstone formation. Gallstones from animals such as the ox and pig contain only a small amount of cholesterol and are composed mainly of bile pigment, calcium, and bile acids. Their bile compositions are quite different from those of man (Nakayama, 1967). Futhermore, commonly occurring human gallstones, i.e., cholesterol stones, dissolve when placed in the gallbladders of dogs (Labes, quoted by Naunyn, 1892) or in pig, sheep, and goat bile (Lutton and Large, 1957). Bile from pig, dog, and ox is less saturated with cholesterol (Figure 20) (Nakayama, 1967). Human cholesterol stones are less soluble in the gallbladder of phylogenically closer rhesus and cebus monkeys (Figure 21) (Nakayama and Johnston, 1960). Twenty animal models for gallstone formation have been described since the turn of the century (Schoenfield, 1972). Gallstones can be produced in experimental animals including hamsters (Dam and Christensen, 1952), mice (Tepperman et al., 1964), rats (Palmer, 1965), Mongolian gerbils (Bergman and Van der Linden, 1971), Tupaias (tree shrews) (Schwaier, 1979), prairie dogs (Patton et al., 1961), guinea pigs (Okey, 1942), ground squirrels (Patton et al., 1961), rabbits (Bevans and Mosbach, 1956), dogs (Englert et al., 1969), sheep (Schoenfield, 1972), pigs (Schoenfield, 1972), cattle (Schoenfield, 1972), and nonhuman primates. Various chemical agents, dietary alterations, infectious agents, implantation of foreign bodies, and surgical procedures have been used. Dietary manipulation includes feeding of cholesterol, 3β-cholestanol, dihydrocholesterol, progesterone and diethylstilbesterol. Excellent reviews on experimental gallstone formation are available (Freston and Bouchier, 1968; Dam, 1969; Dam et al., 1971; Schoenfield, 1972; Portman and Osuga, 1975; Van der Linden et al., 1977b; Gurll and Den Besten, 1978; Van der Linden, 1979; Hofmann, 1984a; Holzbach, 1984; Malet, 1985; Rege and Nahrwold, 1987). Freston and Bouchier defined certain desirable characteristics for the ideal experimental model, against which available models should be selected to meet specific aims (Freston et al., 1968). The criteria are as follows (1) the method should be simple; (2) gallstones should form quickly and in every animal; (3) gallstone composition should resemble that of man; (4) ample amounts of bile, stones, blood, and tissue should be available for analysis; and (5) apart from biliary tract pathology, there should be no toxicity which would cause the animals to differ from control animals. Different kinds of gallstones can be produced in animals, including cholesterol stones, black pigment stones, brown pigment stones (calcium bilirubinate stones), fatty acid calcium stones, inorganic stones, and bile acid stones. They will be discussed consecutively. It should be emphasized that the source of animals, weight, time of the year, sex, age, diet, and total nutrition are important for replication of the results from experiment to experiment (Cohen et al., 1991).

## Cholesterol stones

### Hamsters

In 1952, Dam and Christensen found gallstones containing 51–90 % cholesterol in the gallbladder of Syrian golden hamsters (Mesocricetus auratus suratus) during study on diet and atherosclerosis (Dam and Christensen, 1952). Two main types of gallstones can be produced in hamsters: (1) white or light yellow crystalline stones, consisting entirely or almost entirely of cholesterol, i.e., cholesterol stones and (2) amorphous, more or less pigmented (brown or green) stones containing no cholesterol but having a high content of calcium, phosphate, and glycine conjugated bile acids and a low content of pigment (Dam, 1971), which are structurally and compositionally similar to human black pigment stones (Freed et al., 1986; Malet et al., 1989). Unsaturated fat, especially at levels greater than 10 % favors the development of amorphous stones, while the total incidence of gallstones decreases (Christensen et al., 1964). Essential fatty acid seems to protect against cholesterol stone formation but not against amorphous pigmented stone formation (Shioda, 1965). An intermediate type, mixed gallstones, may also occur. Cholesterol stones can be produced as the only or almost the only type of gallstones in 80–100 % of the animals within 6 or 7 weeks by feeding young hamsters of 4 to 6 weeks of age a fat-free diet in which the carbohydrate is supplied by an easily absorbable sugar such as glucose or sucrose (Hikasa et al., 1980). The incidence of cholesterol stones is decreased or abolished by substituting uncooked starch for sugar (Prange et al., 1962), by adding bulk-forming agents such as carboxymethyl cellulose or clofibrate (Dam et al., 1972a), or by adding fat especially rich in polyunsaturated fatty acids (Dam and Christensen, 1961). When cholesterol

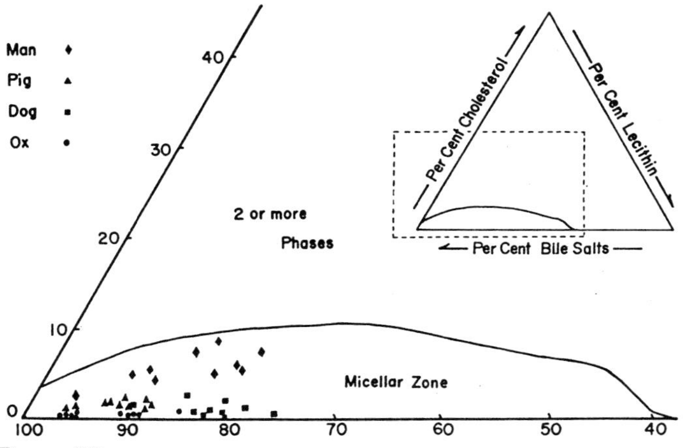


Figure 20

Bile Composition: Species Difference

Only the line of metastable-labile limit of cholesterol solubility (Admirand and Small 1968) is shown.

Source: Nakayama 1969

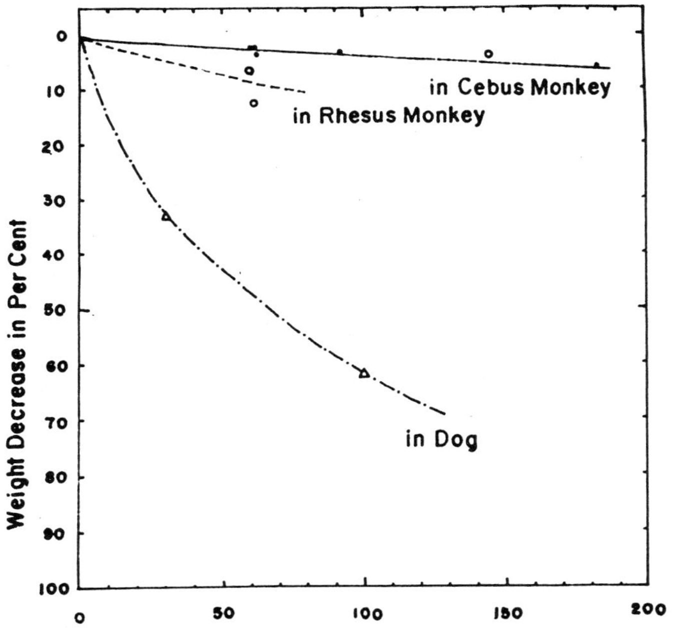


Figure 21

Dissolution of Human Cholesterol Stones in Primate Gallbladder

Source: Nakayama and Johnston (1960)

is added to the diet, the incidence of cholesterol stones decreases and that of amorphous pigmented gallstones increases (Dam et al., 1968). Hyodeoxycholic acid markedly inhibits (Dam and Christensen, 1962) and chenodeoxycholic acid increases (Dam et al., 1972b) the formation of cholesterol stones; by contrast, the other bile acids tested including cholic, deoxycholic, dehydrocholic, and lithocholic acids, have little, if any, inhibitory effect (Dam and Christensen, 1962). Addition of 3 % cholestyramine, a bile acid-binding agent, dissolves cholesterol stones induced (Bergman and Van der Linden, 1967). The effect of dietary protein on gallstone formation in hamsters has been studied. Casein- and bovine albumin-fed hamsters exhibited the highest relative concentration of biliary cholesterol and the highest incidence of gallstones (Redinger and Small, 1972). Substitution of casein by soy bean protein in Dam's diet increases the incidence of gallstones, while vegetable protein decreases it. The lysine : arginine ratio of experimental diets alters their lithogenicity. Addition of arginine decreases the lithogenic potential of lysine (Kritschevsky and Klurfeld, 1983). An experimental diet containing 20 % protein of animal and vegetable origin increases the incidence of gallstones, except for egg albumin (Sullivan et al., 1985). Substitution of soybean protein is associated with a low incidence of gallstones, but addition of lysine increases the lithogenicity of bile. Although this model has been extensively used to study the pathogenesis of cholesterol gallstones, the animals tolerate the diet poorly and the diet is not applicable to other species, such as mice and chicks (Christensen et al., 1962) or mystromys, the South African equivalent of the hamster belonging to the Muridae-Cricetinae (Lorentz, 1966). Because rabbits and guinea pigs refuse to eat the diet even when it is furnished in pelleted form, gallstones do not form (Dam, 1969).

Recently, a new hamster model of experimental formation of cholesterol stones has been developed, with a success rate of 55–65 % (Cohen et al., 1989a). This model has some advantages. The diet used seems to be nutritionally adequate (the animals grow rapidly). It consists of casein, corn starch, soluble starch, butter fat, corn oil, cellulose, and 0.3 % cholesterol but no other additives. Significant differences in cholesterol metabolism and rate of gallstone formation exist among hamsters of differing origins. The hamster seems to be an adequate model for the study of cholesterol and bile acid metabolism (Scheibner et al., 1994) because of the low capacity of hepatic cholesterol synthesis, regulation of cholesterol balance by the modulation of LDL transport (Spady et al., 1985b, Malavolti et al., 1987), much like that in man, increase in biliary cholesterol output by excess dietary cholesterol intake (Kajiyama et al., 1981) and gallbladder and bile acid patterns similar to those of man (Kuroki et al., 1983).

### Mice

A systematic analysis of many of the factors in the atherogenic diet of mice revealed that the combination of cholesterol and cholic acid is necessary and sufficient for cholesterol stone formation if food intake remains adequate and liver function is unimpaired (Tepperman et al., 1964). Gallstones start to appear after 2 months; their incidence increases to 75 % after 8 months. The highest incidence is achieved in mice which gain weight satisfactorily and show no obvious impairment of liver function. There is no sex difference in the cumulative incidence, but gallstones seem to appear earlier in females (Tepperman, 1965). Elimination of other potentially contributory factors, such as thiouracil, low-protein diet, or high-fat diet does not prevent gallstone formation. By changing the salt mixture, gallstone formation can be prevented (Tepperman et al., 1964). A very high cholesterol level achieved in gallbladder bile in the face of an ordinary level in hepatic bile indicates that a large volume of secreted bile is being concentrated in the gallbladder. The bile salt concentration in gallbladder bile, after an initial increase, falls, resulting in an increase in the cholesterol : bile salts ratio (Caldwell et al., 1965). The increased ratios of cholesterol : bile salts and of cholesterol : phospholipids remained below the precipitation point for cholesterol in hepatic bile but not in gallbladder bile (Caldwell and Levitsky, 1967). This may be explained by the abnormal absorption of bile salts by the gallbladder induced by diet, since the acute inflammatory response produced in the gallbladder coincides with the change in bile acid concentration (Caldwell et al, 1965). Riegel et al. demonstrated that bile acid and cholesterol are not absorbed from normal dog gallbladder and that the concentration of bile in the gallbladder is an iso-osmolar process. In the presence of inflammation, absorption of bile acid, but not of cholesterol, takes place (Riegel et al., 1931). Abnormal gallbladder function seems to be essential for the formation of gallstones in mice. Yellin et al. compared the effect of cholic acid and chenodeoxycholic acid on the composition of bile in mice (Yellin et al., 1973). Feeding of cholic acid increased biliary PC but this did not change with chenodeoxycholic acid, suggesting that they differ in their regulation of PC secretion and synthesis by the liver and may help explain why cholic acid is not cholelitholytic in man. The mixture of bile salt and PC ultimately solubilizes more cholesterol than does bile salt alone; the rapidity of dissolution is determined by the bile salt (Small, 1970). When the accumulation of solid cholesterol in supersaturated bile is considered as a dynamic process governed by changing biliary composition and consisting of alternating periods of precipitation and dissolution, it is conceivable that an excess of PC might drive the process in the direction of stone formation (Yellin et al., 1973). After stone-forming mice are returned to the control chow diet for several months, the stones disappear. Cholesterol gallstones can be induced in mice by feeding a diet supplemented with dehydrocholic acid (Besançon et al., 1967). Christensen et al. could not induce gallstones in mice with the diet which is successful in hamsters (Christensen et al., 1962), underlining the species difference in experimental gallstone formation.

### Mongolian gerbils

Cholesterol stones can also be produced in Mongolian gerbils by feeding a cholesterol- and cholic acid-enriched diet (Bergman and Van der linden, 1971). Small, whitish cholesterol stones occurred in five of seven surviving animals. A marked rise in cholesterol concentration in bile coupled, with a slight rise in bile acid and phospholipids, resulted in increased ratios of cholesterol to bile acid and cholesterol to phospholipids in bile similar to the increase in the mice fed on the cholesterol-cholic acid diet (Tepperman et al., 1964). Reactions of these two species to the cholesterol-cholic acid diet are quite similar, including a reduction of chenodeoxycholic acid in bile and marked distention of the gallbladder, with signs of inflammation. However, a marked difference is noted in the disposal of excess cholesterol accumulated after discontinuance of the diet. Because of the poor tolerance to the diet given over a long period, Mongolian gerbils seem to be a less suitable model for study (Bergman and Van der Linden, 1971). The glucose-rich, lithogenic diet of the hamster is not effective in Mongolian gerbils (Bergman and Van der Linden, 1971).

### Tupaias (tree shrews)

With 20% butter, 20% sucrose, and 1% cholesterol added, the standard diet was found to cause massive gallstone formation in tupaias (tree shrews) (Schwaier, 1979). This rat-sized animal has a unique phylogenic position between insectivores and primates. It closely resembles the squirrel monkey in its reaction to fat-, cholesterol- and sucrose-rich diets and its tendency to develop gallstones. The gallstones thus produced are composed almost totally of cholesterol and closely resemble those in squirrel monkeys on a similar diet (Osuga and Portman, 1971). This animal has been used to study cholesterol metabolism under different dietary conditions (Schwaier et al., 1979; Van der Linden et al., 1980) because of its availability, genetic uniformity, defined health state, ease of handling, and reasonable cost. The success rate of gallstone formation is about 75%. Sand-like concrements and loose aggregates 1 to 3 mm in diameter are produced within 4 months. In longer-fed tupaias, variations of the stones in shape, size, and color between individual animals are more pronounced and the stones produced are more compact. However, the incidence of gallstones remains the same, probably due to the well-maintained gallbladder function, with stones passing via the cystic duct.

### Prairie dogs

Since the discovery in 1961 of gallstone formation in prairie dogs (Patton et al., 1961), this animal has been used extensively to study lithogenesis. All prairie dogs fed a 36.6% egg yolk diet with added cholesterol to a total of 1.2% formed multiple stones in the gallbladder containing 77% cholesterol in 2 to 6 months (Brenneman et al., 1972). The concentration of cholesterol in both hepatic and gallbladder bile increased. Increased secretion of cholesterol and bile flow have been noted. There is a shift from predominantly cholic acid before to predominantly chenodeoxycholic acid after the commencement of the lithogenic diet. This prairie dog model provides a unique instance of experimental cholesterol gallstone formation but it is not completely analogous to human cholelithiasis. Since the caloric distribution of the diet is equivalent to the regular diet in the United States, with high prevalence of gallstones, a natural source such as egg yolk is used for the cholesterol source, and no additives or unusual diets are used. However, this model is often accompanied by fatty liver and atherosclerosis, which do not conform to the criteria defined by Freston and Bouchier (1968) (page 142). Seventy per cent of the cholesterol accumulated in gallstones is found to originate from the diet. Apparently, the hepatobiliary system is overloaded by cholesterol and causes the deposition (Holzbach et al., 1976).

### Guinea pigs

As early as in 1942, Okey reported the effect of the intake of B vitamins on the formation of gallstones consisting of calcium phosphate and some cholesterol in guinea pigs fed a diet rich in riboflavin, pantothenate, cholesterol, and fat (Okey, 1942). The incidence of gallstones exceeded 80 %. Later, parenteral injection of Klebsiella polysaccharide induced flocculant precipitates and a small mass composed of 85 % cholesterol, with some pigment in guinea pig gallbladder bile (Jones and Peric-Golia, 1962). Gallstones containing 50 % cholesterol are induced in 86 % of guinea pigs given a pellet diet containing 1 % cholestyramine, a bile acid-binding resin, for 1 month (Schoenfield and Sjövall, 1966)—a situation similar to that of ileal disease or resection in man, in which a large loss of bile acid from the enterohepatic circulation occurs. Hypovitaminotic C guinea pigs fed a high cholesterol-diet produced gallstones containing 81 % cholesterol in 5 weeks, while vitamin C-repleted animals did not (Jenkins, 1977). It was thought that the impaired conversion of cholesterol to chenodeoxycholic acid due to the vitamin C-related effect on the cytochrome P-450-dependent cholesterol $7\alpha$-hydroxylase system in hypovitaminotic guinea pigs leads to cholesterol precipitation and cholesterol stone formation.

### Ground squirrels

Ground squirrels also produces gallstones under certain dietary manipulations (Patton et al., 1961; Fridhandler et al., 1983; MacPharson et al., 1987). All of Richardson's ground squirrels, fed a 2 % cholesterol-enriched rat chow diet, developed cholesterol stones within 3 weeks (MacPharson et al., 1987). The cholesterol saturation index increased to the theoretical saturation level after 2 weeks, and macroscopic stones appear after 6 weeks on a 1 % cholesterol-enriched diet. The crystals grew by appositional layering into microliths and then, by aggregation, into mulberry-shaped stones. Mucus secretion in the gallbladder increased before the precipitation of rhomboidal cholesterol monohydrate crystals. Five days after the introduction of the diet, a thick, discontinuous sludge-like layer was observed overlying large regions of the epithelial sheet. In later stages, this layer embedded cholesterol crystals into the surface of stones. The nature and pattern of stone formation closely resemble those in man. In this experimental model, an in vitro defect in gallbladder contractility, as demonstrated by the reduced isomeric tensions generated in response to cholecystokinin-octapeptide, acetylcholine, or potassium depolarization, is present and is associated with the early changes in bile lithogenicity (Fridhandler et al., 1983). Tension in response to CCK-octapeptide decreases significantly as the stages of gallstone formation progress. Thus, stasis caused by impaired contractility of the gallbladder may well be the critical permissive event and plays a deleterious role in all stages of gallstone formation. At the early stage when bile lithogenicity is increasing, gallbladder stasis may exacerbate the primary metabolic defect by decreasing the flux of bile acid through the liver. Once bile becomes supersaturated, stasis in the gallbladder may provide the time required for cholesterol nucleation and may retain precipitated microcrystals, allowing them to grow macroscopically recognizable gallstones.

### Nonhuman primates

Gallstones can be produced experimentally in nonhuman primate. In 1970, Mann induced gallstones in Cebus monkeys (Cebus albifrons) by feeding them a cholesterol-rich diet (Mann, 1970). The squirrel monkey (Saimiri sciureus) on an atherogenic diet is highly susceptible to experimental gallstone formation (Osuga and Portman, 1971), but the African green monkey is only moderately susceptible (Lofland, 1976). Macaques are moderately resistant, but gallstones can be induced (Lofland, 1976; Geistfeld et al., 1977). Most, if not all, gallstones induced in nonhuman primates are cholesterol stones. A female preponderance of gallstones occurs in nonhuman primates (Kessler, 1982). However, Portman et al. found no clear sex difference in gallstone incidence in Brazilian squirrel monkeys, and in neither biliary function nor plasma lipoprotein (Portman et al., 1980).

In squirrel monkeys fed a semipurified diet in which 45 % of calories are supplied as butter plus crystalline cholesterol (0.1 g/100 kcal), gallstones appear within 3 months; the incidence increases to as much as 83 % at 9 months or more (Osuga and Portman, 1971). The gallstones produced are greenish-white, and in shape are round, ovoid, or polyhedral. The size, number, and total mass increase with time. The largest has been 3.3 mm in diameter. When the diet is changed after 3 months to a basal diet, no stones are found. The gallstones are composed totally or almost totally of cholesterol. Microcrystals of cholesterol also appear (Osuga and Portman, 1972). Fine black pigment stones are found in a few monkeys. The cholic acid pool is smaller in animals on a lithogenic diet with gallstones than in those without gallstones (Osuga et al., 1976). The diet does not affect the pool size of chenodeoxycholic acid as much as that of cholic acid. Thus squirrel monkeys with a plasma cholesterol level similar to that of man, producing gallstones on the dietary regimen, seem to be a good experimental model to study human cholelithiasis. However, this model is consistently associated with hypercholesterolemia and atherosclerosis (Osuga et al., 1974) and no parallel can be drawn between the lithogenic diet used and the diet of men with gallstones. Unlike human bile, taurine-conjugated bile acids predominate in squirrel monkeys (Schoenfield, 1972).

## Black pigment stones (Black stones)

Several animal species are available for the experimental production of black pigment stones. The American deer mouse, Peromyscus maniculatus, suffers from spherocytosis which is very similar to that in man. The incidence of gallstones in American deer mice is as high as 41 % when spherocytosis is present; these are mostly black pigment stones (Fitzpatrick et al., 1963). Susceptibility to cholelithiasis is inherited in American deer mice. The concentration of gallstones in certain lines and a higher incidence of gallstones in offspring of mice with gallstones, as well as the presence of gallstones in nonspherocytic animals without apparent etiological factors, favor this contention. Mice with a hereditary hemolytic disease, i.e., normoblastic anemia genotype nb/nb, offer good examples of the experimental formation of black pigment stones (Trotman et al., 1980). In 1980 a laboratory mouse in Jackson Laboratory, Bar Harbor, Maine, developed a genetic mutation, genotype nb/nb, leading to congenital hemolytic anemia and spontaneous production of black pigment stones with an incidence of 57 % (Trotman et al., 1980). Spontaneously formed gallstones in this strain are nearly identical to black pigment stones formed in men with sickle cell anemia. Female nb/nb mice formed gallstones twice as frequently as males. The incidence increases with age 6 months after birth. Hematocrit, reticulocyte count, and total plasma bilirubin values are not useful in distinguishing gallstone-bearing and non-gallstone-bearing mice. Gallbladder bile of nb/nb mice with gallstones has higher than normal hydrogen ion, total bilirubin, calcium, and bile acid. The output and concentration of total and unconjugated bilirubin increase (Trotman et al., 1981), while the concentration of bile salt, an important solubilizer of bilirubin, decreases or unchanged (Trotman et al., 1980), thus setting a stage for the formation of black pigment stones. Total unconjugated bilirubin is similar, but the ionized fraction of unconjugated bilirubin is higher in bile from nb/nb mice without gallstones than in those with gallstones. Neutral mucin plugs and pigment concretons with increased gallbladder mucin secretion are observed histologically in the glandular crypts of the gallbladder in 80 % of nb/nb mice with stones compared to 33 % of those without gallstones. Glandular concretions within the gallbladder are present at least twice as often in nb/nb mice (Trotman et al., 1982). Bile pigment concretions occur only in nb/nb mice gallbladders and are three times more frequent in those with luminal gallstones. The glandular density of nb/nb mice gallbladder is higher than that of control gallbladders, and nb/nb gallbladders with luminal gallstones have a higher glandular density than nb/nb gallbladders without gallstones. These findings indicate that luminal gallstones in mice with hemolysis are preceded by microscopic precipitation of calcium bilirubinate in the glandular crypts of the gallbladder, which migrate into the lumen and grow by accretion. Enhanced secretion of [$^3$H]-glucosamine-labeled glycoprotein at the neck of the gallbladder in nb/nb mice with gallstones favors precipitation of pigment-mucin concretions in the gallbladder neck glands (LaMont et al., 1983a), and precipitation of mucin-pigment aggregates may be an initial step in the formation of black pigment stones. Calcium bilirubinate can precipitate from solutions in the physiological pH range of 7.0 to 8.4 (Sutor and Wilkie, 1977b). Thus genotype determines glandular density and formation of concretion within the gallbladder prior to luminal gallstone formation. Microscopic pigment concretions are incorporated in mucin plugs, which may be the initial microscopic features of hemolysis-induced black pigment stones in mice (Trotman et al., 1980).

The proportion of black pigment and cholesterol stones induced in hamsters can be changed by dietary manipulation (Shioda, 1965; Hashimoto, 1966; Soloway et al., 1977). Cholesterol stones can be produced in all young hamsters fed 60 % glucose, 20 % casein, and 10 % butter, while in older hamsters on the same diet, black pigment stones occur in 20 % (Hikasa et al 1980). Those fed on a diet consisting of 54.3 % glucose, 20 % starch, 20 % casein, and 5.7 % salts and vitamins produce black pigment gallstones (Freed et al., 1986; Malet et al., 1989). Eight percent of animals have black pigment stones after 3 weeks and 23 % after 5 weeks. The first precipitation of pigment crystals occurs in the mucus layer in bile or on the gallbladder surface, with evidence of hypersecretion of mucin

(Malet et al., 1989). Black pigment stones seem to grow by agglomeration of pigment crystals enmeshed in mucus. The production of mucin by the gallbladder mucosa, as detected by the incorporation of $^{3}$H-glucosamine in mucin glycoproteins using gallbladder explant, increases significantly before the actual formation of black pigment stones. Thus mucin seems to play an important role in the growth of black pigment stones. Black pigment stones are more common in female hamsters (Nagase et al., 1978; Hikasa et al., 1980), in female hamsters treated with progesterone, and in castrated male hamsters, suggesting the influence of hormones (Dam and Christensen, 1965). The incidence of black pigment gallstones in hamsters is enhanced by the addition of carbon tetrachloride (Bergman et al., 1971), thyroxine (Bergman and Van der Linden, 1966) or ethanol (Bergman et al., 1971), in addition to the occurrence of liver cirrhosis. A newer model of pigment stone formation has been introduced by feeding a nutritionally adequate, semipurified diet containing a moderate amount of cholesterol and ethinyl estradiol (Cohen et al., 1987). The stones induced contained calcium phosphate 26.7 %, calcium bilirubinate 12.8 %, cholesterol 15.1 % and protein 45.5 %. When the diet is supplemented with cholic acid and/or calcium as calcium carbonate, no cholesterol stones are formed and the incidence of black pigment gallstones is not affected (Cohen et al., 1989b).

Prairie dogs with ileal resection or bypass of the distal one-third of the small intestine fed on a trace cholesterol diet formed black smooth and brittle gallstones, with bilirubin as a major component, but these may not be identical to the black pigment stones in man (Bickerstaff and Moossa, 1983). Significant elevation of total bilrubin and calcium is noted in gallbladder bile with the appearance of pigment stones, indicating that the defect lies in bilirubin metabolism (Pitt et al., 1984). Feeding of a carbohydrate-rich diet (35 % sucrose and 32 % starch) to prairie dogs resulted in the formation of pigment crystals, sludge, and microscopic black pigment gallstones, and coincided with the increased concentrations of phospholipids, calcium, and bilirubin in bile (Conter et al., 1986a). A nonlithogenic diet supplemented with calcium, in the form of calcium lactate in drinking water, induced black pigment stones in prairie dogs (Magnuson et al., 1989b). Prairie dogs maintained on a high-carbohydrate, iron-deficient diet develop crystals and pigment gallstones composed mainly of calcium bilirubinate (Conter et al., 1986a; Roslyn et al., 1987b). An increased biliary concentration of calcium, cholesterol, and phospholipids was noted. A positive linear relationship was found between the calcium concentration in gallbladder bile and the biliary concentration of total bile acid and taurochenodeoxycholic acid, but an inverse relation with taurocholic acid existed (Abedin et al., 1989). Such a relationship is absent in hepatic bile. Altered bile acid composition may modify calcium solubility, as bile acid acts as an important buffer for free calcium in bile (Moore et al., 1982). Furthermore, the bile acid composition may influence biliary secretion of calcium (Cummings and Hofmann, 1984).

Guinea pigs given lincomycin (60 mg/kg/day) show a striking increase in the renewal of gallbladder epithelium after 48 hours of treatment (Scott, 1976). Calcium bilirubinate precipitates are formed after 8 days. Guinea pigs surviving beyond 34 days had gallstones. Changes in gallbladder epithelium preceded the formation of precipitates and initiated histological changes which culminated in impressive glandular metaplasia and led to the formation of gallstones. Multiple black pigment stones consisting of calcium, carbonate and bilirubin were produced in the gallbladder. Their composition was similar but not identical to that of human black pigment stones (Lee and Thomsen, 1982). Guinea pigs fed a diet supplemented with 0.5 % cholesterol formed black pigment gallstones in 6 to 20 weeks (LaMorte et al., 1985b). The gallstones formed are fine granular crystals resembling calcium bilirubinate. Lower hematocrit values suggest hemolytic anemia induced by cholesterol (Okey and Greaves, 1939). An increased resting gallbladder volume was noted. Increased secretion of mucus, and desquamation and rapid replacement of epithelial cells, occur. However, the underlying mechanism for the induction of inflammation and subsequent gallstone formation is not well understood.

A gallstone model has been developed in dogs fed a diet compounded from normal dietary constituents consisting of low protein, high sugar, very deficient in methionine, low total and unsaturated fat, and 1 % cholesterol added (Englert et al., 1969, 1977). Gallstones appeared in all 21 dogs ingesting the diet. Substitution of glucose for sucrose, increase in protein, or elimination of the added cholesterol delayed the appearance of gallstones. These stones range from dark specks to irregular brown to black structures $10 \times 10$ mm in size—the largest reaches to the size of microspherolith. They are gelatinous, rubber-like or firm in consistency (Englert et al., 1969) and contain mainly protein, mucus, bile salts, bilirubin, and insoluble black residue after acid hydrolysis, with only traces of cholesterol (Englert et al., 1977). Whether these stones are structurally and compositionally identical or similar to black pigment stones in man is uncertain. Increased numbers of secretory vesicles in gallbladder mucosal epithelium, large amounts of mucus in epithelial crypts, hypersecretion of gallbladder mucin, and a heavy layer of mucus coating over the gallbladder epithelium are present. Therefore, biliary protein and mucus substances are important for lithogenesis in this model. An increase of calcium in gallbladder bile is observed in the experimental formation of pigment stones in dogs (Dawes et al., 1989). However, its etiological significance is uncertain.

Although several animal models are available for the formation of black pigment stones, interpretation of the results requires caution, since the majority of men with black pigment stones have neither hemolysis nor elevation of total and unconjugated bilirubin in bile.

## Brown pigment stones (Calcium bilirubinate stones)

Incomplete obstruction of the terminal common bile duct produced by wrapping cellophane sealing tape dusted with dicetyl sodium phosphate, which causes inflammation, around just before it enters the duodenum produced gallstones in 25 % of dogs and 87 % of rabbits (Imamoglu et al., 1957). Gallstones appear mostly in the gallbladder and, in some cases, in the common bile duct. The stones are soft and crumble upon slight external pressure, resembling human brown pigment stones. Those are composed of bilirubin and cholesterol. They suggest that anatomical narrowing of the terminal common bile duct is a precursor of gallstone formation rather than the end result. Bisgard et al. produced gallstones by placing the ligature low on the common duct, permitting reflux of pancreatic juice into the biliary system in the goat (Bisgard and Baker, 1940). Bacteria were recovered from the gallbladders in all cases with the formation of gallstones. Prairie dogs fed on corn and alfalfa produced gallstones composed of cholesterol 45 %, bile pigment 30 % and calcium bilirubinate 25 % (Strichartz et al., 1989b). A decreased transepithelial potential difference and short-circuit indicate changes in gallbladder mucosal function similar to those in men with gallstones.

## Inorganic stones

Inorganic stones can be produced in animals (Phemister et al., 1932). A solid, coarse, sand-like deposit of practically pure calcium carbonate was produced experimentally in the dogs by ligation of the cystic duct, injection of streptococci, and implantation of a human gallstone in the gallbladder. Small calcium deposits were obtained by similar procedures in rabbits. Stones composed of calcium phosphate with small amounts of cholesterol are produced in guinea pigs on a cholesterol-enriched diet supplemented by vitamin B (Okey, 1942).

## Bile acid stones

Gallstones composed mainly of bile acid which are not known to occur in man can be produced in several species of animals by various dietary manipulations. For bile acid with relatively insoluble calcium salt or with a high critical micellar concentration (CMC), an increase in pH causes anions to reach the solubility product of calcium salt before reaching the CMC, so that precipitation of calcium salt occurs instead of the formation of micelles (Hofmann and Mysels, 1992). In 1956 Bevans et al., studying sterol metabolism in rabbits, succeeded in producing gallstones in rabbits by feeding cholestanol, which is easily absorbed from the intestinal tract and stored in tissues (Bevans and Mosbach, 1956). In contrast to cholesterol and $\beta$-sitosterol, cholestanol has a specific irritating effect on the biliary tract of rabbits. Rabbits on a diet containing 250 to 1,000 mg cholestanol per day for 2 to 6 weeks consistently develop biliary concrements and inflammatory lesions of the biliary tract. The gallstones thus produced contain very few digitonin-precipitable sterols. These gallstones are composed mainly of calcium or sodium salts of allodeoxycholic acid, an allo-stereoisomer of deoxycholic acid (Hofmann and Mosbach, 1964; Hofmann et al., 1968). Allodeoxycholic acid, a $5\alpha$-isomer of normally occurring $5\beta$-bile acid, is poorly soluble and has a high propensity to complex with the calcium present in bile to form insoluble concretions. Cholecystitis has been noted in this model (Mosbach and Bevans, 1960). Inflammatory changes and a rise in the labeling index in gallbladder mucosa of rabbits, mice, and guinea pigs studied by autoradiography (Scott, 1978) are often observed even before stones are formed. These morphological changes coincide with a rise in the biliary concentration of allodeoxycholic acid (Hofmann et al., 1968), which may well have caused the injuries observed in the gallbladder mucosa. Gallstone formation is preceded by early increase in mucus production (Hayward et al., 1968) and increased proliferation of epithelial cells (Scott, 1978). When the gallbladder is excluded from the enterohepatic circulation of bile acid by ligation of the cystic duct, no increase of mucus secretion is noted even on a lithogenic diet (Freston et al., 1969). Gallstones are formed in cholecystectomized rabbits by cholestanol feeding, but not in rats, which lack a gallbladder. Only 10% of guinea pigs develop gallstones by cholestanol feeding (Caira et al., 1957).

A similar kind of gallstones can also be produced by feeding rabbits with a diet containing 20% semipurified oleic acid for 12 weeks (Borgman, 1964, 1965). Feeding of oleic acid results in increased hepatic cholesterogenesis, using oleic acid as a carbon source (Kyd and Bouchier, 1971; Lee et al., 1986, 1987b). Hypercholesterolemia develops rapidly and hepatic HMG-CoA reductase increases, resulting in accumulation of cholesterol and cholestanol in the liver and progressive saturation of cholesterol in bile. Hepatic cholesterol accumulated in the liver is metabolized to form cholestanol by a pathway probably through bile acid intermediates, 7$\alpha$-hydroxycholesterol and 7$\alpha$-hydroxy-4-cholesten-3-one (Skrede et al., 1985), followed by synthesis of (5$\alpha$)-glycoallocholic acid, which is excreted in bile. (5$\alpha$)-Allocholic acid is transformed in the gut by intestinal flora to (5$\alpha$)-allodeoxycholic acid, reabsorbed, transported to the liver, and excreted in bile, leading to the formation of gallstones composed mainly of allodeoxycholic acid but with only traces of cholesterol (Kyd and Bouchier, 1971). Absorption of water and bilirubin is unimpaired, but that of glycodeoxycholate absorption from the gallbladder is impaired. The highest percentage of 5$\alpha$-deoxycholic acid in bile attained is 32.4% in 16 weeks on the diet (Kyd and Bouchier, 1972). Administration of kanamycin abolishes gallstone formation mediated by the activity of intestinal flora by inhibiting bacterial dehydroxylation of (5$\alpha$)-allocholic acid to (5$\alpha$)-allodeoxycholic acid, dramatically reducing the proportion of 5$\alpha$-dihydroxy bile acids and increasing that of 5$\beta$-dihydroxy bile acids in bile (Lee et al., 1986, 1987b). In this rabbit model on an oleic acid-rich diet, the changes in gallbladder function does not occur, as determined by the everted sac method (Kyd and Bouchier, 1971).

Spontaneous formation of gallstones in rats is extremely uncommon, presumably due to the absence of a gallbladder in this species. However, gallstones composed of 70% bile acids consisting of free and glycine-conjugated lithocholic acid and 3$\alpha$, 6$\beta$-dihydroxy-5$\beta$-cholanoic acid with a small amount of hyodeoxycholic, chenodeoxycholic and cholic acids, 12% ash, 0.7% lipid including cholesterol, and 0.14% bilirubin are produced in rats by feeding a diet containing 1% lithocholic acid for 8 weeks (Palmer, 1965; Palmer and Hruban, 1966). The color of the gallstones produced is mostly yellow, but some vary from green to black. Free or glycine-conjugated lithocholic and 3$\alpha$, 6$\beta$-dihydroxy-5$\beta$-cholanoic acid, which lack a strongly polar taurine sulfate group and are less soluble than taurine-conjugated bile acid, precipitate in the small bile duct, grow, and accumulate in the common duct. This situation is similar to that of gallstone formation in rabbits given cholestanol, in which the major factor is the precipitation of calcium salt of glycoallodeoxycholic acid in the gallbladder (Hofmann and Mosbach, 1964). Increase of dietary protein or supplementation by taurine- or sulfur-containing amino acids inhibits gallstone formation (Palmer, 1965), as rat liver preferentially conjugates bile acid with taurine possessing a strongly polar sulfonic acid group (Norman, 1954), making the stones more water soluble. Cellular debris resulting from the intense desquamative and cytotoxic effects of lithocholic acid apparently facilitates gallstone formation in this model, although rat liver can hydroxylate lithocholic acid to $\beta$-muricholic acid, via chenodeoxycholic, $3\alpha$, $6\beta$-dihydroxy-$5\beta$-cholanoic and $\alpha$-muricholic acids, to inactivate lithocholic acid (Thomas et al., 1964).

# Liability to Other Diseases

## Gallbladder carcinoma

Gallbladder carcinoma is frequently associated with gallstones, i.e., in 59–88 % (Cooke et al., 1953), 93 % (Kozoll et al., 1959), and 82 % of cases (Torvik and Hølvik, 1960). On the other hand, the incidence of gallbladder carcinoma in gallstone patients is only 1.3–7 % (Torvik and Hølvik, 1960), 1–3 % (Piehler and Crichlow, 1978), or less than 1% (Russell and Brown, 1950). Patients with large gallstones have a greater risk of gallbladder carcinoma (Diehl, 1983; Lowenfels et al., 1989). Although some advocate 'prophylactic cholecystectomy for cholelithiasis because of the risk of developing gallbladder carcinoma, a causative role for gallstones in the formation of gallbladder carcinoma has not been proven (Collier and Blumgart, 1994). Some argue against removing the gallbladder prophylactically (Wenckert and Robertson, 1966). Lund followed 526 patients with gallstones and reported that one-third to one-half of them developed severe symptoms or complications. He maintain that prophylactic cholecystectomy should be performed only in patients who are a good surgical risk (Lund, 1960). Whether or not the risk of cholecystectomy outweighs the benefits of preventing gallbladder carcinoma is a matter of conjecture except in high-risk populations.

## Colorectal carcinoma

An association between cholelithiasis or cholecystectomy and colon carcinoma has been noted by many investigators ( Lowenfels et al., 1982; Weiss et al., 1982; Hill, 1983). The presence of cholelithiasis (or cholecystectomy) may lead to colon carcinoma, but not vice versa. A positive correlation was found between the age-adjusted prevalence of colorectal carcinoma and cholecystitis as a measure of frequency of gallstones in 28 countries, suggesting that cholelithiasis and colorectal carcinoma share similar, perhaps metabolic, factors (Lowenfels, 1980). However, the results of such correlations are often contradictory at best. Although cholecystectomy is implicated in carcinoma of the right side of the colon (Linos et al., 1981; Vernick and Kuller, 1981), Castleden et al. maintain that since the prevalence of gallstones is higher in females and since carcinoma of the right colon is predominat, random sampling may have led to a finding of more gallstones in women and more carcinoma of the right colon (Castleden et al., 1985). It was indicated that 2,085 cases of cholelithiasis and cholecystectomy were found in 11,828 autopsies (Breuer et al., 1988). A positive correlation between gallstones and colorectal carcinoma was found in men but not in women. An elevated risk of developing proximal colon carcinoma was found in both sexes. An increased risk of distal colon carcinoma was found in men but not in women. It is suggested that cholelithiasis may be linked through diet with colorectal carcinoma (Burkitt and Tunstall, 1975). An low-fiber diet is linked to both colon carcinoma (Trock et al., 1990) and gallstones (Bennion and Grundy, 1978). Since cholesterol secretion is increased in cholelithiasis and since cholesterol is a major source of bile acids, a cholesterol/bile acid hypothesis is suggested for the etiology of colorectal carcinoma. Excessive exposure of colon mucosa to degraded bile acid, especially deoxycholic acid, is considered to be responsible (Pomare and Heaton, 1973b; Malagelada et al., 1973; Hepner et al., 1974), not as initiators but as promotors of the adenoma-carcinoma sequence (Narisawa et al., 1974; Reddy et al., 1976; Hill, 1985). However, several reports refute the association between cholelithiasis or cholecystectomy and colon carcinoma (Hoare, 1974; Adami et al., 1983; Ichimiya et al., 1986; Moorehead et al., 1986). We followed 1,238 cholecystectomized cases and found no appreciable excess mortality for colorectal carcinoma when observed death was compared with the expected values calculated from the death rates in Japan, i.e., 5 versus 3.19 during the whole observation period and 5 versus 4.66 for a 10-year period (Ichimiya et al., 1986). Therefore, we concluded that cholecystectomy does not play an important role in the subsequent occurrence of colorectal carcinoma and subsequent colon carcinoma should not ordinarily be a factor when cholecystectomy is considered (Friedman 1993). A recent cohort study by Ekbom et al. in Sweden describes 62,615 cases of cholecystectomy followed up for as long as 23 years; no excess risk of colorectal carcinoma was found except for a modest increase in right-sided colon carcinoma in women (Ekbom et al., 1993). Meta-analysis conducted to quantify the risk of colorectal carcinoma after cholecystectomy by reviewing large numbers of cohort and case-control studies also shows an increased risk of right-sided colon carcinoma in women (Giovannucci et al., 1993).

The underlying reason for the increased risk of right-sided colon carcinoma in cholecystectomized women is not well understood but the risk is considered to be small. Absence of the gallbladder due to cholecystectomy induces greater exposure of bile acids to intestinal flora because of the resultant continuous enterohepatic circulation and increased dehydroxylation of primary to secondary bile acids (Malegelada et al., 1973) such as deoxycholic acid. Such acids can damage the colonic epithelium in the presence of carcinogen when their concentration exceeds a certain level, and they may induce a presumably compensatory proliferative response (Bull et al., 1983). Malagelada (Malagelada et al., 1973), Pomare (Pomare and Heaton, 1973b), and Hepner (Hepner et al., 1974) showed increased secondary bile acids in bile when the biliary bile acid patterns in cholecystectomized patients and controls were compared. This work was criticized because it involved two variables, i.e., one with or without the gallbladder and the other with or without gallstones.

In contrast increased deoxycholic acid was not found in the bile of colon carcinoma patients (Van der Linden et al., 1983; Castleden et al., 1985). Van der Linden et al. analyzed the bile acid composition of duodenal bile sampled before and after cholecystectomy from patients with gallstones in a well-functioning gallbladder (Van der Linden et al., 1983). Cholecystectomy resulted in a shift from cholic acid to chenodeoxycholic acid, i.e., mean cholic acid values fell, chenodeoxycholic acid values rose, and the ratio between chenodeoxycholic acid and cholic acid increased after cholecystectomy. This may explain the relative rarity of recurrent common bile duct stones. In contrast, the percentage of secondary bile acids showed little change. It is suggested that if an association between cholelithiasis and colon carcinoma indeed exists, both diseases may be associated with a high level of secondary bile acids, especially deoxycholic acid, as increasing evidence suggests that this acid in bile is increased in gallstone patients (Marcus and Heaton, 1988). In animal experiments, the carcinogenic effect of cholecystectomy on the colon is inconsistent at best (Werner et al., 1977; Schattenkerk et al., 1980). Populations on a high-fat diet appear to have a higher amount of secondary bile acid in feces. A higher incidence of strains of intestinal anaerobes degrading cholic acid to deoxycholic acid may be responsible (Hill, 1974). However, no case-control study investigating fecal bile acid has been done. Because of the presence of several uncontrollable factors, such as stool homogeneity, transit time, fecal bulk, fecal pH, and water content, in the investigation of fecal bile acids, the serum bile acid concentration of patients with colorectal adenomas was studied (Bayerdörffer et al., 1993). Deoxycholic acid concentration is significantly higher in sera of men with colorectal carcinomas and also in a combined analysis of both sexes. In 6- and 12- month follow-up studies an increase in the serum deoxycholic acid level was found in men with adenomas, which may be considered a precancerous stage. The promoting effect of secondary bile acids in experimentally induced colon carcinoma has been shown (Narisawa et al., 1974; Reddy and Wynder, 1977). Incorporation of cholic acid into the diet resulted in an increased number of colorectal tumors in animals (Galloway et al., 1986; McSherry et al., 1989).

# CHAPTER FIVE

# Clinical Perspective

## Symptoms

Upper abdominal pain, fever, and jaundice constitute the classical triad of cholelithiasis. However, because of the advent of advanced techniques resulting in the diagnosis of cholelithiasis in its early stage, patients with all three symptoms are less and less frequently encountered.

## Abdominal pain

Abdominal pain, in the form of biliary colic, is considered a symptom of cholelithiasis. A recent controlled study by Diehl et al. (1990) on 122 patients with gallstones and 178 controls confirmed the previous contention that upper abdominal pain is the symptom most closely associated with gallstone disease. Biliary colic is usually unremitting, begins suddenly, and lasts for a few minutes or for period ranging from a few hours to 24 hours, radiating to the right shoulder region or the back and subsiding gradually. In some cases, prodromal symptoms such as upper abdominal discomfort and nausea, accompanied occasionally by vomiting, are present. The pain occurs after a fatty meal, but no such relation can be elicited in some cases. It usually occurs more than 1 hour after the meals (Diehl et al., 1990). It is located in the right upper quadrant or the epigastrium and frequently radiates to the right shoulder and/or right side of the back. However, in a certain proportion of cholelithiasis cases, no discernible abdominal pain is attributable to the presence of gallstones, i.e., gallstones are silent or asymptomatic. Whether or not true silent stones are present is a matter of conjecture (Mayo, 1911; Gracie and Ransohoff, 1982; Weiss and Hanis, 1984). A careful follow-up study revealed that about one-third to one-fifth of silent stone cases eventually become symptomatic. A total of 781 surgically untreated gallstone patients were followed in Malmö, Sweden, for 11 years, where 60% of deaths occur in the General Hospital. A remarkable follow-up rate of 99% was achieved (Wenckert and Robertson, 1966). Of this group, 254, or 33% eventually developed severe symptoms necessitating cholecystectomy, and 144, or 18% developed complications. Gracie and Ransohoff followed 123 patients with gallsotnes for 15 years (Gracie and Ransohoff, 1982).

The cumulative probability of developing biliary pain or complications was 18 %. Friedman et al found that the rate of symptom development over 25 years of follow-up was twice that of Gracie and Ransohoff (Friedman et al., 1989). McSherry et al. followed 135 asymptomatic gallstone patients and found 10% developed symptoms within 4 years (McSherry et al., 1985). In a prospective study using real-time ultrasonography in Rome, only one-third of those with gallstones were found to have or have had biliary pain. If all women with cholecystectomy are assumed to have been symptomatic, at least 40 % were asymptomatic (Rome Group for the Epidemiology and Prevention of Cholelithiasis, 1984). Dyspepsia, including fat intolerance, flatulent dyspepsia, aerophagy, heartburn, and acid regurgitation are not considered specifically attributable to gallstone disease. Cases of silent stones have been more and more frequently encountered in recent years because of the advent of various accurate, minimally invasive imaging techniques. In some cases, sludge produces abdominal pain (Lee, 1990).

During the interval, epigastric fullness and discomfort and right upper quadrant pain may persist, usually without a specific complaint pointing to the presence of gallstones. Dyspepsia, indigestion, heartburn, flatulence, nausea, and eructation may be present, but they are not specific.

## Fever

Low-grade fever may accompany abdominal pain, but not frequently. High intermittent or interrupted fever points to the advent of acute cholecystitis, common bile duct stone with cholangitis, or concomitant acute pancreatitis.

## Jaundice

Jaundice appears, as a rule, only when gallstone(s) are present in the bile duct. However, in case of acute cholecystitis or cystic duct stone, slight jaundice may appear even in the absence of stones in the bile duct, probably due to the spread of inflammation toward the bile duct. In older persons, jaundice more frequently accompanies cholelithiasis because of the increased involvement of the common bile duct. Jaundice appearing in cholelithiasis fluctuates, in contrast to progressive jaundice due to malignant obstruction of the bile duct.

In Mirizzi's syndrome (Mirizzi, 1948), with gallstone(s) impacted in the neck of the gallbladder or in the cystic duct, causing obstruction of the common hepatic duct by compression, jaundice is the main feature.

## Nonspecific abdominal symptoms

A feeling of fullness and pressure or slight pain in the right upper abdomen, flatulence, nausea, or food intolerance sometimes occur. An interesting prospective analysis of cholelithiasis patients before and after extracorporeal shock wave lithotripsy (ESWL) and oral bile acid treatment has been conducted by Stölzel et al. (1994). They found that, after complete stone disappearnce, 72 of 100 patients lost symptoms they had before the treatment. The remaining 28 patients with persisting symptoms have unspecific symptoms, although the anatomical structure is left intact, preserving their physiological function.

# Signs

**Tenderness**: Present in the right upper quadrant (Head's gallbladder point) and/or in the upper abdomen (solar point).

**Abdominal spasm**: Elicited by light palpation, but usually absent unless inflammation spreads to the pericholecystic area and the parietal peritoneum.

**Murphy's inspiratory arrest sign**: Arrest of deep inspiration while palpating under the right costal margin because of the sudden onset of pain.

**Palpable gallbladder**: Usually not palpable even in the presence of gallbladder hydrops or empyema. Gallbladder with gallstone is not capable of marked distention because of recurrent cholecystitis and resulting fibrosis of the gallbladder wall. Some patients with acute cholecystitis have a palpable gallbladder.

# Diagnosis

The most important initial step in diagnosing cholelithiasis is to elicit precisely clues to pointing the presence of cholelithiasis among the anamnesis, symptoms, and signs. When the presence of gallstone is suspected, the patient should be subjected to the various biliary tract imaging studies.

## Biliary Tract Imaging

Recent introduction of an array of hepatobiliary imaging techniques has changed radically the diagnostic steps to be taken in establishing the presence of gallstones in the biliary tract and its pathology, i.e., the diagnosis of cholelithiasis.

### Ultrasonography

The most useful screening procedure for the diagnosis of cholelithiasis is ultrasonography. It is noninvasive; simple to perform, as it does not require special preparation or contrast medium; and can be performed in the presence of jaundice or liver dysfunction, giving a wealth of informations. A sensitivity of more than 95 % together with an approximately 99 % specificity can be achieved in the detection of gallbladder stones. The presence of gallstones; their location; state of the biliary tract, including the size, shape, and thickness of the gallbladder wall; pericholecystic accumulation of fluid; and dilatation of intrahepatic and extrahepatic ducts can be elicited by ultrasonography, although information on the distal common duct is frequently obscured by gas present in the adjacent duodenum. Occasionally, sludge may be encountered in the most dependent portion of the gallbladder, but sludge usually does not cast acoustic shadows. Gallstones often produce acoustic shadows (Figure 22). Compared with intravenous cholecystography, ultrasonography is definitely superior, especially in detecting gallstones less than 5–10 mm in diameter. Thus, ultrasonography is the most effective screening procedure for those suspected of having cholelithiasis, as well as for population studies.

## Endoscopic ultrasonography

Endoscopic ultrasonography is quite effective in diagnosing common duct stones (Figure 23). It avoids interference from gas in the overlying duodenum, it is less invasive than endoscopic retrograde cholangiography, and it may avoid unnecessary sphincterotomy (Denis et al., 1993). The sensitivity of endoscopic ultrasonography for common duct stones (97 %) is far greater than that of abdominal ultrasonography (25 %) and computed tomography (75 %) (Amouyal et al 1994). However, its use is not wide spread, since it was introduced just a few years ago.

## Plain abdominal X-ray

The next most commonly used and time-honored diagnostic procedure is routine abdominal X-ray or abdominal scout film. This gives information on the calcification of gallstones as a radiopaque shadow in the right upper abdomen (15–20 % of the cases),

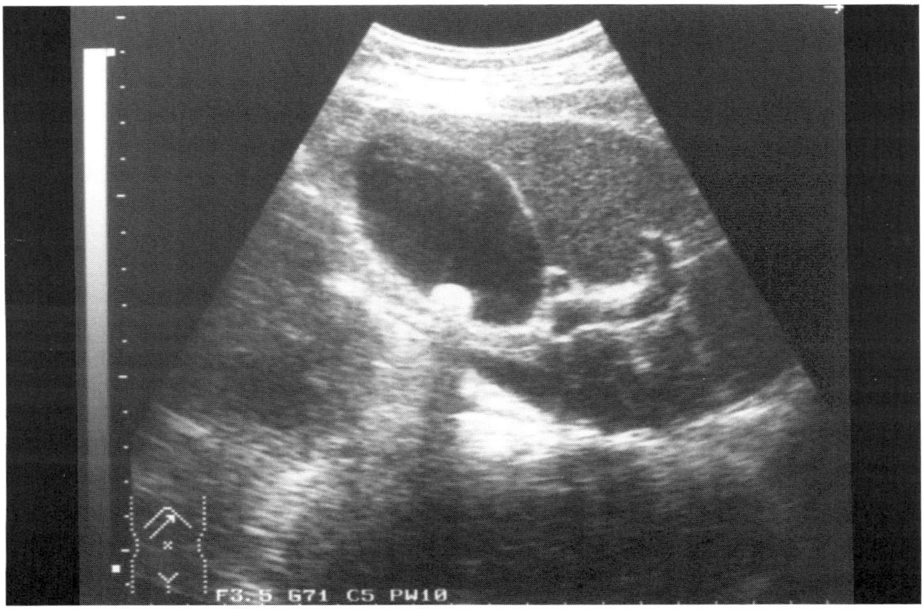


**Figure 22**

Gallstones with Acoustic Shadowing on Ultrasonogram

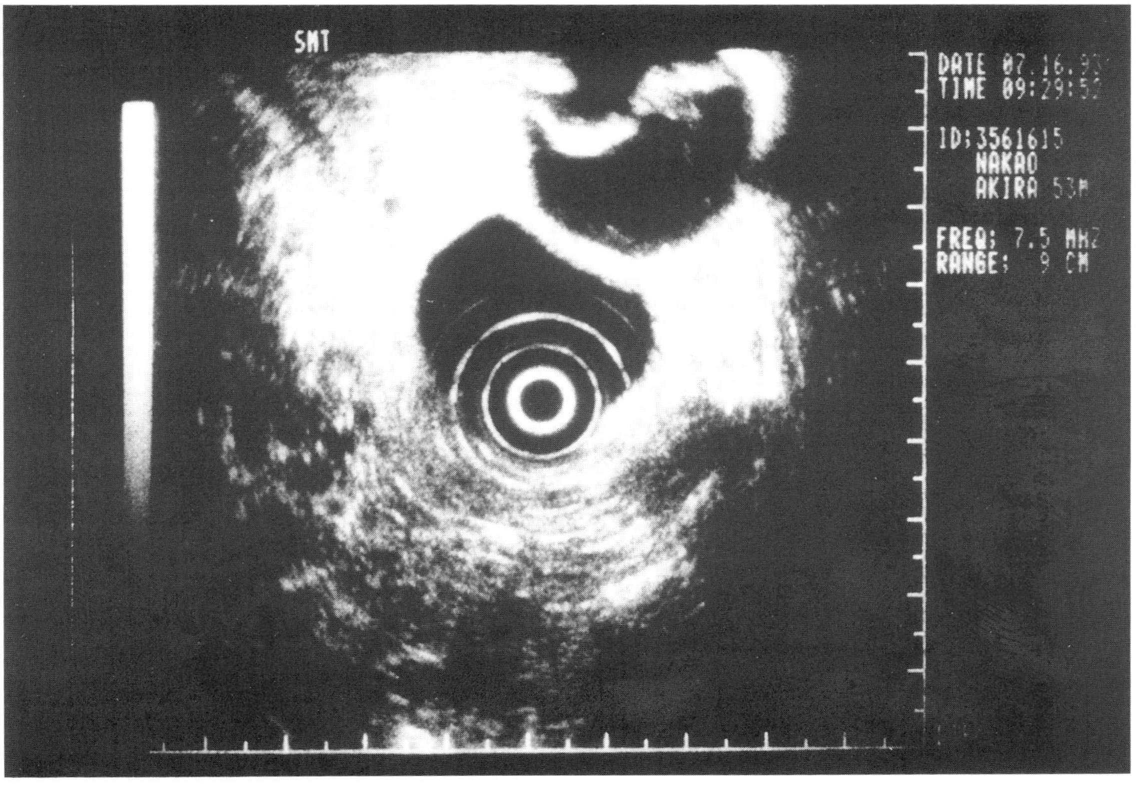


**Figure 23**

Endoscopic Ultrasonogram

The endoscope is within the stomach. The gallstone is visible in the gallbladder on the left.

which provides important clues for the contraindication to oral cholelitholytic treatment. Stellate radiolucencies in the right upper quadrant—the so-called Mercedes-Benz sign—due to the fissure within stones may be seen.

## Computed tomography

Computed tomography, although cost ineffective and not always available, adds information on the site and size of gallstones and the state of the biliary tree. When calcium content exceeds 1%, it gives distinct images. However, in case of brown pigment stones, the Hounsfield value is close to that of surrounding body tissues, hence detection of stones is difficult, if not impossible, unless the ducts are considerably dilated and the stones are surrounded by bile. In general, information on intra- and extrahepatic bile ducts is scanty unless the ducts are considerably dilated.

## Cholecystocholangiography

### Indirect cholecystocholangiography

**Oral and/or intravenous cholecystocholangiography**: Oral and/or intravenous cholecystocholangiography are still the mainstay in the diagnosis of cholelithiasis, since they are noninvasive, apart from X-ray exposure, and give functional information about the gallbladder which is otherwise unobtainable. This is important in establishing the need for oral cholelitholytic treatment. Although visualization of the gallbladder by oral cholecystography depends on absorption from the intestine, uptake and secretion of the contrast medium by the liver, and patency of the cystic duct leading to the gallbladder, most diseases of the gallbladder reduce its absorption capacity; therefore, nonvisualization of the gallbladder indicates gallbladder disease. Floating stones (Åkerlund phenomena) (Åkerlund 1933) can be seen by oral or intravenous cholecystography in the upright position. With the accompanying use of X-ray tomography with intravenous cholangiography, this gives a fairly clear picture of the extrahepatic bile duct. Combined use of oral and intravenous cholecystography (Figure 24) is recommended. Oral cholecystographic agents such as Biloptin (Schering) or Telepaque (Iopanoic acid—Winthrop) are given the previous evening. After an overnight fast, an X-ray film is taken to reveal the gallbladder with gallstones in situ. Visualization of the gallbladder at this stage indicates a functioning gallbladder—an important factor in determining the need for oral cholelitholytic treatment. Thereafter, an intravenous cholecystographic agent such as Biligrafin (Schering) is injected, either in bolus form or by drip infusion (40 ml of 60 % Biligrafin mixed with 160 ml of a 5 % glucose soluton is injected over a 10-minutes period). After completion of the injection, X-ray films are taken at 30, 60, and 120 minutes to follow the visualization of the gallbladder. For assessment of the contractility of the gallbladder, egg yolk is given orally and an X-ray film is taken after 30 and 60 minutes.

When the presence of stones in the bile duct is suspected because of the rise of serum alkaline phosphatase, fever, and jaundice or even due to the past history alone, the patient is subjected to direct cholangiography.

### Direct cholangiography

Direct cholangiography in the form of endoscopic retrograde cholangiography (ERC) and percutaneous transhepatic cholangiography (PTC) is most useful in demonstrating the exact pathology of the biliary tract.

**Endoscopic retrograde cholangiopancreatography (ERCP)**: Contrast medium is injected through a cannula inserted into the duodenal papilla by means of duodenal fiberscope. It gives an extremely clear picture of the biliary tract, including occasionally the gallbladder. When jaundice is absent, endoscopic retrograde cholangiography (ERC) is the procedure of choice when an expertise is available. It gives information on the presence of gallstone(s) in the bile duct, especially the distal common bile duct. It was shown that ERCP would have been avoided in 61 % of the cases, without overlooking stones, by employing a

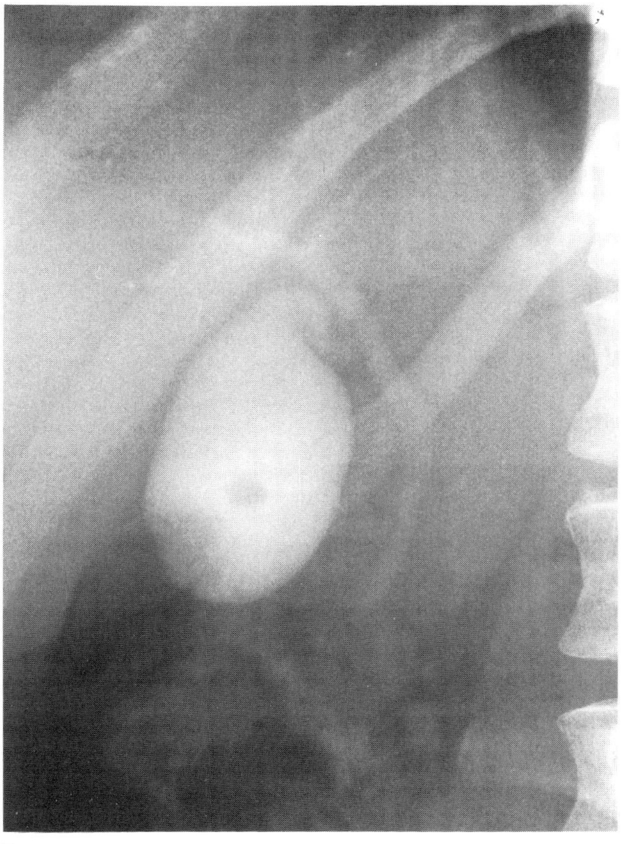

Figure 24

Combined Peroral and Intravenous Cholangiogram

sensitive biochemical index in predicting the presence of ductal stones, i.e., alkaline phosphatase, alanine transferase, aspartate transferase, and bilirubin (Qureshi et al., 1993a). In a few cases with gallstones, ultrasonography and oral and intravenous cholangiography fail to elicit the presence of gallstones because of interference from overlying gas in the duodenum. Therefore, patients in whom stones in the extrahepatic bile duct are strongly suspected should be subjected to ERC. When a stricture is present in the upper portion of the bile duct, injection of a contrast medium may induce severe cholangitis. This should be avoided.

**Percutaneous transhepatic cholangiography (PTC)**: Contrast medium is injected directly into the dilated intrahepatic bile duct through a Chiba skinny needle inserted through the skin and the liver tissue. Side and frontal approaches are available. Due to the recent introduction of ultrasonographic guidance, this procedure has become much simpler and safer.

### Examination of duodenal fluid

A time-honored method of examining duodenal fluid aspirated via Lyon's duodenal tube placed in the duodenum for the presence of various particles, including cholesterol and calcium bilirubinate crystals, should not be totally discarded, as it gives a clue to the nature of gallstones present (Juniper and Burson, 1957). A rapid method of introducing the duodenal tube is available. Aspiration of duodenal bile through a cannula inserted into the duodenal papilla during ERC before the injection of a contrast medium can be substituted.

## Differential diagnosis

When the main symptoms remain vague, such as epigastric discomfort, diagnosis becomes difficult. Differential diagnosis includes neurogenic dyspepsia, gastric ulcer, gastritis, duodenal ulcer, chronic pancreatitis, appendicitis with anomalous location, and urolithiasis. Use of extensive diagnostic procedures presently available is of great help in establishing the diagnosis.

## Treatment

The aim of the treatment of cholelithiasis is not only to remove the gallstones present but also to prevent their recurrence. Cholecystectomy, introduced by a young surgeon, Dr. Karl Langenbuch, of Lazarus Krankenhaus in Berlin in 1882, permanently cures the disease by removing the gallstones as well as the site of their formation, i.e., the gallbladder (Langenbuch, 1882). Cholecystectomy has been and still is the gold standard for the treatment of cholelithiasis (McSherry, 1989). However, operative intervention, although quite effective, inevitably causes pain and therefore is best avoided if possible. Spontaneous disappearance of gallstones is rare. Wolpers in a painstaking study of 188 cases of radiologically proven gallstones followed for up to 17 years, stone shrinkage occur only in 5 cases, i.e., 2.6 % (Wolpers, 1968). Such changes in gallstones were found to differ depending on the kind of gallstones present. No disappearance occurred in solitary cholesterol stones and in (black) pigment stones. However, Wolpers found stone shrinkage in 5 out of 67 cases of multiple (mulberry) cholesterol stones, i.e., 7.5 %, and in all 171 cases of cholesterol stones, i.e., 2.9 % (Wolpers, 1968). In one case, the size of the gallstones decreased but, after 4 years, again started to increase during the 10 years of follow-up. In the National Gallstone Cooperative Study (NCGS), the spontaneous disappearance rate was reported to be less than 1.4 % during the 2-year study period, and, partial and complete dissolution in 8 out of 204 cases, or 3.9 % (Thistle et al., 1984). Using ultrasound examinations conducted 5 years apart in the same age- and sex-stratified random Danish population, Jensen et al found the spontaneous disappearance of gallstones to occur in 4.5 %; this was seen only with small gallstones (Jensen and Jørgensen, 1991).

Numerous oral litholytic agents have been tried, including Karlsbaderwasser, oral intake of water from a spa in Germany (Leo, 1914). The only effective agents known are chenodeoxycholic acid (Danzinger et al., 1972b), its isomer ursodeoxycholic acid (Sugata and Shimizu, 1974), and possibly HMG-CoA reductase inhibitor (Smit et al., 1992). However, the indication for chenodeoxycholic and ursodeoxycholic acids is limited. It requires a fairly long time and is effective in less than half of the cases, even when partial dissolution is included. Stones recur sooner or later in one-third to one-half of the cases. As a result, some patients remain diseased for life. In 1986 a new method, extracorporeal shock wave lithotripsy (ESWL), was introduced (Sauerbruch et al., 1986) to fragment gallstones in vivo by shock waves generated by various means. However, the apparatus required is extremely expensive and therefore not readily available. After their successful disappearance, gallstones recur in one-third to one-half of the cases.

Several solvents have been used in vivo to dissolve gallstones by direct contact, including methyl tert-butyl ether (Thistle et al., 1989). However, because of their low success rate and side effects, such as injury to the epithelial lininig of the biliary tract, this method does not enjoy wide acceptance.

## Oral cholelitholysis

Although disappearance of gallstones after the ingestion of bile salts in man has occasionally been reported (Rewbridge, 1937), ideal characteristics for an effective oral cholelitholytic agent were first proposed by Johnston et al. in 1957. The agent must (1) solubilize cholesterol readily, (2) flow continuously over the stones, (3) be nontoxic, and (4) be introduced into the biliary tree (Johnston and Nakayama, 1957). Several preparations containing bile acid were tried clinically including desiccated ox and hog gallbladder bile without success (Johnston and Irvin, 1947, Johnston and Nakayama, 1957). The use of chenodeoxycholic acid is planned but not tried clinically because enough supply could not be secured (Johnston and Nakayama, 1957). So far, the compounds meeting these requirements are chenodeoxycholic acid (Danzinger et al., 1972b) and its isomer, urosodeoxycholic acid (Sugata and Shimizu, 1974). The advantages of oral cholelitholysis are that (1) it does not require a special route of approach to the gallstones and (2) does not cause direct pain to the patient. Drawbacks are the fairly long period of time necessary to effect dissolution and the high rate of recurrence, as the site of gallstone formation, i.e., the gallbladder, remains.

### Chenodeoxycholic acid

Since the discovery of the disappearance of cholesterol crystals after the administration of chenodeoxycholic acid, but not cholic acid (Thistle and Schoenfield, 1971), and the introduction of chenodeoxycholic acid clinically as an effective oral cholelitholytic agent (Danzinger et al., 1972b), its efficacy has been repeatedly verified (Figure 25). Open as well as double-blind studies have been conducted (Schoenfield et al., 1981). A double-masked, placebo-controlled study, the National Cooperative Gallstone Study (NCGS), has been conducted to find a dose of chenodeoxycholic acid with an acceptable balance of dissolution and safety, and to identify the patients characteristics that predict dissolution.

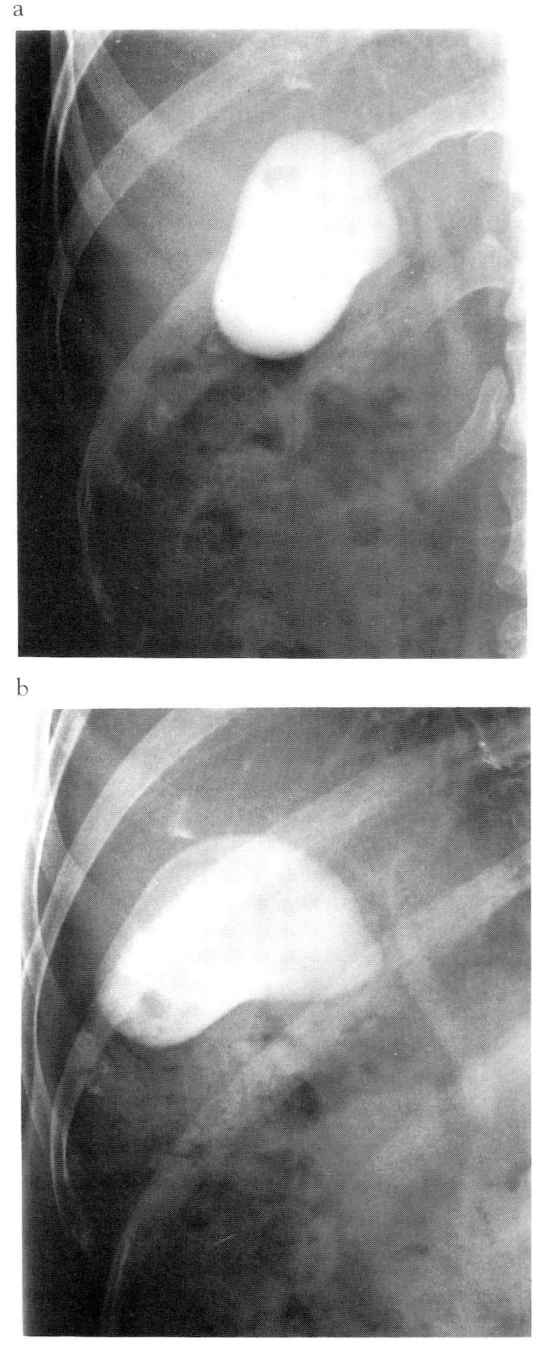

**Figure 25**

Oral Cholelitholysis

a: Cholecystogram before treatment; b: 4 months after chenodeoxycholic acid administration. Rapid disappearance of the stones is apparent.

Efficacy and safety were determined by randomly allocating chenodeoxycholic acid—750 mg/day or 375 mg/day or placebo administered for 2 years—to 916 patients for dissolution of radiolucent gallstones at 10 treatment centers in the United States. Complete dissolution occurred in 14 % and partial or complete dissolution in 41 % of those on 750 mg/day doses. Dissolution occurred more often in women, in patients with less than ideal body weight, in those with small stones (less than 17 mm, in diameter), and in those with floating stones or with high normal levels of serum cholesterol. Further, 23 % of those treated for more than 2 years had complete dissolution (Schoenfield et al., 1983). Efficacy has been reported to be slightly lower in Japan—around 35 % including partial dissolution (Nakayama, 1980). The difference in the success rates is probably due to the higher calcium content of gallstones in Japan compared with those in the United States and Europe (Miyake Jr et al., 1963). The optimal dose of chenodeoxycholic acid is suggested to be 15 mg/kg/day (Hofmann et al., 1978). Coupling of biliary lipids to different bile acids varies considerably. Cholic acid induces more biliary cholesterol secretion than does chenodeoxycholic acid; hence only the latter is an effective cholelitholytic agent (Einarsson and Grundy, 1980). There is a striking species difference. Chenodeoxycholic acid is not effective in squirrel monkeys (Tanaka et al., 1976). A spontaneous increase in chenodeoxycholic acid does not seem to reduce the cholesterol saturation of bile.

### Ursodeoxycholic acid

Gall of the bear, Kuma-no i, has been used for dyspepsia and biliary colic since ancient times in Japan and was probably derived from the Chinese pharmacopeia. Ursodeoxycholic acid is found to be present in the bile of the genus ursidae, including the Giant panda, Red panda, and 11 related carnivores, constituting 1–39 % of total bile acid (Hagey et al., 1993). In the 1950s, when bulk synthesis of ursodeoxycholic acid via chenodeoxycholic acid became possible (Kanazawa et al., 1954), ursodeoxycholic acid preparations, though still crude, became widely available in Japan and were used as cholagogues in a dose of 150 to 300 mg/day. A diminishing number of gallstones in 1967, followed by their disappearance after long-term administration of ursodeoxycholic acid, was reported by Sugata and Shimizu in four cases in 1974 (Sugata and Shimizu, 1974). Since then, open (Makino et al 1975, Nakagawa et al., 1977) as well as double-blind trials (Tokyo Cooperative Gallstone Study Group, 1980) have been conducted in Japan as well as in Belgium and France (Erlinger et al., 1984), Germany (Fromm et al., 1983), and Italy (Roda et al., 1982). The efficacy of ursodeoxycholic acid in dissolving gallstones is partial and complete dissolution occurred in 25.8 % of cases in open clinical trials with doses of 150 to 600 mg/day (Nakagawa et al., 1977); in multicenter cooperative, double-blind studies, dissolution occurred in 34.5 % on 600 mg/day and 17.4 %/day on 150 mg/day (Tokyo Cooperative Gallstone Study Group 1980). Higher doses result in earlier desaturation of bile and are likely to be more effective. Efficacy rose to 83.3 % in noncalcified floating stones less than 15 mm in diameter. Ursodeoxycholic acid administration prevents lithogenic changes of bile and subsequent formation of gallstones during weight loss (Broomfield et al., 1988). Practically no diarrhea or hepatotoxicity occurs. Liver histology remains normal (Maton et al., 1977).

Fasting gallbladder volume becomes even greater and gallbladder emptying further decreases compared with that in untreated gallstone patients (Festi et al., 1990). However, the mechanism by which ursodeoxycholic acid interferes with gallbladder motility is not known.

### Chenodeoxycholic acid versus ursodeoxycholic acid

Comparison of chenodeoxycholic and ursodeoxycholic acids was made with comparable doses collected from contemporary publications (Nakayama, 1980), since the cholelitholytic effect of both acids is dose dependent. Cases with a dose of 600 mg/day were chosen because that dose offered the largest number of cases for comparison and, at the same time, fell into the effective range of both chenodeoxycholic acid and ursodeoxycholic acid. Overall efficacy of ursodeoxycholic acid was 40.7 % in the open trials and 32.6 % in the double-blind trials, which seems comparable to that of chenodeoxycholic acid. Roda et al. studied 223 patients, comparing two different doses: 7–8 mg/kg and 14–15 mg/kg (Roda et al., 1982). They found that ursodeoxycholic acid is more efficacious than chenodeoxycholic acid after 3 and 6 months, but the difference disappeared after 12 months of treatment. This finding was in agreement with that of Fromm et al., who, in their double-blind, controlled trial, found the efficacy of ursodeoxycholic acid to be 60 % including complete and partial dissolution, compared to 47 % for chenodeoxycholic acid at 12 months. However, the difference disappeared after 24 months (Fromm et al., 1983). Most of the total dissolutions occurred during the first 6 months of treatment with ursodeoxycholic acid. They concluded that ursodeoxycholic acid is equally effective with both small and large stones and that chenodeoxycholic acid is effective at higher doses and on smaller stones. A Franco-Belgian double-blind, randomized, multicenter study showed that ursodeoxycholic acid is equally effective and induces diarrhea less frequently than chenodeoxycholic acid at an optimal dose of 8 mg/kg/day, achieving 55.2 % efficacy, including complete and partial dissolution (Erlinger et al., 1984). The optimal dose of ursodeoxycholic acid is 7–8 mg/kg/day, based on the findings of Roda et al. (1982) and Maton et al. (1977). The total bile acid pool expanded significantly in both groups (Fromm et al., 1983). The level of ursodeoxycholic acid is significantly lower than that of chenodeoxycholic acid. This may be attributable to the lower intestinal absorption of ursodeoxycholic acid; the rate of intestinal absorption of chenodeoxycholic acid is 77.6 % in man, while that of ursodeoxycholic acid varies considerably according to the dosage given, from 20.8 % to 60.3 % (Walker et al., 1992). Therefore, to achieve absorption of adequate amounts of ursodeoxycholic acid, higher and/or multiple doses are recommended. **Mechanism of action**: Chenodeoxycholic acid administration lowers both biliary cholesterol secretion and HMG-CoA reductase (Key et al., 1980). Chenodeoxycholic acid is a more potent inhibitor of hepatic HMG-CoA reductase than cholic acid (Ahlberg et al., 1981a). With hydrophobic bile acids such as chenodeoxycholic acid, gallstone dissolution proceeds largely via micelles (Park et al., 1984). On the other hand, with hydrophilic bile acid such as ursodeoxycholic acid, dissolution proceeds via two mechanisms (Salvioli et al., 1983), i.e., formation of micelles and vesicles. Chenodeoxycholic acid reduces the pool size as well as the synthesis rate of cholic acid. Ursodeoxycholic acid reduces the hepatic secretion of cholesterol more than does chenodeoxycholic acid (Nilsell et al., 1983). Enhanced conversion of cholesterol to bile acids may explain why ursodeoxycholic acid reduces biliary cholesterol output without suppressing cholesterol synthesis. Recently, ursodeoxycholic acid administration was found to increase nucleation time (Jüngst et al., 1989; Tazuma et al., 1989; Hirota et al., 1992). In a comparative study (Hirota et al., 1992), although both chenodeoxycholic acid and ursodeoxycholic acid prolonged nucleation time during oral cholelitholysis treatment, ursodeoxycholic acid extended nucleation time, mainly by decreasing the saturation index of bile. Chenodeoxycholic acid does so by lowering the cholesterol saturation index and shifting cholesterol from vesicles to micelles (Hirota et al., 1992). Thus, the distribution of cholesterol between vesicles and micelles is important in distinguishing the underlying mechanisms of these two oral cholelitholytic agents, as the vesicles are shown to play an important role in the crystallization of cholesterol in bile and nucleation occurs from vesicles (Halpern et al., 1986a, 1986b; Harvey et al., 1987; Peled et al., 1988; Schriever and Jüngst, 1989). Ursodeoxycholic acid seems to slow down the growth of cholesterol monohydrate crystals (Tazuma et al., 1989). Ursodeoxycholic acid lowers the cholesterol saturation index of bile without changing the total lipid concentration but has no effect on hepatic HMG-CoA reductase activity (Angelin et al., 1983, 1986). However, others found some effect on HMG-CoA reductase activity (Carulli et al., 1980; Salen et al., 1980; Maton et al., 1980). Ursodeoxycholic acid elevates the serum concentration of apolipoprotein A-I, one of the antinucleating factors (Tazuma et al., 1989), which is transported from plasma to bile. Changes in serum apolipoprotein A-I reflect those in bile (Sewell et al., 1983). Recently ursodeoxycholic acid was found to reduce gallbladder bile mucin and immunoglobulin, both potent pronucleating factors (Brugge et al., 1993). Ursodeoxycholic acid is as effective as chenodeoxycholic acid. Although the micellar solubility of ursodeoxycholic acid is poor, it solubilizes cholesterol by a nonmicellar mechanism, i.e., as aggregated vesicles or liquid crystals composed of PC and cholesterol (Halpern et al., 1986b). This is compatible with the finding that cholesterol gallstone dissolution by ursodeoxycholic acid occurs in spite of the rise in biliary cholesterol saturation (Fromm et al 1983), while chenodeoxycholic acid dissolves cholesterol stones by micellar solubilization (Hofmann, 1984b).

Obese subjects have supersaturated bile during weight maintenance as well as during rapid weight reduction (Bennion and Grundy, 1975) and are resistant to oral cholelitholytic agents (Iser et al., 1978). Chenodeoxycholic acid and ursodeoxycholic acid are effective in lowering the cholesterol saturation index of bile by reducing cholesterol output (Nilsell et al., 1983). Ursodeoxycholic acid is no more effective in obese subjects than during weight reduction (Mazzella et al., 1991). In obese subjects, markedly increased hepatic cholesterol secretion induces cholesterol saturation of bile during weight maintenance but also in the initial stage of weight reduction, probably because of a decrease in bile acid secretion which is not paralleled by a decrease in cholesterol secretion (Bennion and Grundy, 1975). The high level of cholesterol secretion is sustained because of the biliary secretion of cholesterol mobilized from the adipose tissue. This is also apparent from a study in which chenodeoxycholic acid became more effective when the obese subjects were placed on a hypocaloric diet (Mazzella et al., 1991). Ursodeoxycholic acid in a dose of 10 mg/kg/day is suitable during both weight-maintenance and weight reduction. Similar effects could probably be obtained with chenodeoxycholic acid by increasing it beyond the currently recommended dosage of 15 mg/kg/day (Thistle et al., 1977). However, this would involve an increase in the potential hepatotoxicity and enterotoxicity of chenodeoxycholic acid, with the appearance of frequent, usually mild, diarrhea and a slight transient elevation of serum transaminases (Schoenfield et al., 1981).

**Side effects**: During chenodeoxycholic acid treatment, clinically significant but reversible injury to the liver occurs in 3 % of patients. Serious liver damage can be avoided by careful monitoring of liver function. This marked difference in hepatotoxicity between chenodeoxycholic acid and ursodeoxycholic acid seems to be due to the difference in degradation to the potentially hepatotoxic metabolite (Palmer, 1972), i.e., lithocholic acid. Chenodeoxycholic acid and ursodeoxycholic acid are 7-dehydroxylated to lithocholic acid by intestinal flora (Danielsson et al., 1963). Ursodeoxycholic acid is more slowly converted to lithocholic acid than chenodoxycholic acid when incubated with intestinal flora because the $7\beta$-hydroxyl group of ursodeoxycholic acid is removed more slowly than the $7\alpha$-hydroxyl group of chenodeoxycholic acid (Fedorowski et al., 1979). However, no correlation was found between the hepatic function tests and the biliary level of lithocholic acid (Fromm et al., 1983). Lithocholic acid is considered to be a potential co-mutagen (Reddy and Watanabe, 1979). Sulfation of lithocholic acid protects against hepatic injury and is inversely related to the elevation of serum transaminase (Marks et al., 1981). The other possibility is the difference in the direct toxic effect on hepatocytes (Miyazaki et al., 1984). Chenodeoxycholic acid has a drastic effect on isolated human hepatocytes by reducing the number of microvilli and disrupting cell membranes, with a marked release of glutamic-oxaloacetic transaminase (GOT). In contrast, ursodeoxycholic acid produces only slight morphological changes and limited enzyme release. Electron paramagnetic resonance spectroscopy (EPR) shows that chenodeoxycholic acid solubilizes lipids in membranes, and permits water to permeate plasma membranes, producing increased polarity in the apolar domain of the membrane (Güldütuna et al., 1993b). In contrast, the steroid nucleus of ursodeoxycholic acid is bound to the apolar domain and that of its conjugates to the interface of the membrane, stabilizing membrane structure. Chenodeoxycholic acid damages mitochondria mainly by disrupting membrane proteins and releasing glutamate dehydrogenase (GLDH), while ursodeoxycholic acid prevents its occurrence in rat studies (Güldütuna et al., 1993a). Conjugation of the respective bile acids has a moderating effect.

The difference in the occurrence of diarrhea is probably due to the difference in the effect of the acids on the colon such as altered permeability and mucosal damage (Chadwick et al., 1976). The paucity of side effects permits the use of higher doses in ursodeoxycholic acid treatment. By contrast, diarrhea, although mostly transient, induces discontinuation of chenodeoxycholic acid at the initial stage of treatment. Ursodeoxycholic acid is preferable because of the near absence of side effects, such as diarrhea and a rise in hepatic transaminases. Ursodeoxycholic acid achieves a comparable or even superior dissolution rate (Nakayama, 1980; Roda et al., 1982; Fromm et al., 1983). Thus ursodeocycholic acid dissolves cholesterol stones faster, with fewer side effects at lower doses than does chenodeoxycholic acid.

**Indications:** Oral bile acid cholelitholysis may be indicated for radiolucent gallstones less than 15 mm in the largest diameter in the well-functioning gallbladder. Differentiation of would-be responders and nonresponders may be done by determining the lucency of gallstones on plain abdominal X-ray, computed tomography, saturation index, and the presence of cholesterol crystals in bile obtained endoscopically or by nasoduodenal intubation (Delchier et al., 1986; Van Erpecum et al., 1988; Janowitz et al., 1990; Agarwal et al., 1994). Relative contraindications include extreme obesity, choledocholithiasis (Thistle et al., 1978), obstruction of the cystic duct, severe symptoms, presence of liver disease, and fertility in women. Although radiopaque gallstones have been considered resistant to oral cholelitholysis (Tint et al., 1992), dissolution of calcified gallstones does occur (Nakayama, 1980). When a solitary gallstone with a calcified rim is first fragmented by ESWL, stone fragments become amenable to dissolution by bile acid treatment (Sackmann et al., 1992).

Clearly, chenodeoxycholic and ursodeoxycholic acids have a role in the treatment of selected patients with gallstones, such as those with a high probability of success and an increased operative risk. However, apart from the high dropout rate among those on chenodeoxycholic acid (Thistle et al., 1978; Schoenfield et al., 1981), the relatively low success rate, high recurrence rate after successful treatment, and slowness of dissolution hinder the wide acceptance of oral bile acid cholelitholytic treatment, especially given the recent introduction of other modalities of treatment such as ESWL and laparoscopic cholecystectomy.

### Bile acid analogues

In view of the limited success of chenodeoxycholic acid and ursodeoxycholic acid, we must develop new cholelitholytic agents with greater efficiency and less potential hepatotoxicity. Prevention of gallstone formation with highly hydrophilic hyodeoxycholic acid, murideoxychoic acid, and their $6\beta$-epimer is due to inhibition of the phase transition from vesicular cholesterol to crystalline cholesterol (Singhal et al., 1984b). In the prairie dog (Cohen et al., 1986) and the hamster (Cohen et al., 1990b), hyodeoxycholic acid and muricholic acid are more effective than ursodeoxycholic acid probably due to their greater capacity to form the liquid crystalline phase (Singhal et al., 1984a). Hyodeoxycholic acid is not suitable in man because this bile acid does not participate in the enterohepatic circulation; instead it is glucuronidated and excreted (Almé et al., 1978; Sacquet et al., 1983). Nonphysiological bile acids carry even less cholesterol during biliary secretion. Therefore, they may be better cholelitholytic agents, provided they are good micelle formers. Bile acid analogues modified at position C24 of the side chain, bile acid oxazolines, have been tried, as they were resistant to bacterial 7-dehydroxylation (Hylemon et al., 1982). Chenodeoxycholic acid oxazoline did not prevent gallstone formation or the appearance of cholesterol crystals in prairie dogs, while ursodeoxycholic acid oxazoline did (Cohen et al., 1984). 7-methyl analogue of chenodeoxycholic acid, $3\alpha$, $7\alpha$-dihydroxy-$7\beta$-methyl-$5\beta$-cholanoic acid (7-Me-CDCA), and of cholic acid, $3\alpha$, $7\alpha$, $12\alpha$-trihydroxy-$7\beta$-methyl-$5\beta$-cholanoic acid (7-Me-CA), were synthesized to avoid 7-dehydoxylation by intestinal flora during enterohepatic circulation (Matoba et al., 1989a). The former was effective in inhibiting gallstone formation in prairie dogs, but the latter was not. Both became predominant bile acids in bile. In the hamster, 7-methyl analogues of chenodeoxycholic acid, ursodeoxycholic acid, cholic acid, and ursocholic acid are well absorbed, efficiently extracted by the liver, and secreted in bile as glycine and taurine conjugates (Une et al., 1985; Kuroki et al., 1987a, 1987b). 7-Methylation effectively inhibits bacterial dehydroxylation of 7-hydroxyl groups. Next, 6-methyl analogues of hyodeoxycholic acid, $3\alpha$, $6\alpha$-dihydroxy-$6\beta$-methyl-$5\beta$-cholanoic acid, and muricholic acid, $3\alpha$, $6\beta$-dihydroxy-$6\alpha$-methyl-$5\beta$-cholanoic acid, were synthesized (Matoba et al., 1989b) and tried in the hamster (Cohen et al., 1990b), as hyodeoxycholic acid is effective in preventing cholesterol stone formation in the hamster (Dam et al., 1972b; Wheeler, 1973) and in the prairie dog (Singhal et al., 1984b, Cohen et al., 1986) and muricholic acid in the hamster (Cohen et al., 1990b) and prairie dog (Cohen et al., 1993). These bile acid analogues are absorbed rapidly, efficiently extracted by the liver, resecreted, and become major bile acids in bile (Matoba et al., 1989b). Introduction of the methyl group at the 6 position effectively prevents 6-dehydroxylation. Bile acid analogues with a modified side chain which is resistant to deconjugation by intestinal bacteria have been tried by Mosbach and his colleagues to avoid 7-dehydroxylation, which requires free carboxyl group in the side chain (Coleman et al., 1988), i.e., $3\alpha$, $7\alpha$-dihydroxy-24-nor-$5\beta$-cholan-23-sulfonate and $3\alpha$, $7\alpha$-dihydroxy-25-homo-$5\beta$-cholan-25-sulfonate (Miki et al., 1992), but with limited success. However, no transformation is noted during the enterohepatic circulation, and such bile acids became major biliary bile acids. Cholylsarcosine, a synthetic conjugate of cholic acid and sarcosine, is not metabolized, is resistant to deconjugation and dehydroxylation during enterohepatic circulation, and is nontoxic in man but increases biliary cholesterol and phospholipids secretion and is therefore not cholelitholytic (Schmassmann et al., 1993). Ornithine-conjugated bile acid, ornithocholanoic acid, which has been described in bile (Peric-Golia and Jones, 1962, 1963), with polarity characteristics intermediate between those of taurine- and glycine-conjugated bile acid, may have therapeutic potential.

One of the most serous drawbacks of oral bile acid cholelitholytic therapy is the high rate of gallstone recurrence (O'Donnell and Heaton, 1988; Villanova et al., 1989). It is suggested that the administration of erythromycin, a motilin receptor agonist, may prevent recurrence by eliminating a gallbladder motility defect frequently found in some gallstone patients (Catnach et al., 1992). Oral bile acid cholelitholytic agents are not effective with pigment gallstones.

### Modifier of cholesterol-bile acid metabolism

As early as in 1971, the cholesterol biosynthesis inhibitor AY 9944, trans-1,4-bis-(2-chlorobenzyl-aminomethyl)cyclohexane dihydrochloride, was shown to prevent gallstone

Table 10

**Prevention of Gallstone Formation in the Hamster by Cholesterol Biosynthesis Inhibitor AY-9944***

| | Number of animals | Cholesterol stones | Pigment stones | No stones |
|---|---|---|---|---|
| Without AY-9944 | 34 | 18 | 0 | 16 |
| With AY-9944 | 34 | 3 | 0 | 31 |

* Trans-1,4-bis-(2-chlorobenzylaminomethyl)cyclohexane dehydrochloride

Source: Van der Linden et al. (1971).

formation in hamsters (Table 10) (Van der Linden et al., 1971). Later, HMG-CoA reductase inhibitors such as simvastatin and pravastatin decreased biliary cholesterol saturation in patients with familial hypercholesterolemia (Duane et al., 1988a; Hoogerbrugge van der Linden., et al 1990; Reinhér et al., 1990b). In healthy volunteers, Mitchell et al. found that inhibition of cholesterol synthesis by lovastatin, a competitive inhibitor of HMG-CoA reductase, lowers biliary cholesterol saturation in bile by selective reduction of cholesterol secretion in bile; bile acid and perhaps PC secretions are also reduced (Mitchell et al., 1991a) or not altered (Duane, 1994). Bile acid pool size and perhaps bile acid synthesis are also reduced. Thus, they may constitute the direct evidence of an association between cholesterol synthesis and secretion in man by using an inhibitor to induce primary inhibition of cholesterol synthesis. Combined use of lovastatin and chenodeocycholic acid was found to lower biliary cholesterol saturation significantly more than either agent used alone (Hanson and Duane, 1994). The first case of gallstone disappearance after the administration of pravastatin was recently reported (Smit et al., 1992). Successful treatment with an HMG-CoA reductase inhibitor, such as lovastatin or simvastatin in conjunction with ursodeoxycholic acid has been reported (Logan and Duane, 1990; Bateson, 1990). This combination seems to be more effective than ursodeoxycholic acid used alone. Thus HMG-CoA reductase inhibitor may be of value when an additional indication is present, such as in hypercholesterolemia. However, the proportion of chenodeoxycholic acid in gallbladder bile is found to be reduced during the treatment with pravastatin, one of the HMG-CoA reductase inhibitors (Reinhér et al., 1990b). There is a reciprocal relationship between percent deoxycholic acid and percent chenodeoxycholic acid in bile (Pomare and Low Beer, 1975). Thus, this effect of HMG-CoA reductase inhibitor on bile acid compostion in bile may have adverse effect in terms of gallstone formation as the increase of deoxycholic acid in bile is associated with gallstone disease (Marcus and Heaton, 1988). Recently cisapride, a prokinetic agent, has been tested in ground squirrels on a 1 % cholesterol diet. It prevented cholesterol crystal formation and markedly reduced cholesterol saturation by shifting biliary composition toward normal. This was accomplished by enhancing gallbladder (and possibly intestinal) motility and cycling of bile acid pool, thereby increasing bile salt secretion (Xu and Shaffer, 1993b). Theoretically, gallstone formation could be prevented by reducing the cholesterol available for biliary cholesterol secretion, increasing of the enzyme activity for conversion of cholesterol to bile acid, and increasing biliary bile acid secretion, thus enhancing the cholesterol solubility of bile. The lack of understanding of the metabolic basis of gallstone disease is hindering the development of a truly gallstone-specific treatment.

## Contact dissolution agents

Infusion of various solvents into the bile duct has been tried to dissolve gallstones. Monooctanoin (Capmul 8210, predominantly glyceryl mono-octanoate) has been used successfully to dissolve gallstones present in the bile duct by introducing it, via a choledochostomy tube or retrograde biliary catheter through a duodenal fiberscope, when nonoperative extraction through a tube tract or endoscopic extraction, crushing, or sphincterotomy is impossible or unsuccessful (Hofmann et al., 1981). The side effects are limited to pain, nausea, vomiting, and diarrhea; efficacy is 66 % including partial dissolution. In 1985, methyl tert-butyl ether (MTBE), an octane enhancer, aliphatic ether with low viscosity, was introduced as a gallstone-dissolving agent (Allen et al., 1985). MTBE is less viscous than monooctanoin and dissolves cholesterol stones more readily. In 75 patients treated with MTBE instilled through a percutaneous transhepatic catheter and aspirated from the gallbladder four to six times per day for an average 5 hours daily for 1 to 3 days (Thistle et al., 1989), the success rate was 95 % with debris remaining in 68 % of the cases. Of these 29 % the residual debris eventually cleared spontaneously. As calcium bilirubinate and calcium carbonate are the principal components of MTBE-insoluble debris, radiological criteria of radiolucency should be met (Nelson et al., 1990). However, post-MTBE debris has been successfully cleared by infusion of two solvents, i.e., EDTA/sulfobetain-12/urea/1,4-dithioerythritol solvent adjusted to pH 9.5 and citric acid and sulfobetain adjusted to pH 3.95 to 4.15 were used to decrease stone recurrence after MTBE treatment (Wosiewitz and Sabinski, 1993). The latter achieved a success rate of as much as 100 %. Addition of dimethylsulfoxide (DMSO) to MTBE accelerates gallstone dissolution from 220 to 130 minutes (Bergman et al., 1994), as DMSO is miscible with aqueous media such as bile and enhances stone-solvent contact; furthermore, it is capable of dissolving stone-matrix bilirubin (Bergman et al., 1994). MTBE and MTBE/DMSO are superior to ethyl propionate used alone (Esch et al., 1993) as solvents for cholesterol gallstones. An automatic pump system for delivery and recovery of MTBE has been developed (Zakko et al., 1989); however, some contend that it offers no advantage over the use of hand syringe and raising the temperature of MTBE to 37°C (Lauffer et al., 1993). A percutaneous transhepatic catheter can be placed with ultrasound guidance, without serious complications, and substantial leakage of bile after removal of the catheter is infrequent. Radiolucency of gallstones on CT scan is another criterion for MTBE treatment, as the calcification of stones resists the dissolution. It was concluded that MTBE dissolution treatment is a useful alternative to surgery in selected patients with symptomatic cholesterol gallstones. The effect of MTBE on gallbladder in man has been critically examined by Van Sonnenberg et al (1991). Typical inflammatory findings of chronic cholecystitis are observed, with acute changes superimposed . The changes are most conspicuous in the submucosal layer; the mucosa and serosa are almost intact. Mild acute inflammatory changes are noted in the submucosal layer 1 to 2 weeks after instillation, but these are transient and reversible. No ulceration of the mucosa and no unusual wall thickening or fibrosis are observed. There seems to be reasonable patient tolerance. Therefore, it was concluded that MTBE has an acceptable margin of safety when instilled at controlled and appropriate volumes or pressure and removed properly from the gallbladder after the procedure. However, gallstone recurrence occurred in 20% of the cases 6 to 16 months after complete dissolution (Thistle et al., 1989), as the site of cholesterol stone formation, i.e., the gallbladder, remains in situ. In contrast, infusion of MTBE into the bile duct had little success, probably because the solvent escaped into the duodenum, causing duodenitis and possible ulceration (DiPadova et al., 1986; Van Sonnenberg et al., 1988).

Since cholesterol stones contain an organic matrix composed of macromolecular complexes of mucin and bile pigment forming a structural part of the gallstones (Sutor and Wooley, 1974a; Smith and LaMont, 1985), mucolytic thiol reducing agents such as 2-mercaptoethanol (2ME) and N-acetylcysteine (NAcCys) have been tried in conjunction with monooctanoin, i.e., the former to dissolve gallstone matrix and the latter cholesterol. Both agents partially solubilize isolated organic matrix and accelerate gallstone dissolution by monooctanoin two to threefold by releasing a high molecular weight mucin-bilirubin complex and unbound pigment from the insoluble matrix (Smith and LaMont, 1985). During dissolution, concentric layers of organic matrix are exposed. N-acetylcysteine, a mucolytic agent, significantly increases the frequency of complete gallstone dissolution, but only a minority of patients achieve this (Niu and Smith, 1990). Similarly, streptokinase has been suggested to be an effective adjuvant to bile acid therapy, affecting PAS-positive material present in gallstones (Sanchez and Esquivel, 1991). Thus mucolytic agents may constitute adjuvant therapy to increase the efficacy of contact cholelitholysis. Pigmented shell of the organic matrix on the surface of gallstones and calcification hinder complete gallstone dissolution. However, since N-acetylcysteine administered orally is not excreted in bile in the concentration required to accelerate stone dissolution, it cannot be used as an additive to the oral bile acid cholelitholysis treatment of cholesterol stones (Kohse et al., 1992).

Brown pigment stones are often resistant to contact dissolution agents designed for cholesterol stones, as their compositions differ considerably. Recently, buffered 1% ethylenediaminetetraacetic acid (EDTA) 2Na was used for dissolution of pigment stones (Wosiewitz et al., 1989). The maximum effect is achieved by the addition of sodium taurocholate and N-acetylcysteine. Addition of the latter greatly facilitates the dissolution of brown pigment stones but not of black pigment stones. Other solvent mixtures have been tried for the dissolution of brown pigment stones (Dai et al., 1989). One is a mixture of EDTA, sodium deoxycholic acid, monoolein and DMSO, which is effective in dissolving calcium and bilirubin. The other solvent is a mixture of DMSO and MTBE effective for dissolution of cholesterol and bilirubin. Alternate perfusions by these two solvents are more effective than either one used separately. Histotoxicity to the gallbladder mucosa is claimed to be slight.

## Extracorporeal shock wave lithotripsy (ESWL)

The first successful fragmentation of gallstones by ESWL was reported in 1986 (Sauerbruch et al., 1986). Shock waves produced by ESWL consist of high-amplitude pressure fronts followed by a negative pressure of much lower magnitude but with a longer duration. Shock waves converge on the stones to be fragmented.

### Mechanism of action

Theories pertaining to the mechanism of gallstone fragmentation can be grouped into three categories (Vakil and Everbach, 1991).

**Transient acoustic cavitation:** Microscopic bubbles of gas in the bile around the gallstone expand during the negative pressure portion of the acoustic shock wave. When the cavitation produced by this negative pressure collapses, the effects of the shock wave disappear. The violent collapse of the microbubbles creates a minute jet of bile striking at a velocity capable of reaching 200 m/sec, which damages the surface and fragments the stones.

**Stress fracture:** The incident acoustic shock wave produces a compressional wave within the gallstone which propagates through the stone until it reaches a discontinuity, such as the posterior surface of the stone. The compressional wave, then reflects from the surface as a tension wave which propagates back through the stone. If the magnitude of the tension wave exceeds the tensile strength of the stone, fracture results.

**Flaw theory:** The shock wave induces propagation of the crack and fracture because of the pre-existing structural flaws. The presence of gas within the stone promotes fragmentation, since the energy required for incident shock is less if the material filling the crack is compressive, such as gas, rather than incompressive, such as liquid or solid.

### Systems available

Four different systems are used to generate shock waves for ESWL: (1) the spark-gap system, (2) the piezoelectric system, (3) the electromagnetic system, and (4) the microexplosive system. All are capable of fragmenting gallstones in clinical cases; there seems to be no difference in their efficacy and safety. Although each system generates shock waves by a different method, all of them appear to fragment gallstones. However, no system has demonstrated clear clinical superiority in terms of either efficacy or safety (Chapman et al., 1989). Care must be taken that significant tissue damage does not occur when shock waves pass through body tissues with large air content, such as the lung or a hollow viscus (Sauerbruch et al., 1986; Delius et al., 1987; Chapman et al., 1989; Ell et al., 1990). ESWL has been used for stones both in the gallbladder and in the common bile duct. In the spark-gap shock wave lithotripsy system, high-energy shock waves with pressure amplitudes of up to 1,000 bar and a pulse duration of about 1 msec are generated by high current spark discharge. The waves thus produced converge by a semiellipsoid reflector on the second focal point, where the gallstones to be fragmented are placed (Sauerbruch et al., 1986). Although at the beginning this system necessitated immersion of the patient in a water bath, the second-generation spark-gap system currently in use merely requires attachment of a water bag or small minitank to the generator. In the piezoelectric shock wave lithotripsy system, piezoceramic crystals are used to produce either an ultrasonic wave, which is focused on spherical converging waves, or a plane wave, focused by a lens to convert it to converging waves. Ultrasonic waves produced become shock waves near the focal point (Stephenson et al., 1989; Albert et al., 1990; Ell et al., 1990). In the electromagnetic shock wave lithotripsy system, an electric current is pulsed through a coil placed just beneath a metal plate. The current is accelerated by the force of the magnetic field, producing a high-pressure wave. This plane wave is focused by an acoustic lens, producing a high-intensity focal zone where the stones are placed (Staritz et al., 1990). In the microexplosive shock wave lithotripsy system, the principle is the same as that of the spark-gap shock wave lithotripsy system. A minimal amount of explosive in the form of a silver azide or lead azide pellet is placed at the first focal point of semiellipsoidal reflector. The shock waves produced are reflected to converge on the second focal point, fragmenting the stones (Takayama and Kitayama, 1988). The piezoelectric system produces a smaller, high-intensity focal zone, but the pressure within this zone is greater than that generated by the second-generation spark-gap generator. The total energy per pulse and the width of the high-intensity focal zone of the electromagnetic shock wave system are intermediate between those of the spark-gap and piezoelectric systems (Petersen et al., 1988).

### Indications and results

The indications for ESWL include (1) abdominal pain attributable to gallstones, (2) one to three radiolucent gallstones with a maximum diameter of 25 mm, (3) a functioning gallbladder, as verified by oral cholecystography, (4) technical feasibility of cannulation of the common bile duct, as assessed by ERC, and (5) absence of lung tissue in the path of the shock wave (Sauerbruch et al., 1986). The most useful diagnostic procedure before and during the treatment is ultrasonography, which is noninvasive, giving information on the number and size of gallstones present in the gallbladder and possibly on the kind of gallstones. Only 20 % of gallstones are said to be suitable for ESWL (Neubrand et al., 1986). The newer generations of electromagnetic and piesoelectric apparatuses (Ell et al., 1990) are far better tolerated. Pulverization, an end point of ESWL, i.e., fragmentation into echogenic dust or particles similar to grains of sand, can be achieved by the newer generation of ESWL apparatuses for both noncalcified and calcified gallstones with remarkable frequency, i.e., in 96.1 % (Sohendra et al., 1994). The gallstone clearance rate is somewhat less for calcified stones (89.5 %) than for noncalcified stones (94.3 %) at 18–24 months of follow-up. Clearance of the fragments produced should be judged by either ultrasonography or oral cholecystography. Gallbladder emptying seems to be an important determinant of gallstone clearance (Pauletzki et al., 1994). The indication for ESWL is being expanded to common bile duct stones (Benes et al., 1989; Bland et al., 1989; Groen et al., 1989c; Moody et al., 1989a; Sauerbruch et al., 1989; Ponchon et al., 1990; Brückner et al., 1990), solitary stone with calcified rims (Sackmann et al., 1992), and even intrahepatic calculi (Lointier et al., 1990). ESWL facilitates endoscopic extraction of large bile duct stones (Vandermeeren et al., 1993). Failures are due to inability to focus on the stones or to

Mirizzi's syndrome. Adverse effects of ESWL have been noted, such as biliary colic in one-third and macroscopic hematuria in 4% of the cases (Munoz-Ortiz et al., 1993a). Contraindications include nonfunctioning gallbladder, subcostal gallbladder location, multiple stones occupying more than three-fourths of the gallbladder volume, acute cholecystitis, cholangitis, pancreatitis, bile duct obstruction, pregnancy, coagulopathy, aneurysm, and liver cyst. The rate of recurrence after ESWL is similar to that after the oral cholelitholysis (Sackmann et al., 1990, 1994; Munoz-Ortiz et al., 1993b). Recurrent stones are usually small ($6 \pm 5$ mm) and associated with recurrent biliary pain in more than half of the cases (Sackmann et al., 1994). Repeated ESWL and/or bile acid medication resulted in stone disappearance in half of the cases (Sackmann et al., 1994). After complete clearance of gallstones, supersaturation of bile was found in 8/10 patients in each group, with or without gallstone recurrence; nucleation time was abnormal in one-half of the cases (Berr et al., 1994). Those with recurrent stones had smaller bile acid pools, enhanced conversion of cholic acid to deoxycholic acid, and incomplete emptying of the gallbladder.

## Combined ESWL and oral cholelitholysis

Oral cholelitholytic agents such as ursodeoxycholic acid have been tried in conjunction with ESWL to facilitate dissolution of gallstones, as the disintegration of gallstones allows bile salts to dissolve gallstones and the speed of dissolution may be enhanced. ESWL with the spark-gap shock wave system was tested, with and without ursodeoxycholic acid treatment, on 85 patients with radiolucent gallstones (Tint et al., 1992). Biliary lithotripsy plus ursodeoxycholic acid increases efficacy twofold compared to ursodeoxycholic acid alone, i.e., 47% and 22% respectively, of subjects are gallstone free. Product-limit analysis showed that the efficacy of stone dissolution increases from a low with ursodeoxycholic acid alone, to a higher level with lithotripsy-ursodeoxycholic acid, and to the highest level with lithotripsy-ursodeoxycholic acid pretreated with ursodeoxycholic acid. Similar mean gallstone dissolution constants (stone size/time to disappear) of fragments and whole gallstones during ursodeoxycholic acid treatment suggested that most fragments disappear by dissolution, not by expulsion. Therefore, even partial fragmentation by ESWL is likely to accelerate gallstone clearance. However, during the first days after lithotripsy, small stone fragments can be recovered from feces (Greiner et al., 1990). Gallbladder emptying is also thought to play an important role in mechanical evacuation of the fragment (Pauletzki et al., 1994). Gallstone calcification has been thought to interfere with gallstone fragmentation therapy. However, recently, Sackmann and his colleagues expanded the indication to solitary gallstones with a calcified rim (Sackmann et al., 1992). Using a Dornier water-cushion lithotripter at a high power setting followed by adjuvant ursodeoxycholic acid dissolution therapy, they achieved a fragment clearance rate of 38% after 5 to 8 months and 68% after 13 to 18 months. The speed of dissolution is somewhat less than those reported for radiolucent gallstones (Sackmann et al., 1988, 1991).

## Percutaneous cholecystolithotripsy

Percutaneous extraction of gallstones from gallbladder was carried out in five stages using the transhepatic tract, in 1985 (Akiyama et al., 1985; Kerlan et al., 1985; Nagakawa et al., 1985). Subsequently, Kellett et al. adapted the techniques and instruments of percutaneous nephrolithotomy for the extraction of gallstones to safeguard against the possibly dangerous obstructive complications of ESWL (Kellett et al., 1988). The subcostal approach through a peritoneal cavity is used to avoid the hepatic bleeding on dilation of the track accompanying the transhepatic approach formerly used. The procedure can be carried out in a single stage under general anesthesia or using local anesthesia with intravenous sedation. The advantages of percutaneous cholecystolithotomy lie in the fact that (1) it is applicable to removal of gallbladder stones irrespective of their size, number, and composition; (2) neither a patent cystic duct nor a functioning gallbladder is required; (3) it is a single-stage procedure; (4) the success rate is high—over 90% of the stone removal (Chiverton et al., 1990; Cheslyn-Curtis et al., 1992; Donald et al., 1994); (5) removal of gallstones is done speedily.

Indications for percutaneous cholecystolithotomy include (l) a small but ever-increasing group of medically unfit, frail, elderly, and high-risk patients and (2) unsuccessful cases of ESWL. Contraindications include (1) acute complications of gallstone disease and (2) gallstone impaction in the neck or the cystic duct. Caution is necessary in treating a thickset patient as the gallbladder may be too far from the skin surface; dilators and sheaths ordinarily available may well be not long enough to reach the gallbladder (Kellett et al., 1988). Some authors maintain that even an impacted stone in Hartmann's pouch can be managed by percutaneous cholecystolithotomy, with prior drainage of the gallbladder transperitoneally for 1 week to 10 days to allow the stone to disimpact, making it easier to dislodge (Cheslyn-Curtis et al., 1992). These authors also claim that acute complications of gallstone disease can be managed by drainage of the gallbladder, allowing acute inflammation to subside before stone extraction. There is no doubt that the acute situation can be managed safely by gallbladder drainage before the definitive procedure is undertaken. However, the safety and efficacy of percutaneous cholecystolithotomy in this situation are questionable because of the difficulties involved in dislodging the impacted gallstone; handling the acutely inflamed gallbladder, with its frail wall; and conducting a thorough examination. Standard open cholesycstectomy is recommended as a definitive procedure which permits a good examination of the local anatomic structure under direct vision, followed by careful dissection and safe removal of the gallbladder together with the stones in toto.

Kellett et al. give a good description of the operative procedure (Kellett et al., 1988). After anesthesia is introduced, drapes are placed on the patient to collect the endoscopic irrigant. With the use of ultrasound to localize the gallbladder, a 1-cm puncture is made subcostally and a 152-mm-long indwelling sheathed needle is passed into the gallbladder. A guide wire is introduced through the sheath and a 7-Fr pigtail catheter is advanced to aspirate bile from the gallbladder and minimize spillage. The gallbladder is flushed with saline and filled with dilute contrast medium. Under fluoroscopic control, the tract is dilated with a 28-Fr balloon on a 9-Fr catheter. On removal of the balloon catheter, an Amplatz dilator is passed, followed by a 28-Fr Teflon sheath, which is advanced well into the gallbladder under fluoroscopic control, taking care not to invaginate the muscular wall of the gallbladder. After removal of the dilator, but not the guide wire,—which is maintained in the gallbladder throughout the procedure, a Wolf nephroscope is introduced and small stones are removed with alligator forceps under direct vision. The gallbladder is drained for 7–10 days. Then a cholecystogram is obtained to ascertain the absence of gallstones left behind, the absence of leakage of contrast medium into the peritoneal cavity, and the free flow of contrast medium into the common duct and duodenum.

The advantages of percutaneous cholecystolithotomy are its wider application compared to oral cholelithilysis (Maton et al., 1982) and ESWL (Brink et al., 1988); its shorter convalescence period compared to standard open cholecystectomy, oral cholelitholysis (Schoenfield et al., 1981), and ESWL (Sackmann et al., 1991); and the high success rate of stone removal. The main objection to any method which preserves the gallblader is the gallstone recurrence. Recently, Dempsey reviewed the rate of gallstone recurrence after surgical cholecystolithotomy in 2,053 patients described in 23 reports published during the past 36 years and found it to be 34.6 % (Dempsey, cited by Kellett et al., 1988). Recurrence of gallstones after percutaneous cholecystolithotomy is not inevitable. However, the cumulative proportion of gallstone recurrence was reported to be 19 % after 12 months and 28 % after 24 months, with a plateau after 42 months (Donald et al., 1994), comparable to the rates reported for oral cholelitholysis (O'Donnel and Heaton, 1988; Villanova et al., 1989) and ESWL (Sackmann et al., 1990, 1994; Munroz-Ortiz et al., 1993b). Early recurrence after percutaneous cholecystolithotomy may be a result of incomplete clearance of the gallbladder, which is not detected by radiological examination. Since tiny fragments, adherent to or embedded in the gallbladder mucosa, are difficult to remove completely, adjuvant cholelitholysis with either chenodeoxycholic acid or ursodeoxycholic acid is added (Donald et al., 1994). The recurrence rate is found to be slightly less in those with adjuvant treatment. Ablation of the gallbladder mucosa by thermal or chemical injury has been attempted to forestall later recurrence of stones (Nagakawa, 1989).

## Standard (open)cholecystectomy

### Indications

The absolute indication for standard open cholecystectomy is advanced acute cholecystitis with an inherent danger of perforation due to gangrenous change showing signs of peritoneal involvement, gallbladder empyema, and pericholecystic abscess. In case of choledocholithiasis with clinical jaundice, after careful preoperative evaluation of the possible cause of jaundice, standard open cholecystectomy and the removal of common bile duct stones via choledochotomy and choledochal drainage are indicated. When severe biliary tract infection such as acute supprative cholangitis and liver abscess are present, biliary decompression by direct drainage via the percutaneous transhepatic route or via the duodenal papilla using the endoscopic retrograde approach is in order.

However, there is controversy regarding the relative indications for operative intervention. After careful evaluation of the biliary tract pathology both at present and in the past, and physical examination followed by abdominal ultrasonography, indirect cholecystocholangiography such as oral and intravenous cholecystography and direct cholangiography such as ERCP and PTC, the choice of treatment should be individualized. When jaundice is present, it should be followed up for 2 weeks, unless signs of severe infection are present, for the sign of remission as the jaundice accompanying cholelithiasis often fluctuates. If the gallstone attacks recur frequently, with fever and jaundice, operative intervention is recommended during the remission period. In addition, even if the symptoms are not severe but nevertheless disturb the daily routine, definitive treatment is in order, as the gallstones rarely disappear spontaneously (Wolpers, 1968). Even in silent gallstones, the symptoms eventually appear in one-third to one-half of the cases (Wenckert and Robertson, 1966). Cholecystectomy can best be carried out safely and easily when the disease is confined to a gallbladder with few if any signs of inflammation. There seems to be an added risk of developing gallbladder carcinoma in the course of gallstone disease; the incidence of gallbladder carcinoma is considerably higher than in those without gallstones (Piehler and Crichlow, 1978). Hence earlier removal of the gallbladder is recommended.

Operative procedure is carried out after generous laparotomy in either antegrade or retrograde fashion. Upper midline, pararectal, and transrectal incisions are preferred because of the ease of opening and closing the abdominal cavity and the good operative field obtainable. In extremely obese patients, a right subcostal incision is used to secure good exposure. Upon entering the abdominal cavity, the state of the gallbladder is assessed, including adhesion to the surrounding structure; thickening of the wall; the presence of gallstones; the color, surface, and consistency of the liver, stomach, and duodenum; and the consistency of the pancreas and Douglas cavity.

After a thorough examination of the viscera, attention is focused to the biliary tract. For cholecystectomy, two modes are available. The first is retrograde cholecystectomy, and the second is antegrade cholecystectomy. Dissection proceeds from the cystic duct toward the fundus in the former and in the opposite direction in the latter. For retrograde cholecystectomy, retraction of the inferior surface of the liver upward and downward traction of the duodenum with the assistant's left hand reveal Calot's triangle, i.e., an area surrounded by the inferior surface of the liver, the common hepatic duct, and the cystic duct are exposed to avoid possible injury to the cystic artery and cystic duct at a later stage. To dissect out the cystic duct and cystic artery safely, a small volume of physiological saline is injected into Calot's triangle. After incising the peritoneum covering the triangle in a Y-shape, the fat tissue surrounding the cystic duct and cystic artery is carefully dissected away, using gauze held by a forceps (Zupfer), as anomalies are often encountered. The cystic artery is doubly ligated with nonabsorbable thread and divided. Next the cystic duct is ligated near the infundibulum to avoid inadvertent passing of gallstones into common bile duct and for use as traction to stretch the cystic duct from its usual tortuous course. Subsequently, a nonabsorbable thread is passed behind the cystic duct using right angle forceps. A small incision is made with a small, pointed knife, avoiding division of the cystic duct.

A small-caliber plastic tube is inserted through the cut into the cystic duct for operative cholangiography. X-ray exposure is made toward the end while contrast medium is being injected to reveal the terminal portion of the common bile duct. After evaluation of the operative cholangiogram, the tube is withdrawn, the cystic duct is doubly ligated with non-absorbable thread, and the duct is divided. To effect almost bleeding-free dissection of the gallbladder bed, the lateral portions of the serosa are inflated with physiological saline and the serosa is incised from the cystic duct side toward the fundus. The gallbladder bed is closed by approximating the serosal edges around it. Complications may occur during cholecystectomy, such as bile duct injury, arterial injury, and bleeding (Jones, 1990).

## Laparoscopic cholecystectomy

Dr. Phillipe Mauret, a gynecologist at the Clinique de la Sauvegarde, Lyon, France, initiated cholecystectomy by laparoscopic means in 1987 (Mauret, 1987). The advantage of this method is that it requires four small incisions in the abdominal wall; therefore, only barely visible scars remain postoperatively. Since 1987, this method has spread rapidly worldwide, including the United States, Europe, and Asia. However, it is important to note that it has several drawbacks. Complications range from injuries to neighboring structures to spillage of gallstones into the peritoneal cavity (Lee et al., 1993). It is well known that many anomalies and transpositions occur in the hepatobiliary region (Lindner and Green, 1964). Since the laparoscope offers only a very limited operative field in comparison to the standard open cholecystectomy, with wide generous laparotomy, more injuries are likely to occur to the common bile duct, the right hepatic duct, and even the portal vein. To my knowledge, the last in fact has occurred in a few cases. Accessory ducts draining a portion of the right hepatic lobe occur in 8–18 % of cases (Maingot, 1974). Once injury occurs, leakage of bile ensues, followed by the formation of a bile fistula, which later requires either fistuloenterostomy (Roux-en-Y) or resection of the hepatic segment draining to the injured accessory duct. Bile duct injury during laparoscopic cholecystectomy is reported to occur in 0.5–2.7 % of cases in the United States (Peters et al., 1991; Salky et al., 1991; Berci and Sackier, 1991; Zucker et al., 1991), 0.33 % in Europe (Cushieri et al., 1991), and 1–2 % in Japan (Kimura et al., 1991). These rates are remarkably higher than those reported for standard open cholecystectomy, i.e., 0.1–0.2 % in most institutions (Cosman and Porter, 1960). The incidence reported may seem low, but when a bile duct injury occurs, it is a major catastrophe to the patient and a grave matter for the surgeons concerned. When a bile duct injury is suspected during laparoscopic cholecystectomy, one must revert to standard open cholecystectomy, with wide, generous laparotomy with an excellent operative field, followed by meticulous identification of the anatomic structures, especially around Calot's triangle. Careful bile duct repair should be carried out, hopefully for a permanent cure. For this reason, laparoscopic cholecystectomy should be carried out by surgeons who are experienced in hepatobiliary surgery, especially with a long experience with standard open cholecystectomy.

Furthermore, operative cholangiography is often difficult, if not impossible, to perform during laparoscopic cholecystectomy; therefore, a common bile duct stone may be missed. In addition, no examination can be made around the duodenal papilla, and diseases in the hepatobiliary pancreatic region may be overlooked. The actual procedure takes more time than is usually required by standard open cholecystectomy, i.e., 1 to 1 1/2 half hours, and longer anesthesia time is required. However, one advantage of laparoscopic cholecystectomy is the paucity of recurrence of gallstones postoperatively as for standard open cholecystectomy, since the gallbladder, the site of gallstone formation, is removed. Hence, while choosing the best method of treatment, the advantages and disadvantages of each procedure should be weighed and the method should be individualized to suit the particular case.

## Indication

The indications are essentially the same as those for standard open cholecystectomy, except in malignancy, where the meticulous dissection and identification of the anatomic structures are necessary. They include benign gallbladder diseases such as uncomplicated cholecystolithiasis, gallbladder polyps and adenomyomatosis. Indications are being extended to acute cholecystitis (Qureshi et al., 1993b). A low threshold for conversion to open cholecystectomy reduces the morbidity state. Indications for gallbladder polyps are limited to cases when the size of the polyp exceeds 10 mm. However, even if it is less than 10 mm, if it has a tendency to grow rapidly, removal of the gallbladder is recommended. In this connection, laparoscopic cholecystectomy is not advised when an exact pathological examination is required later, such as for the possible presence of malignancy, as the gallbladder requires manipulation during extraction from the abdominal cavity via the small incision in the abdominal wall.

Laparoscopic cholecystectomy is not indicated for various benign biliary tract diseases such as choledocholithiasis, hepatolithiasis or intrahepatic calculi, acute cholecystitis, and acute cholangitis, as well as severe liver cirrhosis, acute pancreatitis, localized peritonitis, advanced duodenal ulcer, a past history of operative intervention of the upper abdominal cavity, and upper abdominal trauma. The presence of jaundice, pregnancy, a hemorrhagic tendency, abdominal malignancy, portal hypertension, and renal insufficiency, as well as inability to tolerate general anesthesia, constitute contraindications. The above indications for laparoscopic cholecystectomy vary considerably depending on the expertise, advancement of operative techniques, and ability of the surgeons performing the procedure. Complications include bile duct injury, bile leaks, and perihepatic collections (Qureshi et al., 1993b).

Since a variety of treatment modalities for gallstone disease became available recently, and since their cost has mounted, cost-effective analysis (CEA) has been increasingly advocated, such as curtailing the length of the hospital stay required (Bass et al., 1991; Fendrick, 1992). A randomized clinical trial on ESWL versus laparoscopic cholecystectomy in the United States shows that total disability attributable to cholelithiasis was 6.8 days for ESWL and 23 days for laparoscopic cholecystectomy (Barkun et al., 1993). However, the choice of the procedure should be weighed carefully to determine how a complete cure is best attained with the least risk to the patient. It should not be influenced by nonmedical reasons such as requests from the patients, i.e., it should not be "consumer driven" (Cameron and Gadacz, 1991).

## Contact lithotripsy

Mechanical lithotripsy is simplest and is done by specially designed baskets (Rieman et al., 1982; Schneider et al., 1988). However, difficulties are encountered in grabbing either voluminous, impacted, or poorly accessible stones. Pulsed dye laser lithotripsy is used for bile duct stones which cannot be extracted after endoscopic sphincterotomy (Ponchon et al., 1991; Ell et al., 1993). Two different approaches can be used, either directly, through the choledochostomy tract when this is available; or indirectly, via a retrograde approach in cases of common duct stones or via a percutaneous transhepatic approach in cases of intrahepatic calculi. Fragmentation and complete clearance have been obtained when these methods are used under direct vision. Theoretically, the risk of damaging the bile duct wall using a pulsed dye laser should be low, providing it is done under direct vision. Complete clearance has been obtained in 88% of the cases without complications (Ponchon et al., 1991). It is preferably conducted under direct endoscopic vision to avoid the possible risk of inadvertent bile duct injury, with a success rate of 89% (Ell et al., 1993). Major complications encountered are hemobilia and cholangitis, though transient. In difficult cases, blind fragmentation may be tried with due caution under radiologic control, using an integrated automatic stone/tissue detection system.

# CHAPTER SIX

# Hepatolithiasis and Intrahepatic Calculi

Gallstones sometimes found in the intrahepatic bile ducts are called intrahepatic calculi, liver stones, or hepatolithiasis (Figure 26). Until quite recently, these stones attracted very little attention worldwide because of their regional occurrence. This is in sharp contrast to ordinary cholelithiasis, in which stones are usually found in the gallbladder and/or extrahepatic bile duct, mostly consisting of cholesterol stones or black pigment stones. In fewer cases, brown pigment stones are found in the extrahepatic bile duct and/or gallbladder. Operative intervention in the form of cholecystectomy and/or choledocholithotomy usually ensures complete recovery. In hepatolithiasis or intrahepatic calculi, however, complete recovery after operative intervention is exceptional; repeated stone removal and/or operative interventions are the rule. Therefore, this disease has aroused much attention recently, especially in East Asia, where a high prevalence is encountered in daily practice.

## Pathology

Intrahepatic calculi are brown, soft, and friable. Chemical analysis shows that they consist of two groups, i.e., brown pigment stones (calcium bilirubinate stones) and cholesterol stones—the former predominating (Mukaihara, 1981; Yamashita et al., 1988; Strichartz et al., 1991). A patient with so-called primary cholesterol hepatolithiasis observed by Strichartz et al. had a history of xanthoma and a markedly elevated serum cholesterol level suggesting the presence of some undefined derangement of cholesterol metabolism (Strichartz et al., 1991). Bile was supersaturated, with a cholesterol saturation index of 1.76. Brown pigment stones in hepatolithiasis contain less bilirubin and bile acid and more cholesterol than those either in the common bile duct or in the gallbladder (Shoda et al., 1991, 1993a). Therefore, when dealing with the pathogenesis of intrahepatic calculi, not only the formation and precipitation of calcium bilirubinate but also the solubility of cholesterol and the formation of calcium salts of fatty acids should be considered.

Hepatolithiasis exists when stones are present in the right and/or left hepatic ducts and/or in their tributaries, irrespective of the coexistence of gallstones in other parts of the biliary tract, such as the extrahepatic bile duct and/or the gallbladder. Although the confluence of the right and left hepatic ducts is generally located extrahepatically, when the

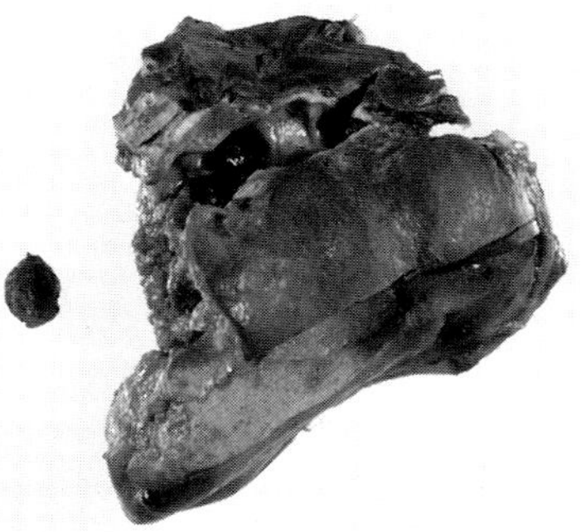

**Figure 26**

Left Lateral Hepatic Segment, Containing Intrahepatic Calculi in the Dilated Duct, Removed

stones are found above the confluence they are considered to be intrahepatic calculi regardless the confluence is located intrahepatically or extrahepatically because the confluence can easily be recognized by hepatobiliary imaging (Nakayama, 1982). The ducts containing gallstones are unevenly dilated, whether saccular or fusiform, with irregularly distributed focal stenosis. The walls of the involved ducts are thickened, mainly by fibrosis (Nakanuma et al., 1988). The parenchyma of the involved liver shows mild to severe atrophy and fibrosis, especially in the peripheral areas and around the bile ducts containing intrahepatic calculi. Atrophic changes just under the liver capsule are frequently seen with an underlying large, dilated bile duct. When these changes are severe, the affected lobe or segment is replaced by fibrous tissue showing thick, saccular ducts filled with intrahepatic calculi. Histologically, numerous glandular elements and inflammatory infiltrates are consistently seen within the ductal wall and in periductal tissue, showing the feature of so-called chronic proliferative cholangitis. Glandular elements within the ductal wall (intramural glands) are mainly composed of simple or branched mucous glands. Those in the periductal connective tissue (periductal glands) are composed of mucous, serous, and mixed mucous-serous acini and are generally arranged in lobules. The mucus is present in the intrahepatic bile ducts with biliary sludge and calculi.

## Classification

Intrahepatic calculi or stones are found in the intrahepatic bile ducts, which are defined as all bile ducts peripheral to the junction of the right and left hepatic ducts, even though the confluence frequently lies outside of the liver substance. Hepatolithiasis is a disease involving gallstones above the confluence. More than 20 classifications have been proposed. This proliferation of classifications has hindered rather than improved the understanding of the disease (Nakayama, 1982). Therefore, in 1982 a more logical and clear-cut classification of hepatolithiasis was proposed (Tables 11–13) based solely on the pathological findings with no unproven assumptions such as those concerning primary and secondary hepatolithiasis.

Since then, this new classification has been increasingly adopted in medical communities not only in Japan but also abroad and seems to be well established. Therefore, a brief description is in order. Hepatolithiasis is defined as gallstones present in the intrahepatic bile ducts (Table 11). The intrahepatic bile ducts are defined as including the right and left hepatic ducts distal to the confluence. The segmental ducts are divided into central and peripheral ducts. The former denote the part between the origin and the first branch. Stricture is defined as a decrease in the diameter of the bile ducts relative to the adjacent parts and is designated as "S". $S_0$" denotes absence of stricture, "$S_1$" slight stricture (>2 mm diameter), and "$S_2$" marked stricture (<2 mm diameter). Dilatation "D" is defined as an increase in the diameter of the bile duct beyond the physiological range. "Do" denotes the absence of dilatation, "$D_1$" slight dilatation and "$D_2$" marked dilatation. In the extrahepatic bile duct, "$D_1$" denotes dilatation of less than 20 mm and $D_2$ dilatation of more than 20 mm. In the intrahepatic bile duct, 10 mm is chosen to divide $D_1$ and $D_2$.

The sites of stricture and dilatation should be described as in Tables 12 and 13 and Figures 27 and 28. When stricture and/or dilatation involves A to B in continuity, they should be connected with the signs "A~B", but if they are present in more than two sites separately, they should be expressed as "A, B". The code describing the pathology is given in large parentheses. The presence or absence of stones in all parts of the biliary tract should be noted and described in codes preceding those describing the pathology. In addition, the kind of gallstone present is noted. "G" denotes gallbladder, "B" extrahepatic bile duct, and "H" intrahepatic bile duct (Figure 27). When no stones are present in the gallbladder, it is expressed as "Go"; if a cholesterol stone is present, it is indicated as "Gc"; if a brown pigment stone or calcium bilirubinate stone is present, it is "Gb". If stones other than cholesterol and brown pigment stones are present, the types are given. When the presence of stone is known but its kind is uncertain, "x" is the designation; "Gx". If the

**Table 11**

**Classification of Hepatolithiasis: Location of Stones***

| Type | Lobe |
|---|---|
| Intrahepatic—I | Left—L |
| Intra- and extrahepatic—IE | Right—R |
| Both locations similar—IE | Left and right—LR |
| Intrahepatic predominant—I̲E | Both lobes similar—LR |
| Extrahepatic predominant—IE̲ | Left predominant—L̲R |
| | Right predominant—LR̲ |

* Predominant location is underlined.

Source: Nakayama (1982).

Table 12

**Classification of Hepatolithiasis: Stenosis of the Bile Duct**

| Grade | Site* |
|---|---|
| No stenosis—$S_0$ | Peripheral<br>Sa-p† Sp-p<br>Sl-p Sm-p |
| Slight stenosis—$S_1$ | Central<br>Sa-c Sp-c<br>Sl-c Sm-c |
| High-grade stenosis—$S_2$ | Hepatic duct—Slh or Srh |
| | Common hepatic duct—Sch |
| | Common bile duct—Scb |

* p: peripheral; c: central; l: lateral segmental duct; m: medial segmental duct; a: anterior segmental duct; p: posterior segmental duct; rh: right hepatic duct; lh: left hepatic duct; ch: common hepatic duct; cb: common bile duct
† Stenosis of peripheral portion of anterior segmental duct

Source: Nakayama (1982).

Table 13

**Classification of Hepatolithiasis: Dilatation of the bile duct**

| Grade | Site* |
|---|---|
| No dilatation—$D_0$ | Peripheral<br>Da-p Dp-p<br>Dl-p Dm-p |
| Slight dilatation—$D_1$ | Central<br>Da-c Dp-c<br>Dl-c Dm-c† |
| High-grade dilataton—$D_2$ | Hepatic duct—Dlh or Drh |
| | Common hepatic duct—Dch |
| | Common bile duct—Dcb |

* p: peripheral; c: central; l: lateral segmental duct; m: medial segmental duct; a: anterior segmental duct; p: posterior segmental duct; rh: right hepatic duct; lh: left hepatic duct; ch: common hepatic duct; cb: common bile duct
† Dilatation of central portion of the medial segmental duct

Source: Nakayama (1982).

presence or absence of stones is uncertain, the postfix "X" is added. The presence or absence of stenosis of the duodenal papilla is treated separately. If absent, it is expressed as "Spo"; if present as "Sp"; and if uncertain as "Spx". Passage of a bougie 3 mm in diameter, ERCP findings, and pressure studies are the criteria for the presence or absence of stenosis

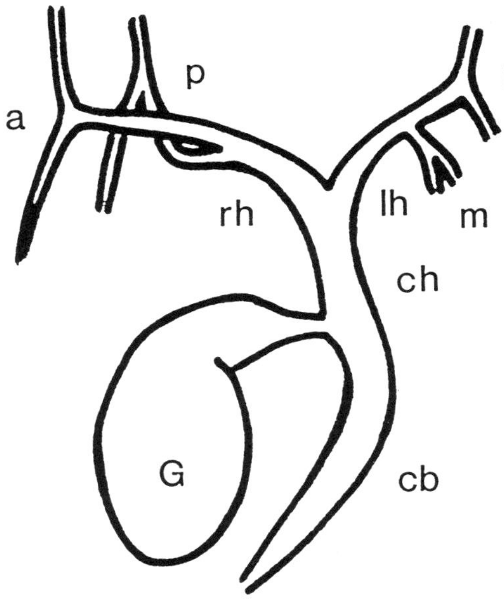


**Figure 27**

Abbreviation of the Biliary Tract

of the duodenal papilla. If cholecystectomy has already been performed, it is expressed as "G̸". In hepatolithiasis cases, multiple operations are not unusual. It is quite possible for the pathology to change as further operative interventions are added. Therefore, it is useful to have previous and present operative interventions listed at the end of the code. The operations are arranged from simpler to the more complicated procedures (Table 14). These are assigned by a letter alphabetically and consecutively. The code denoting the present operation is underlined. Three examples are shown in Figures 29, 30, and 31.

This classification offers several advantages. It is based solely on the exact description of the prevailing pathological findings and is therefore devoid of subjective bias for the designation of stones as primary or secondary, or of conditions such as congenital or acquired. The coding used offers easier compilation of the data, which can be stored in a computer for later retrieval and use.

## Epidemiology

The highest incidence of hepatolithiasis occurs in the fifth to sixth decades and is usually distributed between the 30- and 70-year age groups (Nakayama et al., 1987). Intrahepatic type I is more frequent in the younger age group, while intra- and extrahepatic type IE occur in the older groups. The first sign of hepatolithiasis appears between 30 and 50 but sometimes occurs even earlier.

Hepatolithiasis, or intrahepatic calculi, occurs mainly in East Asia, encompassing China, Korea, Japan, Taiwan, the Philippines, Indochina, Thailand, Malaysia, and Indone-

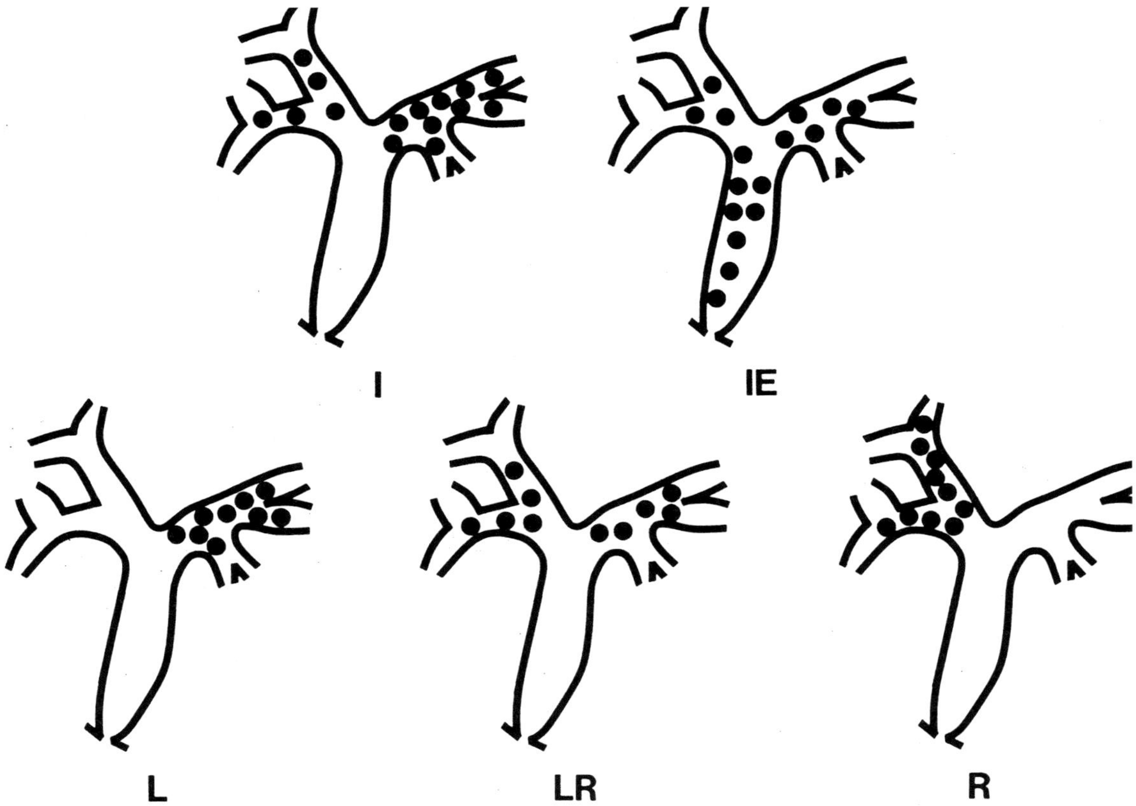


**Figure 28**

Classification of Hepatolithiasis (Nakayama, 1982)

sia (Table 15). It also occurs much less frequently on the Indian subcontinent, in the Middle and Near East, Africa, and the Western countries including Europe and the Americas. The relative proportion of hepatolithiasis to all forms of cholelithiasis varies considerably from area to area within East Asia. For instance, in Japan the prevalence of hepatolothiasis compared to all cholelithiasis cases is highest in the less urbanized Shikoku and Tohoku districts (Figure 32) (Nakayama et al., 1980). In Taiwan it is reported to be over 50 % (Ker et al 1981). Comparable figures for China are 30–38 % (Huang 1959,1976), Republic of Korea 9 % (Kwon, 1986, personal communication), Thailand 15 % (Juttijudata et al., 1984), and Malaya 11 % (King, 1971; Balasegaram, 1972). Our epidemiological survey of the four areas of East Asia from Japan, Taiwan, Hong Kong, and Singapore for hepatolithiasis conducted by the same personnel, using same format, disclosed a striking difference between Taiwan and the other two areas, where the majority, 80–90 %, of the population is also of Chinese descent (Table 16) (Nakayama et al,. 1986). In Taiwan, hepatolithiasis comprises more than 50 % of all cholelithiasis cases, in Hong Kong 3.1 % and in Singapore 1.7 %. Such regional differences also exist within China itself. Our recent survey (Nakayama et al., 1991) shows that Shenyang in northeastern China had a higher relative

Table 14

Code Describing the Operative Procedures Employed

a. Cholecystostomy
b. External cholecystostomy
c. Cholecystectomy
d. Choledochotomy
e. Choledochostomy
f. Transhepatic exploration of intrahepatic bile duct
g. Sphincteroplasty
h. Cholecystoduodenostomy
i. Cholecystojejunostomy
j. Choledochoduodenostomy
k. Choledochojejunostomy
l. Intrahepatic cholangiojejunostomy
m. Hepatic lobectomy
n. Segmental resection of the liver
o. Subsegmental resection of the liver
p. Endoscopic sphinterotomy
q. Percutaneous transhepatic cholangio-drainage
r. Others
x. Procedures employed not known

Source: Nakayama (1982).

proportion of hepatolithiasis to all cholelithiasis cases of, i.e., 21.1 %, while in Beijing it was only 9.2 %. In Chongqing in Sichuan province in central China, the relative proportion was reported to be 30–38 % (Huang, 1959, 1976). In Xinjiang in northwestern China, a much smaller proportion of hepatolithiasis is encountered (Yao, 1990, personal communication). It is estimated that the number of cases occurring in 10 years was approximately 16,000, appearing at the rate of about one case per 100,000 population per year (male:female ratio 0.7:1.0).

A chronological shift in the prevalence of hepatolithiasis has been noted. The relative proportion of hepatolithiasis to all cholelithiasis cases in Japan seems to be declining. For instance, in 1913 Miyake Sr found 20 cases of hepatolithiasis in 257 cases of cholelithiasis among 8,406 autopsy records at the leading universities in Japan (Tokyo, Kyoto, and Kyushu) (Miyake Sr, 1913)—a relative proportion of 7.7 %. A survey conducted in Japan from 1970 to 1977 showed that the relative proportion of hepatolithiasis to all cholelithiasis cases was 4.1 % (Nakayama et al., 1980) and, in the years from 1975 to 1984, 2.7–3.2 % (Nakayama et al., 1987). At present it is variously reported to be 3–4 % (Nakayama et al., 1980). The increase of ordinary cholelithiasis in postwar Japan may have partly contributed to the apparent decrease in the relative proportion of hepatolithiasis. The relative proportion of hepatolithiasis to all cholelithiasis is decreasing in Taiwan (Chang and Passaro Jr, 1983) as well as in Korea (Kwon et al., 1982). The relative proportion of hepatolithiasis to all cholelithiasis in Taiwan has been constant up to 1974 but has gradually fallen to about half, coinciding with the great improvement in the economic status there (Chang and Passaro Jr, 1983). In Republic of Korea the relative proportion of hepatolithasis was 18.3 % in Hur's series (1958–1963) (Hur et al., 1963), 17.0 % in Min's

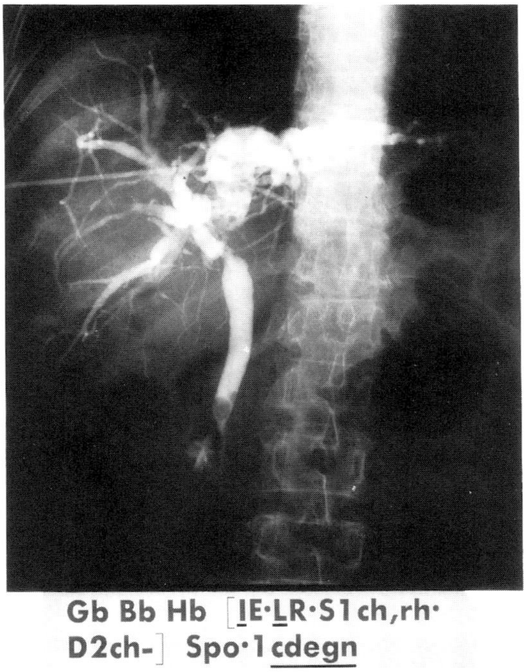


**Figure 29**

Classification of Hepatolithiasis: Example 1

Brown pigment stones in the gallbladder, the extra- and intrahepatic bile duct and the common hepatic ducts. Intra- and extrahepatic ducts are involved, the former predominating. The left and right lobes of the liver are affected, former predominating. Slight stenosis is present from the common hepatic duct and the right hepatic duct. High-grade dilatation is present from the common hepatic duct upward. No stenosis of the duodenal papilla is present. The present operation consists of cholecystectomy, choledochotomy, choledochostomy, sphincteroplasty, and segmental resection of the liver.

(1963–1965) (Min et al., 1966), and 9% in Kwon's (1961–1980) (Park et al (1986) Personal communication). In addition, the pathology of hepatolithiasis seems to be changing. In Japan we no longer see extremely dilated intrahepatic bile ducts filled with large numbers of calculi, as was usual in the immediate postwar period almost 50 years ago.

In contrast, the prevalence of hepatolithiasis in the Western world seems to be much less, as revealed by only occasional reports emerging from the West. Although intrahepatic calculi have long been known to occur in Europe and the United States (Vachell and Stevens, 1906; Phemister et al., 1939), the relative proportion of hepatolithiasis to all cholelithiasis cases has been reported to be 0.6% (Lindström, 1977) and 0.75% (Cetta et al., 1993) to 3% (Simi et al., 1979). A far advanced case of hepatolithiasis in a 23-year-old male was reported long ago in England. Postmortem examination revealed over 600 stones filling both the intra- and extrahepatic bile ducts and as many as 520 stones in the liver; the largest stone weighed 270 g and the total weight of the stones was said to be

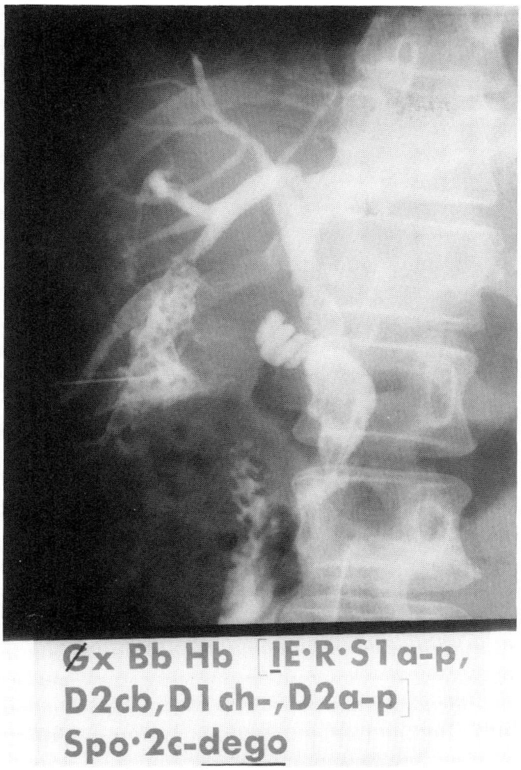


**Figure 30**

Classification of Hepatolithiasis: Example 2

Gallstone(s) were present at the time of cholecystectomy but the nature of the stones was uncertain. Brown pigment stones are present in the intra- and extrahepatic ducts. Both intra- and extrahepatic bile ducts are involved, the former predominating. The right hepatic lobe is involved. Slight stenosis is present in the peripheral part of the anterior segmental duct. High-grade dilatation is present in the common bile duct, slight dilatation from the common hepatic duct up, and high-grade dilatation in the peripheral part of the anterior segmental duct. There is no stenosis of the duodenal papilla. The first operation was cholecystectomy. The present operation consists of choledochotomy, choledochostomy, sphincteroplasty, and segmental resection of the liver involved.

1,378 g (Vachell and Stevens, 1906). Therefore, the pathology of hepatolithiasis must also have changed in the West. Since the number of immigrants from endemic areas entering the West is increasing considerably, the overall relative proportion of hepatolithiasis to all cholelithiasis cases is expected to rise. In fact, most reports on hepatolithiasis appearing recently from the West concern such immigrant populations.

In Latin America the relative proportion of hepatolithiasis to all cholelithiasis cases seems to be relatively high. It is reported to be 2–7 % (Bove et al., 1963; Cobo et al., 1964; Faintuch, 1983, personal communication).

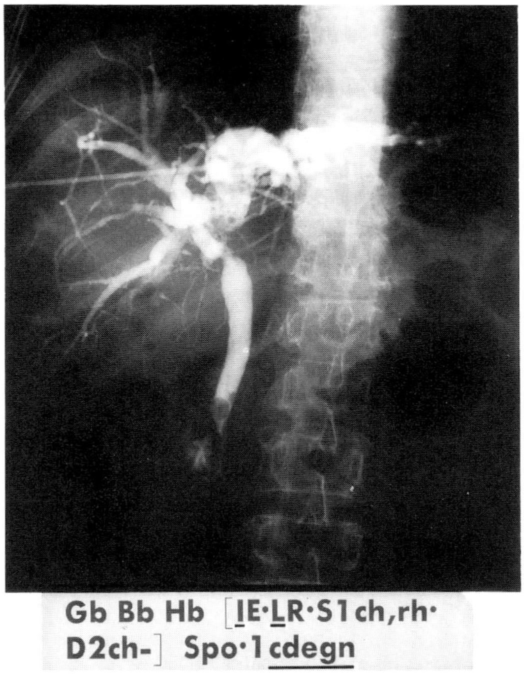


**Figure 31**

Classification of Hepatolithiasis: Example 3

Brown pigment stones were present in the gallbladder, extra- and intrahepatic bile ducts, the last predominating. The left lobe was mostly involved. Slight stricture was present in the common hepatic duct and right hepatic duct. High-grade dilatation appeared from the common hepatic duct upward. No stricture was present in duodenal papilla. The present operation is the first operative intervention consisting of cholecystectomy, choledochotomy, choledochostomy, sphincteroplasty, and segmental resection of the liver (left lateral hepatic segmentectomy).

# Etiology

Possible factors responsible for the geographical differences in the relative proportion of hepatolithiasis to all cholelithiasis cases may be divided into ethnic and environmental factors. In a recent survey conducted in East Asia, the relative proportion of hepatolithiasis in Taiwan, Hong Kong, Shenyang, and Beijing was compared with that in Japan (Nakayama et al., 1986, 1991) (Table 15). In spite of a similar ethnic background, i.e., the majority of the population being Chinese or of Chinese descent, the relative proportion of hepatolithiasis was markedly different, from over 50% in Taiwan to 2–4% in Hong Kong and Singapore. The explanation must therefore be environmental. Infestation with parasites has often been cited as a major cause (Fung, 1961). However, in Taiwan, with the highest prevalence of hepatolithiasis, infestation with Clonorchis sinensis occurs mainly in

Table 15

| Relative Prevalence of Hepatolithiasis in the World* | |
|---|---|
| Taiwan | 50 |
| China | 10—20 |
| South Korea | 10—20 |
| Hong Kong | 10 |
| Malaysia | 10 |
| Japan | 4—5 |
| West | 1 |

*Proportion of hepatolithiasis in all cases of cholelithiasis in percent

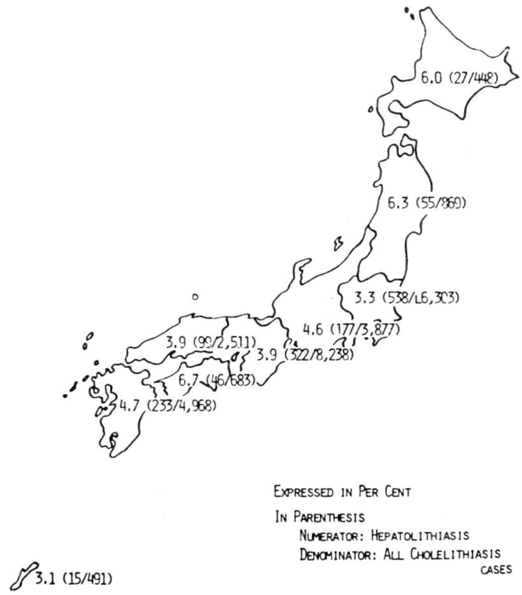


**Figure 32**

Geographical Distribution of Hepatolithiasis in Japan

Source: Nakayama et al., 1980

the southern part of the country (Chow, 1960), and Clonorchis and its ova are found infrequently in cases with intrahepatic calculi. Even the demonstration of Clonorchis ova in intrahepatic calculi does not mean that infestation is responsible for the formation of intrahepatic calculi. They may merely be associated with stones in the endemic areas of infestation, such as Hong Kong and southern China. For instance, in spite of the absence of Clonorchis sinensis infestation, Malaya has a comparatively high relative proportion of hepatolithiasis.

Table 16

**Relative Prevalence of Hepatolithiasis in East Asia***

| | All cholelithiasis | Hepatolithiasis | Relative prevalence (%) |
|---|---|---|---|
| Taiwan | 318 | 170 | 53.5 |
| Shenyang | 394 | 84 | 21.2 |
| Beijing | 422 | 39 | 9.2 |
| Hong Kong | 700 | 22 | 3.1 |
| Singapore | 647 | 11 | 1.7 |
| Fukuoka | 671 | 31 | 4.6 |

*Proportion of hepatolithiasis in all cases of cholelithiasis in percent

Source: Nakayama et al. (1986, 1991).

The factors responsible for the formation of intrahepatic calculi are not well defined but are thought to be due to bacterial infection and stasis of bile. The incidence of bacteria in bile in cases of hepatolithiasis is almost 100% (Tabata and Nakayama, 1984), suggesting a close association between bacterial colonization of bile and the presence of intrahepatic calculi. Among the species of bacteria present, E. coli (Maki, 1966), Clostridium and Bacteroides show $\beta$-glucuronidase activity (Table 9). This is thought to be mainly responsible for the hydrolysis of bilirubin glucuronide, the water-soluble form of bilirubin in bile, to free unconjugated bilirubin (Nakano et al., 1988a). Nonbacterial transformation is also known to take place (Oyabu et al., 1987; Spivak et al., 1987). The free UCB thus formed is water insoluble and combines with ionized calcium present in bile to form calcium bilirubinate, leading to the formation of brown pigment stones (calcium bilirubinate stones), to which the majority of intrahepatic calculi belong. However, a recent analysis of intrahepatic calculi (Yamashita et al., 1988) (Figure 33) shows that in addition to the usual brown pigment stones, stones with a large percentage of cholesterol and less bilirubin, i.e., cholesterol stones, are encountered in about 20% of the cases. Intrahepatic calculi of intermediate composition are also present. Therefore, when considering the etiology of intrahepatic calculi, solubilization not only of bilirubin but also of cholesterol in bile should be taken into account. The composition of bile acids present in gallstones may reflect the etiological process of gallstone formation (Schoenfield et al., 1966; Akiyoshi and Nakayama, 1990). A detailed analysis of the bile acid composition of gallstones present in the intrahepatic duct (intrahepatic calculi) was conducted in comparison to those in the extrahepatic bile duct and in the gallbladder (Shoda et al., 1991, 1993a). Intrahepatic brown pigment stones have a lower total bile acid content, a smaller proportion of unconjugated bile acid, and smaller proportions of secondary bile acid and keto-bile acids compared with those in the extrahepatic bile duct. Complete separation between the two groups was obtained using discriminant analysis with respect to their bile acid composition. In contrast, cholesterol stones in the intrahepatic bile ducts had bile acid composition

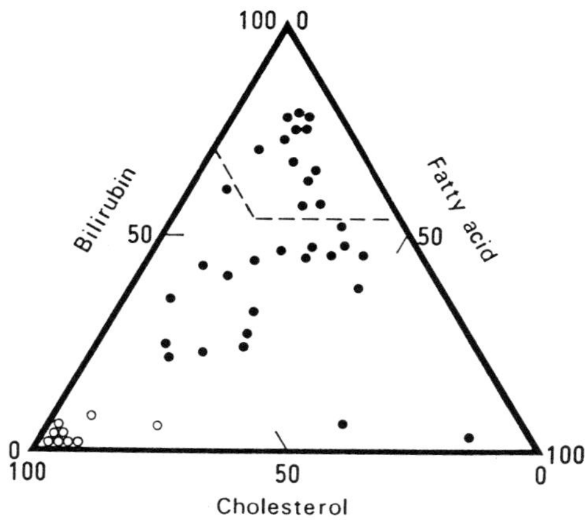


Figure 33

Composition of Intrahepatic Calculi: Triangular Coordinate Diagram

Source: Yamashita et al., 1988

similar to those found in the extrahepatic bile duct and in the gallbladder. Thus, it was concluded that bacterial infection plays a less important role in the formation of intrahepatic brown pigment stones than extrahepatic brown pigment stones. However, bacterial infection no doubt plays a pivotal if not a major role in the formation of intrahepatic calculi, as in a case of brown pigment stones elsewhere, in which over half of the bile acid is present in free unconjugated form. This suggests the prevalence of bacterial deconjugation and the importance of bacterial infection in the formation of brown pigment gallstones (Akiyoshi and Nakayama, 1990; Shoda et al 1993a). Brown pigment stones in the intrahepatic bile duct contain more cholesterol and less calcium bilirubinate than those in the extrachepatic bile duct (Yamashita et al., 1988; Shoda et al., 1993a). Bile from both affected and unaffected hepatic lobes contains an increased molar percentage of cholesterol and less bile acids than controls, diminishing solubiliszation of bilirubin and cholesterol and favoring the formation of cholesterol-rich brown pigment stones.

Bile stasis is caused by stenosis and stricture formation, usually associated with areas of ductal dilatation. Stenosis may occur in either the left or right hepatic duct branches; left hepatic duct involvement predominates for still unknown reasons. Anatomical variation of the right intrahepatic duct joining to the left hepatic duct sometimes found in hepatolithiasis cases was suggested to be of etiological significance (Glenn and Moody, 1961). However, a comparable study on such variation between various diseases, including cholecystolithiasis, choledocholithiasis, and controls, clearly indicated that the incidence of the modes of union of main intrahepatic ducts are not associated with the presence or absence of intrahepatic calculi (Koga et al., 1987). Stenosis is sometimes found at the liver hilum, involving both hepatic ducts. However, in some cases, in spite of the presence of stones not only in the intrahepatic but also in the extrahepatic ducts, no stenosis can be demonstrated in the bile duct. The duodenal papilla may be patulous, and no mechanical stenosis can be demonstrated in such cases.

A recent survey conducted by the Hepatolithiasis Research Group (Director: Professor Fumio Nakayama) with the support of the Ministry of Health of Japan showed that a fair affinity exists between the incidence of hepatolithiasis, on the one hand and possible risk factors, on the other such as (1) being born in the countryside, (2) using water mainly from a well, (3) having a past history of parasite infestation, (4) low hygienic conditions of the present domicile, and (5) consuming the traditional Japanese diet, thus suggesting that older or traditional living habits are associated with a higher incidence of hepatolithiasis (Nakayama et al., 1987).

## Symptoms and Signs

No pathognomonic symptoms exist for hepatolithiasis, but they are similar to the symptoms usually encountered in cholecystocholedocholithiasis, such as upper abdominal pain, occasional fever, and, less frequently jaundice. Liver function tests show some abnormalities, such as elevation of alkaline phosphatase, and $\gamma$-GTP, but they are by no means specific to the disease.

## Diagnosis

The presence of intrahepatic stones can be established by one of the hepatobiliary imaging techniques available. However, additional information including location of the stones, dilatation and stricture of the bile duct, and status of the duodenal papilla should be obtained in order to plan the treatment. Table 17 shows the diagnostic accuracy of the imaging techniques available (Hepatolithiasis Research Group, 1983). The procedure of

**Table 17**

**Diagnositic Accuracy of the Modalities used in Hepatolithiasis***

| Imaging technique | No. of Cases | % |
|---|---|---|
| Percutaneous transhepatic cholangiography (PTC) | 131 | 88.6 |
| Endoscopic retrograde cholangiography (ERC) | 200 | 74.0 |
| Computed tomography (CT) | 89 | 51.7 |
| Ultrasonography | 224 | 40.6 |
| Intravenous cholangiography | 186 | 15.1 |

Source: Hepatolithiasis Research Group (1983).

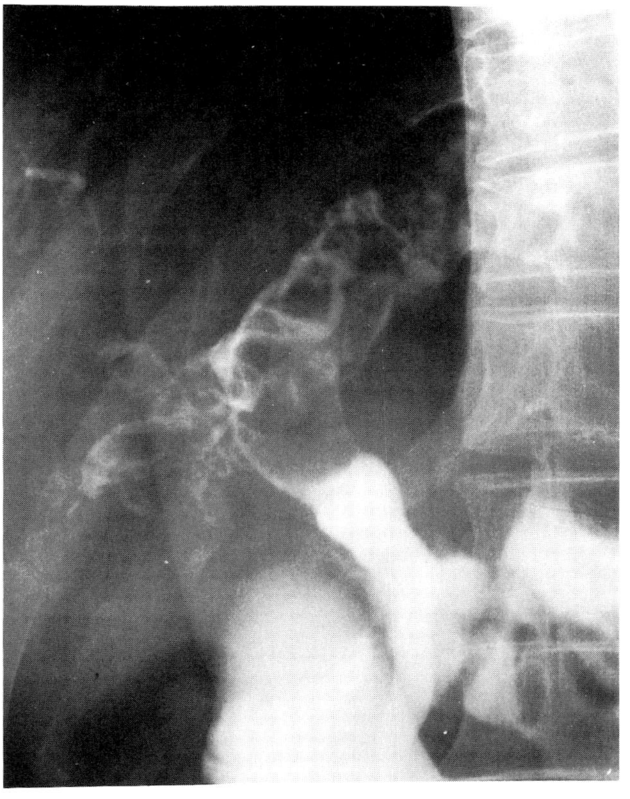

**Figure 34**

Endoscopic Retrograde Cholangiogram Showing Stones in the Right and Left Hepatic Ducts and Common Hepatic Duct

first choice is ultrasonography, which is noninvasive; gives a fair amount of information on the upper abdominal organs, including the liver and intrahepatic ducts; and is considered to be the best screening procedure. Computed tomography is also useful, but it is expensive and requires radiation exposure. It gives a good image of intrahepatic stones when their calcium content is high and they are surrounded by a sufficient amount of bile in the dilated duct. However, when the calcium content is low, it is difficult to differentiate between intrahepatic stones and the presence of cholangiocarcinoma. Magnetic resonance imaging (MRI) does not seem to offer particular advantages. Intravenous cholangiography is less useful, as it is likely to be affected by the excretory function of the liver and by hepatic damage. The presence of jaundice does not always allow a clear image of the intrahepatic bile duct, let alone the peripheral ducts. Final and accurate diagnosis of hepatolithiasis can be obtained by one of the direct cholangiography techniques. When jaundice is absent and expertise is available, ERC is the procedure of choice. It allows direct vision of the duodenal papilla, gives a clear image of the intra- and extrahepatic bile ducts, and causes no bile leakage, which may lead to biliary peritonitis. When the intra-

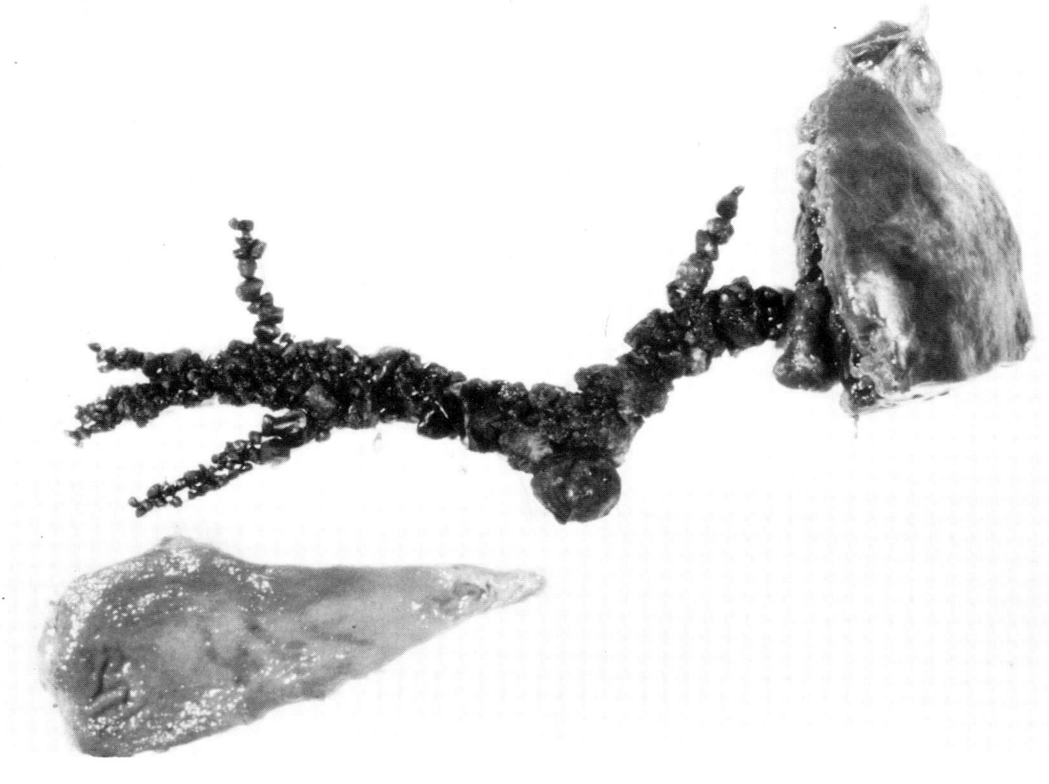

**Figure 35**

Schematic Representation of Intrahepatic Calculi

Same case as in Figure 34. Gallstones were filling both hepatic ducts and the common hepatic duct.

hepatic duct is not well visualized because of the backflow of contrast medium via a patulous duodenal papilla, a balloon catheter can be used to visualize the entire intrahepatic bile duct system (Ikeda et al., 1981) (Figures 34, 35). When jaundice is present, another form of direct cholangiography, namely PTC should be performed; it gives the highest diagnostic accuracy rate, i.e., 88.6% (Hepatolithiasis Research Group, 1983) (Table 17). Although there is a chance of bile leakage from the site of the puncture, this can be alleviated by using a Chiba needle of small caliber (No. 21). With the introduction of ultrasound guidance, the PTC needle can be placed accurately into the dilated bile duct, avoiding complications such as bleeding from inadvertently punctured portal vein branches. In addition, PTC can easily be converted to percutaneous transhepatic bile duct drainage (PTBD), which minimizes bile leakage by effecting biliary decompression.

An algorithm of diagnostic steps for the diagnosis of hepatolithiasis is given in Figure

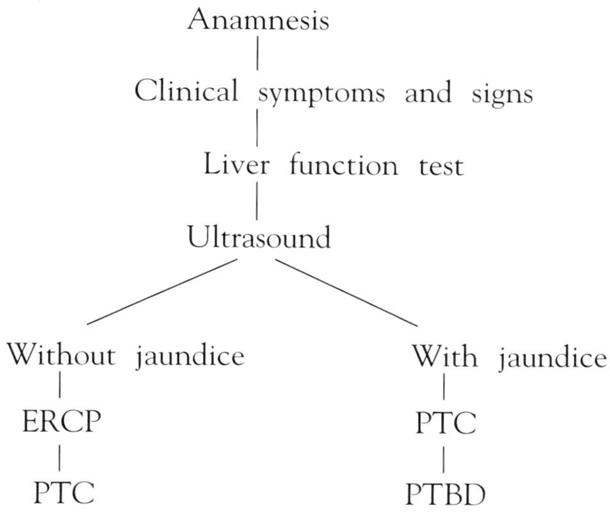


**Figure 36**

Algorithm of the Diagnosis of Cholelithiasis

36. In the first step, the patient's present history, clinical symptoms and signs should be considered, which may lead to a clue to the presence of hepatolithiasis. If there is doubt, upper abdominal ultrasonography should be done. Intrahepatic calculi are mostly brown pigment stones, and their Hounsfield value is close to that of surrounding liver tissues. Therefore, detection is difficult unless the ducts are considerably dilated and the stones are surrounded by bile. In general, information on intrahepatic bile ducts can be obtained only when the ducts are considerably dilated. When the presence of intrahepatic stones is elicited or in doubt, one of the direct cholangiography procedures available should be conducted, depending on the presence or absence of jaundice.

# Treatment

Since hepatolithasis is not infrequently accompanied by obstructive jaundice, severe bacterial infection and biliary cirrhosis, preoperative evaluation should be carefully planned and instituted for safer conduct of operative procedures.

## Preoperative evaluation

It is mandatory to have clear information on the prevailing pathology, using the various examinations previously mentioned. After identifying the disease type and the accompanying pathology, biliary decompression should be done with either percutaneous transhepatic bile duct drainage (PTBD) or endoscopic retrograde bile duct drainage (ERBD), introducing a catheter into the extrahepatic bile duct via a duodenal fiberscope

Table 18

| Purposes of Operative Intervention in Hepatolithiasis |
|---|
| Removal of stones |
| Correction of bile stasis |
| Control of biliary infection |

through the duodenal papilla, which can be kept in place pernasally (Ikeda et al., 1981) . The latter should be used when stricture is absent in the proximal duct. When stricture is present in the upper part of the biliary system, in order to avoid precipitating an episode of acute obstructive cholangitis, PTBD is preferred.

Recently, because of the recognition of the possibile occurrence of cholangiocarcinoma with the presence of hepatolithiasis (Falchuck et al., 1976; Phinney et al., 1981; Koga et al., 1985; Nakanuma et al., 1985), biopsy by percutaneous transhepatic biliary endoscopy via a stepwise enlarged PTBD route and biopsy is advocated preoperatively when malignant involvement is suspected from the direct cholangiographic findings (Nimura et al., 1988).

## Operative treatment

Since intrahepatic stones recur even after their removal, the operative procedure employed should eliminate the causes of hepatolithiasis. Factors responsible for the occurrence of hepatolithiasis include bacterial infection as well as stricture and dilatation of the bile ducts. Therefore, the procedure should aim at (1) complete removal of the stones present, (2) removal of the strictured part of the bile duct causing dilatation of the bile duct and stagnation of bile, and (3) providing good drainage of bile to minimize bacterial infection in situ (Table 18). Furthermore, the possible occurrence of cholangiocarcinoma in cases of long-standing intrahepatic calculi (Falchuck et al., 1976; Phinney at al., 1981; Koga et al., 1985; Nakanuma et al., 1985) can be alleviated by removing the involved liver segment(s) entirely.

Therefore, selection of the operative procedures should be individualized according to the prevailing pathology, i.e., the disease type, according to the classification of hepatolithiasis recently proposed (Nakayama, 1982). For the sake of simplicity, the cases to be operated are divided into intrahepatic (I) and intra- and extrahepatic (IE) types (Table 11), which are considered separately.

### Intrahepatic hepatolithiasis (I)

When stones are found to be located exclusively in the left intrahepatic bile duct, left lateral hepatic segmentectomy or left hepatic lobectomy removes not only the intrahepatic stones and the accompanying bacterial infection but also the involved bile duct (Adson and Nagorney, 1982; Koga et al., 1984). However, the strictured part of the bile duct must be removed completely. Otherwise, local infection and biliary fistula may persist postoperatively.

In the rare cases in which intrahepatic stones are located in the right hepatic lobe exclusively, right hepatic lobectomy is usually not undertaken because of the risks involved. This seems to be unjustified, since hepatolithiasis is essentially a benign disease. Right anterior or posterior segmentectomy may be undertaken when the calculi are located in the respective segment, with accompanying atrophy of the liver parenchyma and fibrosis. If many stones are present in the right hepatic duct and its branches, extended hepaticojejunostomy (Roux-Y) with permanent cutaneous access (Chen et al., 1984; Barker and Winkler, 1985) is indicated (Figure 37). After removal of intrahepatic stones via the choledochotomy opening as much as possible, the common hepatic duct is divided at the liver hilum and the incision is extended to the anterior wall of the left hepatic duct to provide a wide opening for the bilioenteric anastomosis, and a hepatico-jejunostomy (Roux-Y) is constructed. While employing the above procedures, the strictures present at the liver hilum, which are not infrequently encountered in such cases, should be removed as completely as possible to allow wider anastomosis to the jejunal limb. Through the distal limb of the hepaticojejunostomy (Roux-Y) anchored subcutaneously on the abdominal wall, i.e., permanent-access hepaticojejunostomy (Chen et al., 1984; Barker and Winkler, 1984), endoscopic removal of the residual calculi can be attempted using the choledochofiberscope repeatedly (Figure 37).

When hepatolithiasis involves both lobes, i.e., in about one-half of the cases, the procedure of choice is left lateral hepatic segmentectomy or left hepatic lobectomy with permanent-access hepaticojejunostomy (Roux-Y). The stones remaining in the right hepatic lobe should be removed by a choledochoscope inserted via permanent cutaneous access.

### Intra- and extrahepatic hepatolithiais (IE)

Stones originating in the intrahepatic ducts gradually descend into the extrahepatic bile ducts, becoming intra- and extrahepatic hepatolithiasis (IE type). Such hepatolithiasis is known to occur more frequently in older persons with long-standing disease. Some hold that stones formed in the extrahepatic bile ducts accumulate and gradually build up into the intrahepatic ducts; such claim have not been substantiated.

Treatment of intra- and extrahepatic hepatolithiasis consists of two parts. The first is removal of the calculi present in the extrahepatic bile ducts, essentially the same as for choledocholithiasis. The second is the same as for intrahepatic hepatolithiasis (I), as described above. The involved extrahepatic bile duct should be removed, as retaining a dilated bile duct with long-standing inflammation and bacterial infection does not seem to serve a useful purpose. After providing a wide opening, an extended hepaticojejunostomy (Roux-Y) with permanent cutaneous access (Figure 37) is constructed. When the number and size of the intrahepatic stones are not large and removal of the stones is adequately accomplished, instead of removing the extrahepatic bile duct, transduodenal sphincteroplasty with a wide opening may be done. This provides for the residual stone or stones

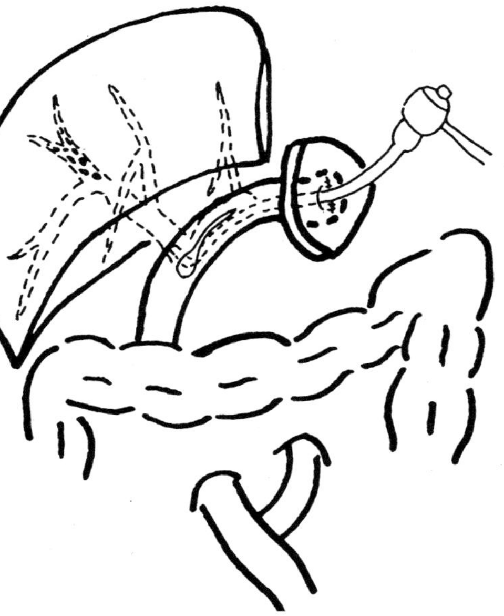

**Figure 37**

Extended Hepaticojejunostomy with Permanent Cutaneous Access

The common hepatic duct is divided at the liver hilum, and the incision is extended to the anterior wall of the left hepatic duct to provide a wide opening for the bilioenteric anastomosis. The distal limb of the hepaticojejunostomy (Roux-Y) is anchored subcutaneously on the abdominal wall for later insertion of the endoscope.

descending into the common bile duct and their eventual evacuation into the duodenum.

## Postoperative treatment

Antibiotic coverage with a wide spectrum for intestinal flora as well as good biliary excretion is usually recommended but not essential, provided good drainage is secured. The outflow from intraabdominal and transjejunal biliary drainage should be carefully monitored. If blood appears from inside or outside the drain, it is essential to determine if it is from the abdominal wall or from a more serious intraabdominal hemorrhage. If it is the former, gauze packing around the drain is sufficient. However, if it is the latter, re-exploration may be necessary. When the bleeding appears to be brisk, accompanied by tachycardia and abdominal distention, celiac angiography followed by transarterial embolization may well be a salvation. Bleeding via the biliary drainage usually ceases after a few days. Bile leakage in and around the intraabdominal drain should be followed carefully, but it gradually diminishes and finally ceases as intestinal movement returns. However, if the bile leakage fails to decrease or even increases, re-exploration and localization of the site of leakage may become necessary to avoid endotoxemia and shock following the intraabdominal accumulation of infected bile.

Hepatic resection is no hindrance to a smooth postoperative recovery. However, the divided surface of the liver should be narrowed as much as possible by placing interrupted mattress sutures at the edge of the liver capsule or covering it with greater omentum to minimize postoperative bleeding, bile leakage, and infection.

## Adjuvant treatment

Operative treatment is the best treatment for hepatolithiasis, as it accomplishes (1) removal of stones, (2) removal of the strictured part of the bile duct causing dilatation of the intrahepatic bile duct and stagnation of bile, (3) providing good drainage of bile and minimizing bacterial infection in situ, and (4) avoiding possible later occurrence of cholangiocarcinoma. The nonoperative approach has certain limitations. Even after the complete removal of intrahepatic stones, recurrence takes place in one-third to one-half of the cases. This is because the conditions for the formation of intrahepatic stones still persist even after successful removal of the stones.

However, there are certain, though limited, cases in which one must rely on the adjuvant treatments presently available, as in cases with severe complications such as cardiovascular and pulmonary and general deterioration. Even after operative intervention, some intrahepatic stones may have to be left in situ because of technical difficulties. In such cases, one must resort to adjuvant treatment for postoperative stone removal.

### Percutaneous transhepatic approach

When jaundice is present and bile duct stricture is suspected, PTC is used to reveal the exact biliary tract pathology present, including the site of the stone, bile duct stricture, and dilatation. Recent introduction of ultrasound guidance has made the procedure much safer and more accurate. Subsequently, the percutaneous transhepatic biliary drainage (PTBD) route is selected to give the best angle for removal of the intrahepatic stones present. After PTBD is established, the sinus tract is gradually enlarged up to 15 to 18 Fr so that the choledochofiberscope (Olympus CHF-P10, P20) can be introduced (Nimura et al., 1988). With the use of a basket catheter (Orii et al., 1983; Cotton et al., 1990), microwave (Inoue at al., 1985), electrohydraulic pressure (Ebbs et al., 1986; Matsumoto et al., 1987; Endo et al., 1990; Bruckner et al., 1990), intrahepatic stones are fragmented and removed piecemeal. This approach has been quite successful, achieving complete to near-complete removal of stones in 84.3 % of the cases (43/51) (Endo et al., 1990). The rate of recurrence was 8 out of 51 cases, or 15.7 %. Dilatation of the strictured part of the bile duct, which may be responsible for stagnation of bile and formation of intrahepatic stones, has been attempted using the Grüntzig balloon catheter, but because of the presence of fibrosis, it is not necessarily successful.

### Endoscopic retrograde route

When jaundice is absent, it is customary to use ERC for the better delineation of biliary tract pathology. Subsequently, removal of extra- and intrahepatic stones can be attempted by introducing a basket catheter, either directly through the duodenal papilla or via a daughter scope inserted into the common bile duct with the aid of a duodenal fiberscope (Saisho et al., 1990; Cotton et al., 1990). However, this route, though having a theoretical advantage of avoiding injury to the hepatic capsule and parenchyma, is indirect and difficult to manage. Even with a daughter scope, the extraction of intrahepatic stones under direct vision is limited because of the narrow vision and restricted angle of the approach provided. Hence, the success rate of the removal of intrahepatic calculi is limited.

### Choledochostomy route

Often the patient undergoes laparotomy and unsuspected hepatolithiasis is found. Such patients are usually referred to larger centers after a T-tube drain is placed in the common bile duct. In such cases, an attempt may be made to insert a choledochofiberscope into the common bile duct via the sinus tract after removal of the T-tube (Yamakawa et al., 1978). However, this route has only limited use because of the fixed angle in which to maneuver. For instance, the right anterior inferior and right posterior inferior ducts are difficult to reach because of the unfavorable angle. Therefore, this approach is limited to stones in the left hepatic duct and its branches and to anterior and posterior superior segmental ducts.

### Extracorporeal shock wave lithotripsy (ESWL)

ESWL is being used to fragment intrahepatic stones in situ (Meyer and Hottenrott, 1986; Bland et al., 1989; Flowers et al., 1990; Lointier et al., 1990; Strichartz et al., 1991) with limited success. Several successful cases of fragmentation have been reported. For this approach to be successful, (1) a route for evacuation of stone fragments should be provided, and (2) the safety of application of shock wave should be assured to avoid damage to the portal vein branches, the inferior vena cava, and the pulmonary tissue. However, because of the frequent presence of stricture of the bile duct and its branches, stone removal remains difficult even after successful fragmentation.

### Oral bile acid therapy for dissolution of stones and prevention of recurrence

After patient with hepatolithiasis is treated with operative intervention, endoscopy and ESWL to remove as many intrahepatic calculi as possible, the calculi are analyzed for their cholesterol content. If intrahepatic calculi are found to have high cholesterol content, i.e. intrahepatic cholesterol stones, adjuvant oral bile acid therapy is in order. This may change the composition of hepatic bile to less lithogenic form which is expected to prevent further stone formation (Strichartz et al., 1991; Ros et al., 1993).

## Prognosis

Compared to ordinary cholelithiasis, the prognosis of hepatolithiasis is far from satisfactory, for the folowing reasons: (1) complete removal of the stones is difficult, if not impossible, (2) recurrence of stones after complete removal occurs in one third of the cases; (3) operative intervention is not always successful because of the presence of extensive pathology, and (4) occurrence of cholangiocarcinoma is seen in 4 % of the cases, precluding a complete cure (Koga et al., 1985).

# References


Abdou MS, Strichartz SD, Abedin MZ, Roslyn JJ (1985) Biliary lipids alter ion transport during cholesterol gallstone formation. *J Surg Res* 44:672–679.

Abedin MZ, Strichartz SD, Festekdijian S, Roslyn JJ (1989) Increased biliary calcium in cholesterol and pigment gallstone disease: the role of altered bile acid composition. *Lipids* 24:572–578.

Abei M, Kawczak P, Nuutinen H, Langnas A, Svanvik J, Holzbach RT (1993a) Isolation and characterization of a cholesterol crystallization promotor from human bile. *Gastroenterology* 104:539–548.

Abei M, Schwarzendrube J, Nuutinen H, Broughan TA, Kawczak P, Williams C, Holzbach RT (1993b) Cholesterol crystallization-promoters in human bile: comparative potencies of immunoglobulins, $\alpha_1$-acid glycoprotein, phospholipase C, and aminopeptidase N[1]. *J Lipid Res* 34:1141–1148.

Abei M, Nuutinen H, Kawczak P, Schwarzendrube J, Pillay SP, Holzbach RT (1994) Identification of human biliary $\alpha_1$-acid glycoprotein as a cholesterol-crystallization promotor. *Gastroenterology* 106:231–238.

Abiru H, Sarna SK, Condon RE (1994) Contractile mechanisms of gallbladder filling and emptying in dogs. *Gastroenterology* 106:1652–1661.

Acalovschi M, Dumitrascu D, Caluser I, Ban A (1987) Comparative prevalence of gallstone disease at 100-year intervals in a large Romanian town, a necropsy study. *Dig Dis Sci* 32:354–357.

Acalovschi M, Badea R, Dumitrascu D, Varga C (1988) Prevalence of gallstones in liver cirrhosis: a sonographic survey. *Am J Gastroenterol* 83:954–956.

Adami HO, Meirik O, Gustavsson S, Nyren O, Krusemo UB (1983) Colorectal cancer after cholecystectomy: absence of risk increase within 11–14 years. *Gastroenterology* 85:859–865.

Adedeji A, Akande B, Olumide F (1986) The changing pattern of cholelithiasis in Lagos. *Scand J Gastroenterol* 21 (suppl 124):63–66.

Admirand WH, Small DM (1968) The physicochemical basis of cholesterol gallstone formation in man. *J Clin Invest* 47:1043–1052.

Adson MA, Nagorney DM (1982) Hepatic resection for intrahepatic ductal stones. *Arch Surg* 117:611–616.

Afdhal NH, Niu N, Gantz D, Small DM, Smith BF (1993) Bovine gallbladder mucin accelerates cholesterol monohydrate crystal growth in model bile. *Gastroenterology* 104:1515–1523

Afdhal NH, Offner GD, Murray FE, Troxler RF, Smith BF (1990) Isolation and characterization of peptides from the core of bovine gallbladder mucin. *Gastroenterology* 98:1633–1641.

Agarwal DK, Choudhuri G, Saraswat VA, Negi TS, Kapoor VK, Saxena R (1994) Duodenal bile examination in identifying potential non-responders to bile salt treatment and its comparison with gall bladder bile examination. *Gut* 35:112–116.

Ahlberg J, Angelin B, Björkhem I, Einarsson K, Leijd B (1979a) Hepatic cholesterol metabolism in normo- and hyperlipidemic patients with cholesterol gallstones. *J Lipid Res* 20:107–115.

Ahlberg J, Angelin B, Einarsson K, Hellström K, Leijd B (1979b) Prevalence of gallbladder disease in hyperlipoproteinemia. *Dig Dis Sci* 24:459–464.

Ahlberg J, Angelin B, Einarsson K, Hellstrom K, Leijd B (1980) Biliary lipid composition in normo- and hyperlipoproteinemia. *Gastroenterology* 79:90–94.

Ahlberg J, Angelin B, Einarsson K (1981a) Hepatic 3-hydroxy-3-methylglutaryl coenzyme A reductase activity and biliary lipid composition in man: relation to cholesterol gallstone disease and effects of cholic acid and chenodeoxycholic acid treatment. *J Lipid Res* 22:410–422.

Ahlberg J, Curstedt T, Einarsson K, Sjövall J (1981b) Molecular species of biliary phosphatidylcholines in gallstone patients: the influence of treatment with cholic acid and chenodeoxycholic acid. *J Lipid Res* 22:404–409.

Ahlberg J, Bergstrand LO, Sahlin S (1984) Changes in gallstone morbidity in a community with decreasing frequency of cholecystectomies. *Acta Chir Scand Suppl* 520:53–58.

Ahmed HA, Petroni ML, Abu-Hamdiyyah M, Jazrawi RP, Northfield TC (1994) Hydrophobic/hydrophilic balance of proteins: a major determinant of cholesterol crystal formation in model bile. *J Lipid Res* 35:211–219.

Aho AJ, Vilhonen E, Peltola S, Lehtonen A (1985) An X-ray diffraction study of the crystalline composition of gallstones. *Scand J Gastroenterol* 20:901–906.

Ahrendt SA, Fox-Talbot K, Kaufman HS, Lillemoe KD, Pitt HA (1994) Cholesterol nucleates rapidly from mixed micelles in the prairie dog. *Biochim Biophys Acta* 1211:7–13

Åkerlund A (1933) Beobachtungen bei Cholecystogrammen in aufrechter Körperstellung: ein neues röntgenologisches Gallensteinsymptom. *Acta Radiol* 14:74–81.

Åkerlund JE, Björkhem I (1990) Studies on the regulation of cholesterol 7$\alpha$-hydroxylase and HMG-CoA reductase in rat liver: effects of lymphatic drainage and ligation of the lymph duct. *J Lipid Res* 31:2159–2166.

Åkerlund JE, Reihnér E, Angelin B, Rudling M, Ewerth S, Björkhem I, Einarsson K (1991) Hepatic metabolism of cholesterol in Crohn's disease. Effect of partial resection of ileum. *Gastroenterology* 100:1046–1053.

Akiyama H, Nagusa Y, Fujita T, Shirane N, Sasao T, Iwamori S, Hidaka T, Okuhara T (1985) A new method for nonsurgical cholecystolithotomy. *Surg Gynecol Obstet* 161:73–74.

Akiyoshi A, Nakayama F (1990) Bile acid composition in brown pigment stones. *Dig Dis Sci* 35:27–32.

Albert MB, Fromm H, Shehan CM (1990) Densely calcified gallstone treated successfully with piezoelectric lithotripsy. *Gastroenterology* 98:777–779.

Alexander M, Portman OW (1987) Different susceptibilities to the formation of cholesterol gallstones in mice. *Hepatology* 7:257–265.

Allen B, Bernhoft R, Blanckaert N, Svanvik J, Filly R, Gooding G, Way L (1981) Sludge is calcium bilirubinate associated with bile stasis. *Am J Surg* 141:51–56.

Allen MJ, Borody TJ, Bugliosi TF, May GR, LaRusso NF, Thistle JL (1985) Cholelitholysis using methyl tertiary butyl ether. *Gastroenterology* 88:122–125.

Almé B, Nordén A, Sjövall J (1978) Glucuronides of unconjugated 6-hydroxylated bile acids in urine of a patient with malabsorption. *Clin Chim Acta* 86:251–259.

Alvaro D, Angelico F, Attili AF, Antonini R, Mazzarella B, Corradini SG, Gentile SG, Bracci F, Angelico M (1986a) Plasma lipid lipoproteins and biliary lipid composition in female gallstone patients. *Biomed Biochem Acta* 45:761–768.

Alvaro D, Cantafora A, Attili AF, Corradini SG, de Luca C, Minervini G, di Biase A, Angelico M (1986b) Relationships between bile salt hydrophobicity and phospholipid composition in bile of various animal species. *Comp Biochem Physiol (B)* 83:551–554.

Ammon HV (1979) Effect of taurine conjugated bile salts with and without lecithin on water and electrolyte transport in the canine gallbladder in vivo. *Gastroenterology* 76:778–783.

Amouyal P, Amouyal G, Lévy P, Tuzet S, Palazzo L, Vilgrain V, Gayet B, Belghiti J, Fékété F, Bernades P (1994) Diagnosis of choledocholithiasis by endoscopic ultrasonography. *Gastroenterology* 106:1062–1067.

Andersen I B, Højgaard L (1991) Whither biliary sludge – Do you exist? *Gastroenterology* 101:1758–1759.

Anderson DL (1972) Acalculous cholecystitis – a possible complication of parenteral hyperalimentation: report of a case. *Med Ann DC* 41:448–451.

Anderson A, James OFW, MacDonald HS, Snowball S, Taylor W (1980) The effects of ethinyl oestradiol on biliary lipid composition in young men. *Eur J Clin Invest* 10:77–80.

Anderson KE, Kok E, Javitt NB (1972) Bile acid synthesis in man: metabolism of 7$\alpha$-hydroxycholesterol-$^{14}$C and 26-hydroxycholesterol-$^{3}$H. *J Clin Invest* 51:112–117.

Andersson H, Bosaeus I, Fasth S, Hellberg R, Hultén L (1987) Cholelithiasis and urolithiasis in Crohn's disease. *Scand J Gastroenterol* 22:253–256.

Andrassy RJ, Treadwel TA, Ralner IA, Buckley CJ (1976) Gallbladder disease in children and adolescents. *Am J Surg* 132:19–21.

Andreini JP, Prigge WF, Ma C, Gebhard RL (1994) Vesicles and mixed micelles in hypothyroid rat bile before and after thyroid hormone treatment: evidence for a vesicle transport system for biliary cholesterol secretion. *J Lipid Res* 35:1405–1412.

Andrews E, Dostal LE, Goff M, Hrdina L (1932) The mechanism of cholesterol gallstone formation. *Ann Surg* 96:615–624.

Angelin B, Einarsson K (1988) Regulation of biliary cholesterol secretion in man. *Agents Actions Suppl (Basel)* 26:83–97.

Angelin B, Einarsson K, Hellstrom K, Kallner M (1976) Elimination of cholesterol in hyperlipoproteinemia. *Clin Sci Mol Med* 51:393–397.

Angelin B, Ewerth S, Einarsson K (1983) Ursodeoxycholic acid treatment in cholesterol gallstone disease: effects on hepatic 3-hydroxy-3-methylglutaryl coenzyme A reductase activity, biliary lipid composition, and plasma lipid levels. *J Lipid Res* 24:461–468.

Angelin B, Nilsell K, Einarsson K (1986) Ursodeoxycholic acid treatment in humans: effects on plasma and biliary lipid metabolism with special reference to very low density lipoprotein triglyceride and bile acid kinetics. *Eur J Clin Invest* 16:169–177.

Angelin B, Olivecrona H, Reihnér E, Rudling M, Ståhlberg D, Ericksson M, Ewerth S, Henriksson P, Einarsson K (1992) Hepatic cholesterol metabolism in estrogen-treated men. *Gastroenterology* 103:1657–1663.

Anver MR, Hunt RD, Chalifoux LV (1972) Cholesterol gallstones in *Aotus trivirgitatus*. *J Med Primatol* 1:241–246.

Apstein MD, Dalecki-Chipperfield K (1987) Spinal cord injury is a risk factor for gallstone disease. *Gastroenterology* 92:966–968.

Arca M, Ciocca S, Montali A, Capocaccia R, Angelico F, Angelico M, Attili AF, Calvieri A, Capocaccia L, Conti R, DeSantis A, Lalloni L, Morisi G, Ricci G, GREPCO (1987) Erythrocyte fatty acid composition and gallstone disease: results of an epidemiological survey. *Am J Clin Nutr* 46:110–114.

Archampong EQ (1969) Cholelithiasis in Accra. *Ghana Med* J 8:134 –139.

Arnesjö B, Bodvall B, Ståhl E (1975) Bile acid pattern of gallbladder and hepatic bile in patients with and without cholesterol gallstones. *Acta Chir Scand* 141:135–138.

Aschoff L, Bacmeister A (1909) *Die Cholelithiasis*. Jena, Verlag von Gustav Fischer.

Axelson M, Björkhem I, Reihnér E, Einarsson K (1991) The plasma level of 7$\alpha$-hydroxy-4-cholesten-3-one reflects the activity of hepatic cholesterol 7$\alpha$-hydroxylase in man. *FEBS lett* 284:216–218.

Axelsson H, Danielsson Å, Henriksson R, Wahlin T (1979) Secretory behavior and ultrastructural changes in mouse gallbladder principal cells after stimulation with cholinergic and adrenergic drugs. A morphometric study. *Gastroenterology* 76:335–340.

Ayyad N, Cohen BI, Mosbach EH, Mikami T, McSherry CK (1993) Biliary phospholipids and gallstones are affected by dietary fat in SASC0 hamsters. *Gastroenterology* 104:A347 (abstract).

Bailey PV, Conners RH, Tracy TF Jr, Sotelo-Avila C, Lewis JE, Weber TR (1989) Changing spectrum of cholelithiasis and cholecystitis in infants and children. *Am J Surg* 158:585–588.

Bainton D, Davies GT, Evans KT, Gravelle IH (1976) Gallbladder disease. Prevalence in a south Wales industrial town. *N Engl J Med* 294:1147–1149.

Balasegaram M (1972) Hepatic calculi. *Ann Surg* 175:149–154.

Balint J A, Kyriakides E C, Spitzer H L, Morrison E S (1965) Lecithin fatty acid composition in bile and plasma of man, dogs, rats and oxen. *J Lipid Res* 6:96–99.

Balint JA, Beeler DA, Kyriakides EC, Treble DM (1971) The effect of bile salts upon lecithin synthesis. *J Lab Clin Med* 77:122–133.

Balzer K, Goebell H, Breuer N, Rüping KW, Leder LD (1986) Epidemiology of gallstones in a German industrial town (Essen) from 1940–1975. *Digestion* 33:189–197.

Barbara L, Sama C, Labate AMM, Taroni F, Rusticali AG, Festi D, Sapio C, Roda E, Banterle C, Puci A, Formentini F, Colasanti S, Nardin F (1987) A population study on the prevalence of gallstone disease: the Sirmione study. *Hepatology* 7:913–917.

Barker EM, Winkler M (1984) Permanent-access hepaticojejunosotmy. *Br J Surg* 71:188–191.

Barkun AN, Barkun JS, Sampalis JS, Fried GM, Meakins JL, Goresky CA, McGill Gallstone Treatment Group (1993) Randomized clinical trial comparing gallbladder stone shock wave lithotripsy to laparoscopic cholecystectomy. *Gastroenterology* 104:A2 (abstract).

Barnett WO, Hilbun GR (1966) Dissolution of human gallstones in the dog's gallbladder after various degrees of vagotomy. *Surgery* 60:840–843.

Barnwell SG, Lowe PJ, Colman R (1984) The effects of colchicina on secretion into bile of bile salts, phospholipids, cholesterol and plasma membrane enzymes: bile salts are secreted unaccompanied by phospholipids and cholesterol. *Biochem J* 220:723–731.

Bass EB, Steinberg EP, Pitt HA, Saba GP, Lillemoe KD, Kafonek DR, Gadacz TR, Gordon TA, Anderson GF (1991) Cost-effectiveness of extracorporeal shock-wave lithotripsy versus cholecystectomy for symptomatic gallstones. *Gastroenterology* 101:189–199.

Bates GC, Brown CH (1952) Incidence of gallbladder disease in chronic hemolytic anemia (spherocytosis). *Gastroenterology* 21:104–109.

Bateson MC (1988) Oral contraceptives and gallstones. *Lancet* I:1115–1116.

Bateson MC (1990) Simvastatin and ursodeoxycholic acid for rapid gallstone dissolution. *Lancet* 336:1196.

Bayerdörffer E, Mannes GA, Richter WO, Ochsenkühn T, Wiebecke B, Köpcke W, Paumgartner G (1993) Increased serum deoxycholic acid levels in men with colorectal adenomas. *Gastroenterology* 104:145–151.

Becker BJP, Chatgidakis CB (1952) Carcinoma of the gallbladder and cholelithiasis in Witwatersrand: autopsy survey of racial incidence. *South Afr J Clin Sci* 3:13–22.

Becker BJP, Chatgidakis CB (1959) Acute cholecystitis and cholelithiasis. *Central Afr J Med* 10:513–519.

Been JM, Bills PM, Lewis D (1979) Microstructure of gallstones. *Gastroenterology* 76:548–555.

Beg ZH, Stonik JA, Brewer HB Jr (1987) Modulation of the enzyme activity of 3-hydroxy-3-methylglutaryl coenzyme A reductase by multiple kinase systems involving reversible phosphorylation: a review. *Metabolism* 36:900–917.

Behar J, Lee KY, Thompson WR, Biancani P (1989) Gallbladder contraction in patients with pigment and cholesterol stones. *Gastroenterology* 97:1479–1484.

Bell CC Jr, McCormick WC III, Gregory DH, Law DH, Vlahcevic ZR, Swell L (1972) Relationship of bile acid pool size to the formation of lithogenous bile in male Indians of the Southwest. *Surg Gynecol Obstet* 134:473–478.

Bell CC Jr, Vlahcevic ZR, Prazich J, Swell L (1973) Evidence that a diminished bile acid pool precedes the formation of cholesterol gallstones in man. *Surg Gynecol Obstet* 136:961–965.

Bell JJ, Sargeant TE, Watson JA (1976) Inhibition of 3-hydroxy-3-methylglutaryl coenzyme A reductase activity in hepatoma tissue culture cells by pure cholesterol and several cholesterol derivatives. Evidence supporting two distinct mechanisms. *J Biol Chem* 251:1745–1758.

Benes J, Chmel J, Dufek V, Kovdac V, Stuka C, Sunka P, Kalab M, Horejsi A (1989) Extracorporeal shock-wave lithotripsy of the common bile duct stone with ultrasound localization. *J Hepatol* 9:95–98.

Bennion LJ, Grundy SM (1975) Effects of obesity and caloric intake on biliary lipid metabolism in man. *J Clin Invest* 56:966–1011.

Bennion LJ, Grundy SM (1977) Effects of diabetes mellitus on cholesterol metabolism in man. *N. Engl J Med* 296:1365–1371.

Bennion LJ, Grundy SM (1978) Risk factors for the development of cholelithiasis in man. First of two parts. *N Engl J Med* 299:1161–1167. Second of two parts 1221–1227.

Bennion L J, Ginsberg R L, Garnick M B, Bennett P H (1976) Effects of oral contraceptives on the gallbladder bile of normal women. *N Engl J Med* 294:189–192.

Bennion LJ, Drobny E, Knowler WC, Ginsberg RL, Garnick MB, Adler RD, Duane WC (1978) Sex differences in the size of bile acid pools. *Metabolism* 27:961–969.

Bennion LJ, Knowler WC, Mott DM, Spagnola AM, Bennett PH (1979) Development of lithogenic bile during puberty in Pima Indians. *N Engl J Med* 300:873–876.

Bennion LJ, Mott DM, Howard BV (1980) Oral contraceptives raise cholesterol saturation of bile by increasing biliary cholesterol secretion. *Metabolism* 29:18–22.

Berci G, Sackier JM (1991) The Los Angeles experience with laparoscopic cholecystectomy. *Am J Surg* 161:382–384 .

Bergman F, Van der Linden W (1964) Influence of D-thyroxine on gallstone formation in hamsters. *Acta Chir Scand* 129:547–552.

Bergman F, Van der Linden W (1966) Further studies on the influence of thyroxine on gallstone formation in hamsters. *Acta Chir Scand* 131:319–328.

Bergman F, Van der Linden W (1967) Diet-induced cholesterol gallstones in hamsters: prevention and dissolution by cholestyramine. *Gastroenterology* 53:418–421.

Bergman F, Van der Linden W (1971) Reaction of the Mongolian gerbil to a cholesterol-cholic acid-containing diet. *Acta Pathol Microbiol Scand Sect* A 79:476–486.

Bergman F, Jaul AH, Van der Linden W (1971) The effect of liver toxins on gallstone formation in Syrian hamsters. *Acta Hepatosplenol* 18:215–223.

Bergman JJGHM, Groen AK, Huibregtse K, Tytgat GNJ (1994) Addition of dimethylsulphoxide to methyl-*tert*-butyl ether and ethyl propionate increases cholesterol dissolving capacity and cholesterol gall stone dissolution in vitro. *Gut* 35:1653–1658.

Bernhoft RA, Pellegrini CA, Broderick WC, Way LW (1983) Pigment sludge and stone formation in the acutely ligated dog gallbladder. *Gastroenterology* 85:1166–1171.

Bernhoft RA, Pellegrini CA, Motson RW, Way L W (1984) Composition and morphologic and clinical features of common duct stones. *Am J Surg* 148:77–85.

Bernstein RA, Werner LH, Rimm AA (1973) Relationship of gallbladder disease to parity, obesity, and age. *Health Serv Rep* 88:925–936.

Berr F, Mayer M, Sackmann MF, Sauerbruch T, Holl J, Paumgartner G (1994) Pathogenic factors in early recurrence of cholesterol gallstones. *Gastroenterology* 106:215–224.

Berr F, Pratschke E, Fischer S, Paumgartner G (1992a) Disorders of bile acid metabolism in cholesterol gallstone disease. *J Clin Invest* 90:859–868.

Berr F, Schreiber E, Frick U (1992b) Interrelationships of bile acid and phospholipid fatty acid species with cholesterol saturation of duodenal bile in health and gallstone disease. *Hepatology* 16:71–81.

Bertolotti M, Abate N, Bertolotti S, Loria P, Concari M, Messora R, Carubbi F, Pinetti A, Carulli N (1993) Effect of aging on cholesterol $7\alpha$-hydroxylation in humans. *J Lipid Res* 34:1001–1007.

Besançon F, Marche C, Souchard M, Debray C (1967) Cholesterol lithiasis and gallbladder injuries by dehydrocholate in mice. *Gastroenterology* 52:1071. (abstract).

Bevans M, Mosbach EH (1956) Biological studies of dihydrocholesterol. Production of biliary concrements and inflammatory lesions of the biliary tract in rabbits. *Arch Pathol* 62:112–117.

Bickerstaff KI, Moossa AR (1983) Effects of resection or bypass of the distal ileum on the lithogenicity of bile. *Am J Surg* 145:34–40.

Bienenstock J, Befus AD (1983) Some thoughts on the biologic role of immunoglobulin A. *Gastroenterology* 84:178–185.

Bilhartz LE, Dietschy JM (1988) Bile salt hydrophobicity influences cholesterol recruitment from rat liver in vivo when cholesterol synthesis and lipoprotein uptake are constant. *Gastroenterology* 95:771–779.

Bills PM, Lewis D (1975) A structual study of gallstones. *Gut* 16:630–637.

Binder HJ, Filburn C, Volpe BT (1977) Bile salt alteration of colonic electrolyte transport: role of cyclic adenosine monophosphate. *Gastroenterology* 68:503–508.

Binns RM (1964) Cholelithiasis causing obstructive jaundice in a Boxer dog. *Vet Rec* 76:239–243.

Bisgard JD, Baker CP (1940) Studies relating to the pathogenesis of cholecystitis, cholelithiasis and acute pancreatitis. *Ann Surg* 112:1006–1034.

Biss K, Ho KJ, Mikkelson B, Lewis L, Taylor CB (1971) Some unique biologic characteristics of the Masai of East Africa. *N Engl J Med* 284:694–699.

Björkhem I (1985) Mechanism of bile acid biosynthesis in mammalian liver. In Danielsson H, Sjövall J, (eds.): Sterols and Bile Acids. Amsterdam, Elsevier, pp 231–278

Björkhem I (1992) Mechanism of degradation of the steroid side chain in the formation of bile acids. *J Lipid Res* 33:455–471.

Björkhem I, Åkerlund JE (1988) Studies on the link beween HMG-CoA reductase and cholesterol 7$\alpha$-hydroxylase in rat liver. *J Lipid Res* 29:136–143.

Björkhem I, Reihnér E, Angelin B, Ewerth S, Åkerlund JE, Einarsson K (1987) On the possible use of the serum level of 7$\alpha$-hydroxycholesterol as a marker for increased activity of the cholesterol 7$\alpha$-hydroxylase in humans. *J Lipid Res* 28:889–894.

Björkhem I, Eggertsen G, Andersson U (1991) On the mechanism of stimulation of cholesterol 7$\alpha$-hydroxylase by dietary cholesterol. *Biochim Biophys Acta* 1085:329–335.

Björkhem I, Andersson U, Sudjama-Sugiaman E, Eggertsen G, Hylemon P (1993) Studies on the link between HMG-CoA reductase and cholesterol 7$\alpha$-hydroxylase on lymph-fistula rats: evidence for both transcriptional and post-transcriptional mechanisms for down-regulation of the two enzymes by bile acids. *J Lipid Res* 34:1497–1503.

Black BE, Carr SH, Ohkubo H, Ostrow JD (1982) Equilibrium swelling of pigment gallstones: evidence for network polymer structure. *Biopolymers* 21:601–610.

Bland KI, Jones RS, Maher JW, Cotton PB, Pennell TC, Amerson J R, Munson JL, Berci G, Fuchs GJ, Way LW, Graham JB, Lindenau BU, Moody FG, Newman RC, Finlayson B, Copeland EM III, Gravenstein N, Hawkins IF, Hocking MP, Kalvaria I, King CE, Ros PR, Vogel SB, Gillenwater JY, McCallum RW, Tegtmeyer CJ, Johlin F, Loening S, Summers R, Weinerth J, McCullough DL, Gelfand D, Gilliam J, Myers RT, Wolf D, Ambrose S, Rossi R, Panish J, Fink A, Tompkins R, Gordon R, Ring E, Shapiro H, Craigs R, Nahrwold D (1989) Extracorporeal shockwave lithotripsy of bile duct calculi: an interim report of the Dornier US bile duct lithotripsy. *Ann Surg* 209:743–755.

Bloch K, Rittenberg D (1942) On the utilization of acetic acid for cholesterol formation. *J Biol Chem* 145:625–636.

Bloch K, Berg BN, Rittenberg D (1943) The biological conversion of cholesterol to cholic acid. *J Biol Chem* 149:511–517.

Bloch HM, Thornton JR, Heaton KW (1980) Effects of fasting on the composition of gallbladder bile. *Gut* 21:1087–1089.

Blomstrand R, Ekdahl P (1960) Fatty acid pattern of human bile under normal and pathological conditions. *Proc Soc Exp Biol Med* 104:205–209.

Bloom AA, Stachenfeld R (1969) Diabetic cholecystomegaly. *J A M A* 208:357–359.

Bodvall B, Övergaard B (1966) The association between ABO blood groups and cholelithiasis with special reference to biliary distress following cholecystectomy. *Acta Chir Scand* 131:334–342.

Bogren H (1983) The polymorphs of calcium carbonate in human gall stones. *Scand J Clin Lab Invest* 43:371–375.

Bogren H, Larsson K (1963) Crystalline components of biliary calculi. *Scand J Clin Lab Invest* 15:457–462.

Bolondi L, Gaiani S, Testa S, Labo G (1985) Gall bladder sludge formation during prolonged fasting after gastrointestinal tract surgery. *Gut* 26:734–738.

Bomzon A, Finberg JPM, Tovbin D, Naidu SG, Better OS (1984) Bile salts, hypotension and obstructive jaundice. *Clin Sci* 67:177–183.

Bond LR, Hatty SR, Horn MEC, Dick M, Meire HB, Bellingham AJ (1987) Gall stones in sickle cell disease in the United Kingdom. *Br Med J* 295:234–236.

Booker ML, Scott TE, LaMorte WW (1989) Effect of dietary cholesterol on phosphatidylcholines and phsophatidylethanolamines in bile and gallbladder mucosa in the prairie dog. *Gastroenterology* 97:1261–1267.

Booker ML, Scott TE, LaMorte WW (1990) Effects of dietary fish oil on biliary phospholipids and prostaglandin synthesis in the cholesterol-fed prairie dog. *Lipids* 25:27–32.

Booker ML, LaMorte WW, Ahrendt SA, Lillemore KD, Pitt HA (1992) Distribution of phosphatidylcholine molecular species between mixed micelles and phospholipid-cholesterol vesicles in human gallbladder bile: dependence on acyl chain length and unsaturation. *J Lipid Res* 33:1485–1492.

Borch K, Chu M, Kullman E, Carlsson B, Rehfeld JF (1994) Endogenous hypercholecystokininemia, but not aspirin, reduces the gallstone incidence in the hamster model. *Scand J Gastroenterol* 29:740–743.

Borgman RF (1964) Fat metabolism as influenced by dietary fatty acids and vitamin E status in the rabbit. *J Food Sci* 29:20–24.

Borgman RF (1965) Gallstone formation in rabbits as affected by dietary fat and protein. *Am J Vet Res* 26:1167–1171.

Bortnichak EA, Freeman DH Jr, Ostfeld AM, Castelli WP, Kannel WB, Feinleib M, McNamara PM (1985) The association between cholesterol cholelithiasis and coronary heart disease in Framingham, Massachusetts. *Am J Epidemiol* 121:19–28.

Boscaini M, Piccinni-Leopardi M, Andreotti F, Montori A (1994) Gall stone pulverisation strategy in patients treated with extracorporeal lithotripsy and follow-up results of maintenance treatment with ursodeoxycholic acid. *Gut* 35:117–121.

Boston Collaborative Drug Surveillance Program (1973) Oral contraceptives and venous thromboembolic disease, surgically confirmed gallbladder disease and breast tumors. *Lancet* l:1399–1404.

Boston Collaborative Drug Surveillance Program (1974) Surgically confirmed gallbladder disease, venous thromboembolism, and breast tumors in relation to postmenopausal estrogen therapy. *N Engl J Med* 290:15–19.

Bouchier IAD (1969) Postmortem study of the frequency of gallstones in patients with cirrhosis of the liver. *Gut* 10:705–710.

Bouchier IAD (1988) Gallstones: formation and epidemiology. In Blumgart LH (ed): Surgery of the Liver and Biliary Tract. Edinburgh: Churchill Livingstone, pp 503–516.

Bouchier IAD, Cooperband SR (1967) Isolation and characterization of a macromolecular aggregate associated with bilirubin. *Clin Chim Acta* 15:291–302.

Bouchier IAD, Cooperband SR, El Kodsi BM (1965) Mucous substances and viscosity of normal and pathological human bile. *Gastroenterology* 49:343–353.

Bove P, de Oliveira MR, Sparanzini M (1963) Intrahepatic lithiasis. *Gastroenterology* 44:251–256.

Boyden E A, Grantham S A Jr (1936) Evacuation of gall bladder in old age. Surg Gynecol Obstet 62: 34–42.

Braverman DZ (1986) The lack of effect of metoclopramide on gallbladder volume and contraction in diabetic cholecystoparesis. *Am J Gastroenterol* 81:960–962

Braverman DZ, Johnson ML, Kern F Jr (1980) Effects of pregnancy and contraceptive steroids on gallbladder function. *N Engl J Med* 302:362–364.

Brenneman DE, Conner WE, Forker EL, DenBesten L (1972) The formation of abnormal bile and cholesterol gallstones from dietary cholesterol in the prairie dog. *J Clin Invest* 51:1495–1503.

Brett M, Barker DJP (1976) The world distribution of gallstones. *Int J Epidemiol* 5:335–341.

Breuer NF, Katschinski B, Mörtl E, Leder LD, Goebell H (1988) Large bowel cancer risk in cholelithiasis and after cholecystectomy. Postmortem study. *Digestion* 40:219–226.

Brill PW, Winchester P, Rosen MS (1982) Neonatal cholelithiasis. *Pediatr Radiol* 12:285–288.

Brink JA, Simeone JF, Mueller PR, Richter JM, Prien EL, Ferrucci JT (1988) Physical characteristics of gallstones removed at cholecystectomy: implications for extracorporeal shockwave lithotripsy. *Am J Roentgenol* 151:927–931.

Brodersen R (1979) Bilirubin. Solubility and interaction with albumin and phospholipid. *J Biol Chem* 254:2364–2369.

Broomfield PH, Chopra R, Sheinbaum RC, Bonorris GG, Silverman A, Schoenfield LJ (1988) Effects of ursodeoxycholic acid and aspirin on the formation of lithogenic bile and gallstones during loss of weight. *N Engl J Med* 319: 1567–1572.

Browman AA, Hastings AB (1937) Solubility of aragonite in salt solutions. *J Biol Chem* 119:241–246.

Browman PC, Kottler RE, Terblanche J, Kingsnorth AN, Krige JE, Marks IN (1988) Does low entry of cystic duct predispose to stones in the common bile duct ? *Br Med J* 297:31–32.

Brown MS, Goldstein JL (1984) How LDL receptors influence cholesterol and atherosclerosis. *Sci Am* 251 (5):52–60.

Bruce LA, Behsudi FM (1979) Progesterone effects on three regional gastrointestinal tissues. *Life Sci* 25:729–734.

Brückner M, Grimm H, Soehendra N (1990) Electrohydraulic lithotripsy of complicated choledocholithiasis. *Endoscopy* 22:234–235.

Brugge WR, Brand DL, Atkins HL, Lane BP, Abel WG (1986) Gallbladder dyskinesia in chronic acalculous cholecystitis. *Dig Dis Sci* 31:461–467.

Brugge WR, Shiffman ML, Furth EL, MacDermott RP, Malet PF (1993) Ursodiol reduces gallbladder bile mucin and immunoglobulins in gallstone patients. *Gastroenterology* 104:A351 (abstract).

Bull AW, Marnett LJ, Dawe EJ, Nigro ND (1983) Stimulation of deoxythymidine incorporation in the colon of rats treated intrarectally with bile acids and fats. *Carcinogenesis* 4:207–210.

Burkitt DP, Tunstall M (1975) Gall-stones: geographical and chronological features. *J Trop Med Hyg* 78:140–144.

Burnstein MJ, Ilson RG, Petrunka CN, Taylor RD, Strasberg SM (1983) Evidence for a potent nucleating factor in gallbladder bile of patients with cholesterol gallstones. *Gastroenterology* 85:801–807.

Busch N, Tokumo H, Holzbach RT (1990) A sensitive method for determination of cholesterol growth using model solutions of supersaturated bile. *J Lipid Res* 31:1903–1909.

Busch N, Matiuck N, Sahlin S, Pillay SP, Holzbach RT (1991) Inhibition and promotion of cholesterol crystallization by protein fractions from normal human gallbladder bile. *J Lipid Res* 32:695–702.

Cahlin E, Jönsson J, Nilsson S, Scherstén T (1973a) Biliary lipid composition in normolipidemic and prebeta hyperlipoproteinemia gallstone patients. Influence of sucrose feeding of the patients on the biliary lipid composition. *Scand J Gastroenterol* 8:449–456.

Cahlin E, Jönsson J, Persson B, Stakeberg H, Björntorp P, Gustafson A, Scherstén T (1973b) Sucrose feeding in man. Effects of substrate incorporation into hepatic triglyceride and phosphoglycerides in vitro and on removal of intravenous fat in patients with hyperlipoproteinemia. *Scand J Clin Lab Invest* 32:21–33.

Caira EG, Skoryna SC, Ritchie AC, Webster DR (1957) Studies on production of biliary concrements with 3$\beta$-

cholestanol in laboratory animals. *Surg Forum* 8:222–225.

Caldwell FT Jr, Levitsky K (1967) The gallbladder and gallstone formation. *Ann Surg* 166:753–758.

Caldwell FT Jr, Levitsky K, Rosenberg B (1965) Dietary production and dissolution of cholesterol gallstones in the mouse. Am J Physiol 209:473–478.

Cameron JL, Gadacz T R (1991) Laparoscopic cholecystectomy. *Ann Surg* 213:1–2.

Cameron JL, Maddrey WC, Zuidema GD (1971) Biliary tract disease in sickle cell anemia: surgical consideration. *Ann Surg* 174:702–710.

Cano N, Cicero F, Ranieri F, Martin J, Di Costanzo J (1986) Ultrasonographic study of gallbladder motility during total parenteral nutrition. *Gastroenterology* 91:313–317.

Cantafora A, Angelico M, Di Biase A, Pieche U, Bracci F, Attili AF, Capocaccia L (1981) Structure of biliary phosphatidylcholine in cholesterol gallstone patients. *Lipids* 16:589–592.

Capron JP, Delamarre J, Herve MA, Dupas JL, Poulain P, Descombes P (1981) Meal frequency and duration of overnight fast: a role in gallstone formation? *Br Med J* 283:1435.

Carey MC (1978) Critical tables for calculating the cholesterol satulation of native bile. *J Lipid Res* 19:945–955.

Carey MC, Cahalane MJ (1988a) Whither biliary sludge? *Gastroenterology* 95:508–523.

Carey MC, Cahalane MJ (1988b) Enterohepatic circulation. In Arias IM, Jacoby WB, Popper H, Schachter D, Shafritz D (eds): The liver: biology and pathobiology. New York, Raven Press, pp 573–616.

Carey MC, Mazer NA (1984) Biliary lipid secretion in health and in cholesterol gallstone diesease. *Hepatology* 4:31S–37S.

Carey MC, Small DM (1978) The physical chemistry of cholesterol solubility in bile. Relationship to gallstone formation and dissolution in man. *J Clin Invest* 61: 998–1026.

Cartmell WB, Edwards HG, Hammonds P (1964) Cholelithiasis in a Dachshund bitch and its surgical treatment. *Vet Rec* 76: 1323–1324.

Carulli N, Ponz de Leon M, Zironi F, Pinetti A, Smerieri A, Iori R, Loria P (1980) Hepatic cholesterol and bile acid metabolism in subjects with gallstones: comparative effects of short term feeding of chenodeoxycholic acid and ursodeoxycholic acid. *J Lipid Res* 21:35–43.

Carulli N, Ponz de Leon M, Loria P, Iori R, Rosi A, Romani M (1981) Effect of the selective expansion of the cholic acid pool on bile lipid composition: possible mechanism of bile acid induced biliary cholesterol desaturation. *Gastroenterology* 81:539–546.

Carulli N, Loria P, Bertolotti M, Ponz de Leon M, Menozzi D, Medici G, Piccagli I (1984) Effects of acute changes of bile acid pool composition on biliary lipid secretion. *J Clin Invest* 74:614–624.

Caselli M, Morsiani E, Aleotti A, Alvisi V (1990) Gall bladder epithelium and cholesterol gall stones. *Gut* 31:1423.

Castleden WM, Detchon P, Misso NLA (1985) Biliary bile acids in cholelithiasis and colon cancer. *Gut* 30:860–865.

Catnach SM, Fairclough PD, Trembath RC, O'Donnel LJD, McLean AM, Law PA, Wickham JEA (1992) Effect of oral erythromycin on gallbladder motility in normal subjects and subjects with gallstones. *Gastroenterology* 102:2071–2076.

Cattey RP, Wilson SD (1989) Cholelithiasis follows total gastrectomy in Zollinger-Ellison syndrome. *Surgery* 106:1070–1073.

Cawein MJ III, Hagedorn AB, Owen CA Jr (1960) Anemia of hepatic disease studied with radiochromium. *Gastroenterology* 38:324–331.

Cetta F (1986) Bile infection documented as initial event in the pathogenesis of brown pigment biliary stones. *Hepatology* 6:482–489.

Cetta F, De Nisi A (1986) Importance of biliary phsopholipase activity in the formation of brown stones. *Hepatology* 6:153–154.

Cetta F, De Nisi D, Petrini C, Bralia A, Campopiano M (1984) Composition and possible pathogenesis of pigment gallstones. *Gastroenterology* 86:1314 (abstract).

Cetta F, Lombardo F (1991) The possible role of phospholipase in gallstone pathogenesis. *Gastroenterology* 101:592–593.

Cetta F, Lombardo F, Giubbolini M, Malet P (1993) Hepatolithiasis: 1. Frequency, stones type and compostion in a consecutive series of 1350 surgical patients. *Gastroenterology* 104:A355 (abstract).

Chadwick VS, Gaginella TS, Debonguie JC, Phillips SF, Hofmann AF (1976) Different effects of chenodeoxycholic and ursodeoxycholic acids on colonic secretion, permeability and morphology. *Gastroenterology* 71:900 (abstract).

Chang TM, Passaro E Jr (1983) Intrahepatic stones: the Taiwan experience. *Am J Surg* 146:241–244.

Chapman WC, Stephens WH, Williams LF (1989) Principles of biliary extracorporeal lithotripsy. Technical considerations and clinical implications. *Am J Surg* 158:179–183.

Chen HH, Zhang WH, Wang SS Caruana JA (1984) Twenty-two year experience with the diagnosis and treatment of intrahepatic calculi. *Surg Gynecol Obstet* 159:519–524.

Cheslyn-Curtis S, Gillams AR, Russell RCG, Donald JJ, Lake SP, Ainley CA, Hatfield ARW, Lees WR (1992) Selection, management, and early outcome of 113 patients with symptomatic gall stones treated by percutaneous cholecystolithotomy. *Gut* 33:1253–1259.

Chevreul HJ (1815) Recherches chimiques sur plusieurs corps gras, et particulierement sur leurs combinations avec les alcalis. Cinqureme Mémoire. Des corps qu'on a appelés adipocire, c'est-a-dire, de la substance cristallisée des calculs biliaires humanis, du spermacéti et de la substance grasse des cadavres. *Ann Chim* 95:5–50.

Chijiiwa K, Ogawa Y, Hirota I, Nakayama F (1990) Biliary lipid and bile acid composition before and after endoscopic sphincterotomy. *Hepatogastroenterology* 37:510–512.

Chijiiwa K, Koga A, Yamasaki T, Shimada K, Noshiro H, Nakayama F (1991) Fibronectin: a possible factor promoting cholesterol monohydrate crystallization in bile. *Biochim Biophys Acta* 1086:44–48.

Chiverton SG, Inglis JA, Hudd C, Kellett MJ, Russell RCG, Wickham JEA (1990) Percutaneous cholecystolithotomy: the first 60 patients. *Br Med J* 300:1310–1312.

Chow LP (1960) Epidemiological studies of clonorchiasis at Meinung township in southern Taiwan. Formosan Sci 14:134–166.

Christensen F, Prange I, Dam H (1962) Composition of the bladder bile of young white mice reared on a diet causing formation of cholesterol gallstones in young hamsters. *Z Ernährungswiss* 3:117–121.

Christensen F, Prange I, Dam H (1964) Alimental production of gallstones in hamsters. 13. Influence of highly unsaturated fats and certain minerals on gallstone production. *Z Ernährungswiss* 4:186–192.

Clarke BF, Ewing DJ, Campbell LW (1979) Diabetic autonomic neuropathy. Diabetologia 17:195–212.

Clave RA, Gaspar MR (1969) Incidence of gallstone disease after vagotomy. *Am J Surg* 118:169–176.

Cobo A, Hall RC, Torres E, Cuello CJ (1964) Intrahepatic calculi. *Arch Surg* 89:936–941.

Cohen DE, Carey MC (1990a) Physical chemistry of biliary lipids during bile formation. *Hepatology* 12:143S–148S.

Cohen DE, Carey MC (1990b) Rapid (1 hour) high performance gel filtration chromatography resolves coexisting simple micelles, mixed micelles, and vesicles in bile. *J Lipid Res* 31:2103–2112.

Cohen DE, Carey MC (1991) Acyl chain unsaturation modulates distribution of lecithin molecular species between mixed micelles and vesicles in model bile. Implications for particle structure and metastable cholesterol solubilities. *J Lipid Res* 32:1291–1302.

Cohen S, Soloway RD (1985) *Gallstones.* New York, Churchill Livingstone.

Cohen S, Kaplan M, Gottlieb L, Patterson J (1971) Liver disease and gallstones in regional enteritis. *Gastroenterology* 60:237–245.

Cohen BI, Singhal AK, Stenger RJ, May-Donath P, Finver-Sadowsky J, McSherry CK, Mosbach EH (1984) Effects of bile acid oxazoline on gallstone formation in prairie dogs. *Lipids* 19:515–521.

Cohen BI, Mosbach EH, McSherry CK, Rzigalinski B, Kuroki S (1986) A hydrophilic bile acid effects partial dissolution of cholesterol gallstones in the prairie dog. *Lipids* 21:575–579.

Cohen BI, Setoguchi T, Mosbach EH, McSherry CK, Stenger R J, Kuroki S, Soloway RD (1987) An animal model of pigment cholelithiasis. *Am J Surg* 153:130–138.

Cohen BI, Matoba N, Mosbach EH, McSherry CK (1989a) Dietary induction of cholesterol gallstones in hamsters from three different sources. *Lipids* 24:151–156.

Cohen BI, Matoba N, Mosbach EH, Stenger RJ, McSherry CK (1989b) Cholelithiasis in hamsters: effects of cholic acid and calcium on gallstone formation. *Lipids* 24:482–487.

Cohen DE, Angelico M, Carey MC (1990a) Structural alterations in lecithin-cholesterol vesicles following interactions with monomeric and micellar bile salts: physical and chemical basis for subselection of biliary lecithin species and aggregative states of biliary lipids during bile formation. *J Lipid Res* 31:55–70.

Cohen BI, Matoba N, Mosbach EH, Ayyad N, Hakam K, Suh SO, McSherry CK (1990b) Bile acids substituted in the 6 position prevent cholesterol gallstone formation in the hamster. *Gastroenterology* 98:397–405.

Cohen BI, Mosbach EH, Ayyad N, Yoshii M, McSherry CK (1991) Aspirin does not inhibit cholesterol cholelithiasis in two established animal models. *Gastroenterology* 101:1109–1116.

Cohen BI, Mosbach EH, Miki S, Mikami T, Infante R (1993) $\beta$-Muricholic acid – a hydrophilic bile acid with cholelitholytic potential. Gastroenterology 104:A889, (abstract).

Coleman R (1987) Biochemistry of bile secretion. *Biochem J* 244:249–261.

Coleman R, Rahman K (1992) Lipid flow in bile formation. *Biochim Biophys Acta* 1125:113–133.

Coleman JP, White WB, Lijewski M, Hylemon PB (1988) Nucleotide sequence and regulation of a gene involved in bile acid 7-dehydroxylation by *Eubacterium* sp. Strain VPI 12708. *J Bacteriol* 170:2070–2077.

Collier NA, Blumgart LH (1994) Tumours of the gallbladder. In Blumgart L H (ed): *Surgery of the Liver and Biliary Tract*, Vol 2 (2nd ed). Edinburgh, Churchill Livingstone, pp 955–965.

Collins JJ, Phillips MC (1982) The stability and structure of cholesterol-rich codispersions of cholesterol and phosphatidylcholine. *J Lipid Res* 23:291–298.

Comess LJ, Bennet PH, Burch TA (1967) Clinical gallbladder disease in Pima Indians. Its high prevalence in contrast to Framingham, Massachusetts. *N Engl J Med* 277:894–898.

Conrad RR, Janes JO, Dietchy J (1979) Significance of low level echoes within the gallbladder. *Am J Roentgenol* 132:967–972.

Conter RL, Roslyn JJ, Pitt HA, DenBesten L (1986a) Carbohydrate diet-induced calcium bilirubinate sludge and pigment gallstones in the prairie dog. *J Surg Res* 40:580–587.

Conter RL, Roslyn JJ, Porter-Fink V, DenBesten L (1986b) Gallbladder absorption increases during early cholesterol gallstone formation. *Am J Surg* 151:184–191.

Conter RL, Washington JL, Liao CC, Kauffman GL Jr (1992) Gallbladder mucosal blood flow increases during early cholesterol gallstone formation. *Gastroenterology* 102:1764–1770.

Cook J, Hou PC, Ho HC, McFadzean AJS (1954) Recurrent pyogenic cholangeitis. *Br J Surg* 42:188–203.

Cooke L, Jones FA, Keech MK (1953) Carcinoma of gall-bladder. A statistical study. *Lancet* 2: 585–587.

Cooper AD (1991) Metabolic basis of cholesterol gallstone disease. Gastroenterol Clin North Am 20:21–46.

Cooperberg PL, Burhenne HJ (1980) Real time ultrasonography. Diagnostic technique of choice in calculous gallbladder disease. *N Engl J Med* 302:1277–1279.

Coronary Drug Project Research Group (1977) Gallbladder disease as a side effect of drugs influencing lipid metabolism. Experience in the Coronary Drug Project. *N Engl J Med* 296:1185–1190.

Cosman B, Porter MR (1960) Benign stricture of the bile ducts. *Ann Surg* 152:730–742.

Costerton JW, Irvin RT (1981) The bacterial glycocalyx in nature and disease. *Ann Rev Microbiol* 35:299–324.

Cotton PB, Kozarek RA, Schapiro RH, Nishioka NS, Kelsey PB, Ball TJ Putnam WS, Barkun A, Weinerth J (1990) Endoscopic laser lithotripsy of large bile duct stones. *Gastroenterology* 99:1128–1133.

Covarrubias C, Valdivieso V, Nervi F (1984) Epidemiology of gallstone disease in Chile. In Capocaccia L, Ricci G, Angelico M, Attili AF (eds): *Epidemiology and Prevention of Gallstone Disease*. London, Lancaster MTP Press, pp

26–30.

Cowie AGA, Clark C G (1972) The lithogenic effect of vagotomy. Br J Surg 59:365–367

Cowie AGA, Sutor DJ, Wooley SE (1973) The calcium palmitate gall-stone. *Br J Surg* 60:16–18.

Cox KL, Cheung ATW, Lohse CL, Iwahashi-Hosoda CK, Walsh EM (1985) Effect of aging on biliary motility and structure. *Fed Proc* 44:1395 (abstract).

Coyne MJ, Bonorris GG, Goldstein LI, Schoenfield LJ (1976) Effect of chenodeoxycholic acid and phenobarbital on the rate-limiting enzymes of hepatic cholesterol and bile acid synthesis in patients with gallstones. *J Lab Clin Med* 87:281–291.

Coyne MJ, Bonorris GG, Chung A, Winchester R, Schoenfield LJ (1978) Estrogen enhances dietary cholesterol induction of saturated bile in the hamster. *Gastroenterology* 75:76–79.

Crawford JM, Berken CA, Gollan JL (1988) Role of the hepatocyte microtubular system in the excretion of bile salts and biliary lipid: implications for intracellular vesicular transport. *J Lipid Res* 29:144–156.

Cripps DJ, Scheuer PJ (1965) Hepatobiliary changes in erythropoietic protoporphyria. *Arch Pathol* 80:500–508.

Crowther RS, Okido M (1994) Inhibition of calcium phosphate precipitation by bile salts: a test of the $Ca^{2+}$-buffering hypothesis. *J Lipid Res* 35:279–290.

Crowther RS, Soloway RD (1990) Pigment gallstone pathogenesis: from man to molecules. *Semin Liver Dis* 10:171–180.

Csendes A, Larach J, Godoy M (1978) Incidence of gallstone development after selective hepatic vagotomy. *Acta Chir Scand* 144:289–291.

Cummings SA, Hofmann AF (1984) Physiologic determinants of biliary calcium secretion in the dog. *Gastroenterology* 87:664–673.

Cuschieri A, Dubois F, Mouiel J, Mouret P, Becker H, Buess G, Trede M, Troidl H (1991) The European experience with laparoscopic cholecystectomy. *Am J Surg* 161:385–387.

Dai K Y, Montet JC, Zhao XM, Amic J, Montet AM (1989) Dissolution of human brown pigment biliary stones. *J Hepatol* 9:301–311.

Daignault PG, Fazekas AG, Rosenthal L, Fried GM (1988) Relationship between gallbladder contraction and progesterone receptors in patients with gallstones. *Am J Surg* 155:147–151.

Dam H (1958) Histroical introduction. In Cook RP (ed): *Cholesterol. Chemistry, Biochemistry and Pathology*. New York, Academic Press, pp 1–14.

Dam H (1969) Nutritional aspects of gallstone formation with particular reference to alimentary production of gallstones in laboratory animals. *World Rev Nutr Diet* 11:199–239.

Dam H (1971) Determinants of cholesterol cholelithiasis in man and animals. *Am J Med* 51:596–613.

Dam H, Christensen F (1952) Alimentary production of gallstones in hamsters. *Acta Pathol Microbiol Scand* 30:236–242.

Dam H, Christensen F (1961) Alimentary production of gallstones in hamster. 8. Influence of dietary fat. *Z Ernährungswiss* 2:36–41.

Dam H, Christensen F (1962) Alimentary production of gallstones in hamsters. 10. The effect of orally ingested bile acids on development of choelsterol gallstones in hamsters fed a fat-free diet with glucose as carbohydrate component. *Z Ernährungswiss* 2:154–159.

Dam H, Christensen F (1965) Alimentary production of gallstones in hamsters. 15. Production of gallstones under varied hormonal conditions. *Z Ernährungswiss* 5:149–160.

Dam H, Kruse I, Prange I, Kallehauge HE, Fenger HJ, Krogh-Jensen M (1971) Studies on human bile. III. Composition of duodenal bile from healthy young volunteers compared with composition of bladder bile from surgical patients with and without uncomplicated gallstone disease. *Z Ernährungswiss* 10:160–177.

Dam H, Prange I, Søndergaard E (1968) Alimentary production of gallstones in hamsters. 20. Influence of dietary cholesterol on gallstone formation. *Z Ernährungswiss* 9:43–48.

Dam H, Prange I, Søndergaard E (1972a) Alimentary production of gallstones in hamsters. 25. Inhibition of production of cholesterol gallstones by 2-(p-chlorophenoxy)-isobutylic acid ethyl ester (Clofibrate). *Z Ernährungswiss* 11:95–104.

Dam H, Prange I, Søndergaard E (1972b) Alimentary production of gallstones in hamsters. 24. Influence of orally ingested chenodeoxycholic acid and hyodeoxycholic acid on formation of gallstones. *Z Ernährungswiss* 11:80–94.

Danalis J, Penny RHC (1967) Cholelithiasis in a sow. *Aust Vet* J 43:119.

Danielsson H, Wikvall K (1981) Evidence for a specific cytochrome P-450 with short half-life catalyzing 7$\alpha$-hydroxylation of cholesterol. *Biochem Biophys Res Commun* 103:46–51.

Danielsson H, Eneroth P, Hellström K, Lindstedt S, Sjövall J (1963) On the turnover and excretory products of cholic acid and chenodeoxycholic acid in man. *J Biol Chem* 238: 2299–2304.

Danon Y L, Dinari G, Garty B Z, Horodniceanu C, Nitzan M, Grunebaum M (1983) Cholelithiasis in children with immunoglobulin A deficiency: a new gastroenterologic syndrome. *J Pediatr Gastroenterol Nutr* 2:663–666.

Danzinger RG, Hofmann AF, Schoenfield LJ, Thistle JL (1971) Altered bile acid metabolism in patients with cholesterol cholelithiasis. *J Clin Invest* 50:24a (abstract).

Danzinger RG, Gordon H, Schoenfield LJ, Thistle JL (1972a) Lithogenic bile in siblings of young women with cholelithiasis. *Mayo Clin Proc* 47:762–766.

Danzinger RG, Hofmann AF, Schoenfield LJ, Thistle JL (1972b) Dissolution of cholesterol gallstones by chenodeoxycholic acid. *N Engl J Med* 286:1–8.

Danzinger RG, Nakagaki M, Hofmann AF, Ljungwe EB (1984) Differing effects of hydroxy-7-oxotaurine-conjugated bile acids on bile flow and biliary lipid secretion in dogs. *Am J Physiol* 246:G166–G172.

Daughaday WH (1990) Octreotide is effective in acromegaly but often results in cholelithiasis. *Ann Intern Med* 112:159–160.

Davidson JF (1962) Alcohol and cholelithiasis: a necropsy survey of cirrhotics. *Am J Med Sci* 244:703–705.

Davis RA, Kern F Jr (1976) Effects of ethinylestradiol and phenobarbital on bile acid synthesis and biliary bile acid and cholesterol excretion. *Gastroenterology* 70:1130–1135.

Davis RA, Highsmith WE, McNeal MM, Schexnayder JA, Kuan JC (1983) Bile acid synthesis by cultured hepatocytes. Inhibition by mevinolin but not by bile acids. *J Biol Chem* 258:4079–4082.

Davis RA, Musso CA, McNeal MM, Lattier GR, Hyde PM, Schexnayder JA, Straka M (1988) Examination of bile acid negative feedback regulation in rats. *J Lipid Res* 29:202–211.

Dawes LG, Nahrwold DL, Rege RV (1988) Increased total and free ionized calcium in a canine model of pigment gallstones. *Surgery* 104:86–90.

Dawes LG, Nahrwold DL, Rege RV (1989) Supersaturation of canine gallbladder bile with calcium bilirubinate during formation of pigment gallstones. *Am J Surg* 157:82–88.

Dawes LG, Moore EW, Rege RV, Shimizu S, Ostrow JD (1991) Canine bile contains anticrystallization factors that inhibit precipitation of calcium carbonate. *Hepatology* 14:701–706.

Decker RA, Krohn AF (1973) Cholelithiasis in an Indian elephant. *J Am Vet Med Assoc* 163:546–547.

de Leon M P, Ferenderes R, Carulli N (1978) Bile lipid composition and bile acid pool size in diabetes. *Am J Dig Dis* 23:710–716.

Delchier JC, Benfredj P, Preaux AM, Metreau JM, Dhumeaux D (1986) The usefulness of microscopic bile examination in patients with suspected microlithiasis: a prospective evaluation. *Hepatology* 6:118–122.

Delius M, Enders G, Heine G, Stark J, Remberger K, Brendel W (1987) Biological effects of shock wave: lung hemorrrhage by shock waves in dogs – pressure dependence. Ultrasound Med Biol 13:61–67.

DenBesten L, Conner WE, Bell S (1973) The effect of dietary cholesterol on the composition of human bile. *Surgery* 73:266–273.

Denis BJ, Bas V, Goudot C, Frederic M, Bigard MA, Gaucher P (1993) Accuracy of endoscopic ultrasonography (EUS) for diagnosis of common bile duct stones (CBDS). *Gastroenterology* 104:A358 (abstract).

DeSantis A, Paganelli R, Stefanoni R, DiSabatino A, Angelico M (1990) Prevalence of gallstones in patients with primary immunoglobulin deficiency. Evidence for lack of association. *Dig Dis Sci* 35:716–720.

Diamond JM (1964) Transport of salt and water in rabbit and guinea pig gallbladder. *J Gen Physiol* 48:15–42.

Diaz-Buxo JA, Hermans PE, Elveback LR (1975) Prevalence of cholelithiasis in idiopathic late-onset immunoglobulin deficiency. *Ann Intern Med* 82:213–214.

Diehl AK (1983) Gallstone size and the risk of gallbladder cancer. *JAMA* 250:2323–2326.

Diehl AK (1987) Trends in cholecystectomy rates in the United States. Lancet 2: 683.

Diehl AK (1991) Epidemiology and natural history of gallstone disease. *Gastroenterol Clin North Am* 20:1–19.

Diehl AK, Elford J (1981) Gallstone disease in diabetics: analysis using multiple-cause mortality tables. *Public Health* 95:261–263.

Diehl AK, Stern MP, Ostrower VS, Friedman PC (1980) Prevalence of clinical gallbladder disease in Mexican-American, Anglo and black women. *South Med J* 73: 438–443.

Diehl AK, Rosenthal M, Hazuda HP, Comeaux PJ, Stern MP (1985) Socioeconomic status and the prevalence of clinical gallbladder disease. *J Chronic Dis* 38: 1019–1026.

Diehl AK, Haffner SM, Hazuda HP, Stern MP (1987) Coronary risk factors and clinical gallbladder disease: an approach to the prevention of gallstones? Am J Public Health 77:841–845.

Diehl AK, Sugarek NJ, Todd KH (1990) Clinical evaluation for gallstone diesease: usefulness of symptoms and signs in diagnosis. *Am J Med* 89:29–33.

Dietel M, Petrov I (1987) Incidence of symptomatic gallstones after bariatric operations. *Surg Gynecol Obstet* 164:549–552.

Dietschy JM (1968) Mechanisms for the intestinal absorption of bile acids. *J Lipid Res* 9:297–309.

Dietschy JM, Turley SD, Spady DK (1993) Role of liver in the maintenance of cholesterol and low density lipoprotein homeostasis in different animal species, including humans. *J Lipid Res* 34:1637–1659.

DiPadova C, DiPadova F, Montorsi W, Tritapepe R (1986) Methyl tert-butyl ether fails to dissolve retained radiolucent common bile duct stones. *Gastroenterology* 91:1296–1300.

Domellöf L, Lowenfels AB, Sipponen P (1984) Prevalence of gallstones in Finland: an autopsy study in the Helsinki area. *Scand J Gastroenterol* 19:761–764.

Domingo N, Grosclaude J, Bekaert ED, Mege D, Chapman MJ, Shimizu S, Ayrault-Jarrier M, Ostrow JD, Lafont H (1992) Epitope mapping of the human biliary amphipathic, anionic polypeptide: similarity with a calcium-binding protein isolated from gallstones and bile, and immunologic cross-reactivity with apoprotein A-1. *J Lipid Res* 33:1419–1430.

Donald JJ, Cheslyn-Curtis S, Gillams AR, Russell RCG, Lees WR (1994) Percutaneous cholecystolithotomy: is gall stone recurrence inevitable? *Gut* 35:692–695.

Donovan JM, Carey MC (1991) Physical-chemical basis of gallstone formation. *Gastroenterol Clin North Am* 20:47–66.

Donovan JM, Jackson AA (1993) Rapid determination by centrifugal ultrafiltration of inter-mixed micellar/vesicualr (non-lecithin-associated) bile salt concentrations in model bile: Influence of Donnan equilibrium effects. *J Lipid Res* 34:1121–1129.

Donovan JM, Timofeyeva N, Carey MC (1989) Cholesterol monohydrate and liquid crystal formation in model biles: effects of bile salt hydrophobicity and phosphatidyl choline (PL) contents. *Hepatology* 10:598 (abstract).

Donovan JM, Timofeyeva N, Carey MC (1991) Influence of total lipid concentration, bile salt : lecithin ratio, and cholesterol content on inter-mixed micellar/vesicular (non-lecithin-associated) bile salt concentrations in model bile. *J Lipid Res* 32:1501–1512.

Donovan JM, Jackson AA, Carey MC (1993) Molecular species composition of inter-mixed micellar/vesicular bile salt concentrations in model bile: dependence upon hydrophilic-hydrophobic balance. *J Lipid Res* 34:1131–1140.

Donovan JM, Leonard MR, Batta AK, Carey MC (1994) Calcium affinity for biliary aggregates in model biles: complementary importance of bile salts and lecithin. *Gastroenterology* 107:831–846.

Doty JE, Pitt HA, Porter-Fink V, Kuchenbecker S, DenBesten L (1982) The pathophysiology of gallbladder disease induced by total parenteral nutrition. *Gastroenterology* 82:1046 (abstract).

Doty JE, Pitt HA, Kuchenbacker SL, DenBesten L (1983) Impaired gallbladder emptying before gallstone formation in the prairie dog. *Gastroenterology* 85:168–174.

Doty JE, Pitt HA, Porter-Fink V, DenBesten L (1984) The effect of intravenous fat and total parenteral nutrition on biliary physiology. *J Parenteral Enteral Nutr* 8:265–268.

Dowling RH, Mack E, Small DM, Picott J (1970) Effects of controlled interruption of the enterohepatic circulation of bile salts by biliary diversion and by ileal resection on bile salt secretion, synthesis and pool size in man. *J Clin Invest* 49:232–242.

Dowling RH, Mack E, Small DM (1971) Biliary lipid secretion and bile composition after acute and chronic interruption of the enterohepatic circulation in the rhesus monkey. IV. Primate biliary physiology. *J Clin Invest* 50:1917–1926.

Dowling RH, Bell GD, White J (1972) Lithogenic bile in patients with ileal dysfunction. *Gut* 13:415–420.

Down RHL, Whitting MJ, Watts JM, Jones W (1983) Effect of synthetic estrogens and progestagens in oral contraceptives on bile lipid composition. *Gut* 24:253–259.

Duane WC (1994) Effects of lovastatin and dietary cholesterol on bile acid kinetics and bile lipid composition in healthy male subjects. *J Lipid Res* 35:501–509.

Duane WC, Hanson KC (1978) Role of gallbladder emptying and small bowel transit in regulation of bile acid pool size in man. *J Lab Clin Med* 92:858–872.

Duane WC, Ginsberg RL, Bennion LJ (1976) Effects of fasting on bile acid metabolism and biliary composition in man. *J Lipid Res* 17:211–219.

Duane WC, Hunninghake DB, Freeman ML, Pooler PA, Schlasner LA, Gebhard RL (1988a) Simvastatin, a competitive inhibitor of HMG-CoA reductase, lowers cholesterol saturation index of gallbladder bile. *Hepatology* 8:1147–1150.

Duane WC, Pooler PA, Hamilton JN (1988b) Bile acid synthesis in man. In vivo activity of 25-hydroxylation pathway. *J Clin Invest* 82:82–85.

Duffy AM, Sullivan MS, DiMarco NM, Liepa GU (1985) Effects of dietary protein on serum and biliary constituents and gallstone formation in hamsters. *Nutr Rep Int* 31:1319–1330.

Dugan RE, Slakey LL, Briedis AV, Porter JW (1972) Factors affecting diurnal variation in the level of $\beta$-hydroxy-$\beta$-methylglutaryl coenzyme A reductase and cholesterol-synthesizing activity in rat liver. *Arch Biochem Biophys* 152:21–27.

Dumont AE, Martelli AB, Schinella RA, Valensi QJ (1982) Transmural fluid movement in the freshly excised human gallbladder. *Surg Gynecol Obstet* 155:203–208.

Ebbs SR, Beckly DE, Hammonds JC, Teasdale C (1986) Percutaneous electrohydraulic lithotripsy of retained bile duct calculus. *Br Med J* 292:94.

Edington GM (1957) Observation on hepatic disease in the Gold Coast: with special reference to cirrhosis. *Trans R Soc Trop Med Hyg* 51:48–55.

Editorial (1973) Diet and cholesterol gallstones. *Lancet* I:471.

Edlund Y, Olsson O (1956) Incidence of biliary tract operations in a town population. Analysis of a 15-year series. Acta Chir Scand lll: 481–489.

Edwards PA, Muroya H, Gould RG (1972) In vivo demonstration of the circadian rhythm of cholesterol biosynthesis in the liver and intestine of the rat. *J Lipid Res* 13:396–401.

Einarsson K, Angelin B (1986) Hyperlipoproteinemia, hypolipidemic treatment and gallstone disease. In Grundy SM (ed): *Bile Acid and Atherosclerosis*, Vol 15. New York, Raven Press, pp 67–97.

Einarsson K, Grundy SM (1980) Effects of feeding cholic acid and chenodeoxycholic acid on cholesterol absorption and hepatic secretion of biliary lipids in man. *J Lipid Res* 21:23–34.

Einarsson K, Hellström K, Kallner M (1974) Bile acid kinetics in relation to sex, serum lipids, body weight, and gallbladder disease in patients with various types of hyperlipoproteinemia. *J Clin Invest* 54:1301–1311.

Einarsson K, Hellström K, Kallner M (1975) Gallbladder disease in hyperlipoproteinaemia. *Lancet* 1:484–487.

Einarsson K, Nilsell K, Leijd B, Angelin B (1985) Influence of age on secretion of cholesterol and synthesis of bile acids by the liver. *N Engl J Med* 313:277–282.

Einarsson K, Angelin B, Ewerth S, Nilsell K, Björkhem I (1986) Bile acid synthesis in man: assay of hepatic microsomal cholesterol 7$\alpha$-hydroxylase activity by isotope dilution-mass spectrometry. *J Lipid Res* 27:82–88.

Einarsson K, Reihnér E, Björkhem I (1989) On the saturation of the cholesterol 7$\alpha$-hydroxylase in human liver microsomes. *J Lipid Res* 30:1477–1481.

Ekbom A, Yuen J, Adami HO, McLaughlin JK, Chow WH, Persson I, Fraumeni JF Jr (1993) Cholecystectomy and colorectal cancer. *Gastroenterology* 105:142–147.

Ell C, Kerzel W, Schneider HT, Benninger J, Wirtz P, Domschke W, Hahn E (1990) Piezoelectric lithotripsy: stone disintegration and follow-up results in patients with symptomatic gallbladder stones. *Gastroenterology* 99:1439–1444.

Ell C, Hochberger J, May A, Mendez L, Bauer R, Fleig WE, Hahn EG (1993) Laser lithotripsy of difficult bile duct stones by means of a rhodamine-6G dye laser with an integrated automatic stone/tissue detection system (STDS). *Gastroenterology* 104:A359 (abstract).

Endo M, Ono K, Sasaki H, Suzuki H, Hada R, Hayashi K, Asakura Y, Yamazaki S, Shida S, Nakuchi H, Inoue S (1990) Cholangioscopic treatment of intrahepatic stones using lithotriptor. *Shokakigeka* (*Gastroenterol Surg*) 13:453–463. (In Japanese)

Englert E Jr, Harman CG, Wales EE Jr (1969) Gallstones induced by normal foodstuffs in dogs. *Nature* 224:280–281.

Englert E Jr, Harman CG, Freston JW, Straight RC, Wales EE Jr (1977) Studies on the pathogenesis of diet-induced dog gallstones. *Am J Dig Dis* 22:305–314.

Epprecht W, Rosenmund H, Schinz HR (1953) Chemische, mineralogische und Röntgenfeinstrukturuntersuchungen an Gallensteinen des Menschen und des Rindes. *Fortschr geb Röntgenstr* 79:1–20.

Erickson RA, Tarnawski A, Krause WJ (1987) 16,16-Dimethyl prostaglandin $E_2$ reduces chenodeoxycholate-induced small intestinal mucosal injury in the rat. *J Lab Clin Med* 110:387–395.

Eriksson M, Berglund L, Rudling M, Henriksson P, Angelin B (1989) Effects of estrogen on low density lipoprotein metabolism in males. Short-term and long-term studies during hormonal treatment of prostatic carcinoma. *J Clin Invest* 84:802–810.

Erlinger S (1988) Bile flow. In Arias IM, Jakoby WB, Popper H, Schachter D, Shaffer EA (eds): *The Liver: Biology and Pathobiology*. (2nd edition). New York, Raven Press, pp 643–661.

Erlinger S, Go AL, Husson JM, Fevery J (1984) Franco-Belgian cooperative study of ursodeoxycholic acid in the medical dissolution of gallstones: a double-blind, radomized, dose-response study and comparison with chenodeoxycholic acid. *Hepatology* 4:308–314.

Esch O, Schteingart CD, Pappert D, Kirby D, Streich R, Hofmann AF (1993) Increased blood levels of methyl tert butyl ether but not of ethyl propionate during instillation with contact dissolution agents in the pig. *Hepatology* 18:373–379.

Esser V, Limbird LE, Brown MS, Goldstein JL, Russell DW (1988) Mutational analysis of the ligand binding domain of the low density lipoprotein receptor. *J Biol Chem* 263:13282–13290.

Esterly JR, Oppenheimer EH (1962) Observations in cystic fibrosis of the pancreas. I. The gallbladder. *Bull Johns Hopkins Hosp* 110: 247–255.

Everhart JE (1993) Contributions of obesity and weight loss to gallstone disease. *Ann Intern Med* 119:1029–1035.

Everson GT (1991) Gallbladder function in gallstone disease. *Gastroenterol Clin North Am* 20:85–110.

Everson GT, Braverman DZ, Johnson ML, Kern F Jr (1980) A critical evaluation of real-time ultrasonography for the study of gallbladder volume and contraction. *Gastroenterology* 79:40–46.

Everson GT, Kern F Jr, McKinley C, Showalter R, DeMark B, Szczepanik-Van Leeuwen P, Klein P (1981) A new technique for measuring storage and concentration of bile acids (BAs) in the gallbladder (GB) in intact subjects: Studies in pregnant women. *Gastroenterology* 80:1144 (abstract).

Everson GT, McKinley C, Lawson M, Johnson M, Kern F Jr (1982) Gallbladder function in the human female: Effect of the ovulatory cycle, pregnancy, and contraceptive steroids. *Gastroenterology* 82:711–719.

Everson GT, Fennessey P, Kern F Jr (1988) Contraceptive steroids alter the steady-state kinetics of bile acids. *J Lipid Res* 29:68–76.

Everson GT, Nemeth A, Kourourian S, Zogg D, Leff NB, Dixon D, Githens JH, Pretorius D (1989) Gallbladder function is altered in sickle hemoglobinopathy. *Gastroenterology* 96:1307–1316.

Everson GT, McKinley C, Kern F Jr (1991) Mechanisms of gallstone formation in women. Effects of exogenous estrogen (Premarin) and dietary cholesterol on hepatic lipid metabolism. *J Clin Invest* 87:237–246.

Everson GT, Daggy BP, McKinley C, Story JA (1992) Effects of psyllium mucilloid on LDL-cholesterol and bile acid synthesis in hypercholesterolemic men. *J Lipid Res* 33:1183–1192.

Fagan BM (1990) The journey from Eden. *The Peopling of Our World*. London, Thames and Hudson.

Falchuck KR, Lesser PB, Galdabini JJ, Isselbacher KJ (1976) Cholangiocarcinoma as related to chronic intrahepatic cholangitis and hepatolithiasis. *Am J Gastroenterol* 66:57–61.

Falls AH, Davis HT, Scriven LE, Talmon Y (1982) Imaging vesicular dispersions with cold-stage electron microscopy. *Biochim Biophys Acta* 693:364–378.

Färkkilä MA, Tilvis RS, Miettinen TA (1988) Cholesterol absorption regulates cholesterol metabolism and plasma lipoprotein levels in patients with gut exclusions. *Gastroenterology* 94:582–589.

Fedorowski T, Salen G, Tint G S, Mosbach EH (1979) Transformation of chenodeoxycholic acid and ursodeoxycholic acid by human intestinal bacteria. *Gastroenterology* 77:1068–1073.

Feldman M, Feldman M Jr (1954) The incidence of cholelithiasis, cholesterolosis and liver disease in diabetes mellitus; autopsy study. *Diabetes* 3:305–307.

Fendrick A M (1992) Cost-effectiveness of symptomatic gallstone management: what exactly are we measuring? *Gastroenterology* 102:745–746.

Festi D, Frabboni R, Bazzoli F, Sangermano A, Ronchi M, Rossi L, Parini P, Orsini M, Primerano AMM, Mazzella G, Aldini R, Roda E (1990) Gallbladder motility in cholesterol gallstone disease. Effect of ursodeoxycholic acid administration and gallstone dissolution. *Gastroenterology* 99:1779–1785.

Feurle GE. Ho AD, Wosiewitz U, Encke A (1980) Cholelithiasis bei einem bisher nicht beschriebenen Fall von Porphyria erythropoietica congenita. Dtsch Med Wochenschr 105:1153–1156.

Filly RA, Allen B, Minton MJ, Bernhoft R, Way LW (1980) In vitro investigations of the origin of echoes within biliary sludge. *J Clin Ultrasound* 8:193–200.

Fischer H (1911) Zur Kenntnis der Gallenfarbstoffe. I. *Z Physiol Chem* 73:204–239.

Fisher MM, Goresky CA, Shaffer EA, Strasberg SM (1979) *Gallstones*. New York, Plenum Press.

Fisher RS, Stelzer F, Rock E, Malmud LS (1982) Abnormal gallbladder emptying in patients with gallstones. *Dig Dis Sci* 27:1019–1024.

Fisher RS, Rock E, Levin G, Malmud L (1987) Effects of somatostatin on gallbladder emptying. *Gastroenterology* 92:885–890.

Fitzpatrick WK Jr, Burdette WJ, Huestis RR (1963) Cholelithiasis and spherocytosis in *Peromyscus*. *Arch Surg* 86:897–903.

Flowers BF, Saslawsky MJ, Mathes GL, Tonkin AK (1990) Use of pulsed dye laser and ultrasonic lithotriptor for removal of multiple intrahepatic gallstones. *Surg Gynecol Obstet* 170:443–444.

Ford EJ (1955) A case of biliary calculus and jaundice in a cow. *Vet Res* 67:634–635.

Fornari F, Civardi G, Buscarini E, Cavanna L, Imberti D, Rossi S, Sbolli G, Di Stasi M, Buscarini L (1990) Cirrhosis of the liver. A risk factor for development of cholelithiasis in males. *Dig Dis Sci* 35:1403–1408.

Fox H (1923) *Diseases in Wild Mammals and Birds*. Philadelphia, Lippincott.

Fox H (1930) *Animals of Special Importance*. *Report of the Laboratory of Comparable Pathology*. Philadelphia, pp12–22. Cited by Martin et al (1973).

Fredrickson DS, Ono K (1956) The in vitro production of 25- and 26-hydroxycholesterol and their in vivo metabolism. *Biochem Biophys Acta* 22:183–184.

Freed LA, Berman JM, Martini D, Malet PF, Cunnane S, Mosbach EH, Cohen B, Soloway RD (1986) Hamster black pigment stones: phosphate and bilirubinate content can be altered by diet to resemble human pigment stones. *Gastroenterology* 90:1789 (abstract).

Freedman DS, Srinivasan SR, Shear CL, Hunter SM, Croft JB, Webber LS, Berenson GS (1986) Cigarette smoking initiation and longitudinal changes in serum lipids and lipoproteins in early adulthood: the Bogalusa Heart Study. *Am J Epidemiol* 124:207–219.

Freel RW, Hatch M, Earnest DL, Goldner AM (1983) Role of the tight junctional pathways in bile salt-induced increases in colonic permeability. *Am J Physiol* 245:G816–G823.

Freston JW, Bouchier IAD (1968) Experimental cholelithiasis. *Gut* 9:2–4.

Freston JW, Bouchier IAD, Newman J (1969) Biliary mucous substances in dehydrocholesterol-induced cholelithiasis. *Gastroenterology* 57:670–678.

Frick MH, Elo O, Haapa K, Heinonen OP, Heinsalmi P, Helo P, Huttunen JK, Kaitaniemi P, Koskinen P, Manninen V, Mäenpää H, Mänkönan M, Mänttäri M, Norola S, Pasternack A, Pikkarainen J, Romo M, Sjöblom, Nikkilä EA (1987) Helsinki heart study: Primary-prevention trial with gemfibrozil in middle-aged men with dyslipidemia. Safety of treatment, changes in risk factors, and incidence of coronary heart disease. *N Engl J Med* 317:1237–1245.

Fridhandler TM, Davison JS, Shaffer EA (1983) Defective gallbladder contractility in the ground squirrel and prairie dog during the early stages of cholesterol gallstone formation. *Gastroenterology* 85:830–836.

Friedman GD (1993) Natural history of asymptomatic and symptomatic gallstones. *Am J. Surg* 165:399–404.

Friedman GD, Kannel WB, Dawber TR (1966) The epidemiology of gallbladder disease: observations in the Framingham study. *J Chronic Dis* 19:273–292.

Friedman GD, Raviola CA, Fireman B (1989) Prognosis of gallstones with mild or no symptoms: 25 years of follow-up in a health maintenance organization. *J Chronic Dis* 42:127–136.

Friesen CA, Roberts CC (1989) Cholelithiasis: clinical characteristics in children. Case analysis and literature review. *Clin Pediatr* 28:294–298.

Fromm H, Roat JW, Gonzalez V, Sarva RP, Farivar S (1983) Comparative efficacy and side effects of ursodeoxycholic and chenodeoxycholic acids in dissolving gallstones. A double-blind controlled study. *Gastroenterology* 85:1257–1264.

Fujihira E, Kaneta S, Ohshima T (1978) Strain difference in mouse cholelithiasis and the effect of taurine on the gallstone formation in C57BL/C mice. *Biochem Med* 19:211–217.

Fujii T, Yanagisawa J, Nakayama F (1988) Absorption of bile acids in dog as determined by portal blood sampling: Evidence for colonic absorption of bile acid conjugates. *Digestion* 41:207–214.

Fujino R (1974) Consequence of selective proximal vagotomy in biliary tract pathology. *Jpn J Surg* 4:104–111.

Fukudome K, Chijiiwa K, Furusawa T, Nakayama F (1987) Effect of albumin on the solubility of cholesterol in bile. *Biochim Biophys Acta* 922:155–161.

Fung J (1961) Liver fluke infestation and cholangio-hepatitis. *Br J Surg* 48:404–415.

Gallinger S, Taylor RD, Harvey PRC, Petrunka CN, Strasberg SM (1985) Effect of mucous glycoprotein on nucleation time of human bile. *Gastroenterology* 89:648–658.

Gallinger S, Harvey PRC, Petrunka CN, Ilson RG, Strasberg SM (1987) Biliary proteins and the nucleation defect in cholesterol cholelithiasis. *Gastroenterology* 92:867–875.

Galloway DJ, Owen RW, Jarrett F, Boyle P, Hill MJ, George WD (1986) Experimental colorectal cancer: the relationship of diet and faecal bile acid concentration to tumour induction. *Br J Surg* 73:233–237.

Garbutt JT, Heaton KW, Lack L, Tyor MP (1969) Increased ratio of glycine- to taurine-conjugated bile salts in patients with ileal disorders. *Gastroenterology* 56:711–720.

Gebhard RL, Prigge WF (1992) Thyroid hormone differentially augments biliary sterol secretion in the rat. II. The chronic bile fistula model. *J Lipid Res* 33:1467–1473.

Geistfeld BL, Bond MG, St Clair RW (1977) Cholelithiasis in a male rhesus monkey (*Macaca mulatta*) fed a cholesterol-containing diet. *J Med Primatol* 6:237–244.

Gerdes MM, Boyden EA (1938) The rate of emptying of the human gallbladder in pregnancy. *Surg Gynecol Obstet* 66:145–156.

Gilat T, Feldman C, Halpern Z, Dan M, Bar-Meir S (1983) An increased familial frequency of gallstones. *Gastroenterology* 84:242–246.

Gilbert J (1955) Absence of coronary thrombosis in Navajo Indians. *Calif Med* 82:114–115.

Gilmore IT, Barnhart JL, Hofmann AF, Erlinger S (1982) Effects of individual taurine-conjugated bile acids on biliary secretion and sucrose clearance in the unanesthetized dog. *Am J Physiol* 5:G40–G46.

Gimmon Z, Kelly R E, Simko V, Fisher JE (1982) Total parenteral nutrition solution increases bile lithogenicity in rat. *J Surg Res* 32:256–263.

Giovannucci E, Colditz GA, Stampfer MJ (1993) A meta-analysis of cholecystectomy and risk of colorectal cancer. *Gastroenterology* 105:130–141.

Gitelson S, Schwartz A, Fraenkell M, Chowers I (1963) Gall bladder dysfunction in diabetes mellitus. The diabetic neurogenic gall bladder. *Diabetes* 12:308–312.

Glambek I, Kvaale G, Arnesjö B, Søreide O (1987) Prevalence of gallstones in a Norwegian population. *Scand J Gastroenterol* 22:1089–1094.

Gleeson D, Murphy GM, Dowling RH (1990) Calcium binding by bile acids: in vitro studies using a calcium ion electrode. *J Lipid Res* 31:781–791.

Gleeson D, Hood KA, Murphy GM, Dowling RH (1992) Calcium and carbonate ion concentrations in gallbladder and hepatic bile. *Gastroenterology* 102:1707–1716.

Glenn F, McSherry CK (1970) The baboon and experimental cholelithiasis. *Arch Surg* 100:105–108.

Glenn F, Moody FG (1961) Intrahepatic calculi. *Ann Surg* 153:711–724.

Goldfarb A, Grisaru D, Gimmon Z, Okon E, Lebensart P, Rachmilewitz EA (1990) High incidence of cholelithiasis in older patients with homozygous beta-thalassemia. *Acta Haematol* 83:120–122.

Goldstein ME, Schein CJ (1964) The significance of biliary tract disease in the diabetic – its unique features. *Am J Gastroenterol* 39:630–634.

Goldstein JL, Brown MS, Anderson RGW, Russell DW, Schneider WJ (1985) Receptor-mediated endocytosis: concepts emerging from the LDL receptor system. *Ann Rev Cell Biol* 1:1–39.

Gollish SH, Burnstein MJ, Ilson RG, Petrunka CN, Strasberg SM (1983) Nucleation of cholesterol monohydrate crystals from hepatic and gall bladder bile of patients with cholesterol gallstones. *Gut* 24:836–844.

Goodchild MC, Murphy GM, Howell AM, Nutter SA, Anderson CM (1975) Aspects of bile acid metabolism in cystic fibrosis. *Arch Dis Child* 50:769–778.

Goodhart GL, Levison ME, Trotman BW, Soloway RD (1978) Pigment vs. cholesterol cholelithiasis. Bacteriology of gallbladder stone, bile, and tissue correlated with biliary lipid analysis. *Am J Dig Dis* 23:877–882.

Gordon T, Castelli WP, Hjortland MC, Kannel WB, Dawber TR (1977) High density lipoprotein as a protective factor against coronary heart disease. The Framinham study. *Am J Med* 62:707–714.

Govers MJAP, Termont DSML, Van Aken GA, Van der Meer R (1994) Characterization of the adsorption of conjugated and unconjugated bile acids to insoluble, amorphous calcium phosphate. *J Lipid Res* 35:741–748.

Gracie WA, Ransohoff DF (1982) The natural history of silent gallstones. The innocent gallstone is not a myth. *N*

*Engl J Med* 307:798–800.

Green TW, Conley CL, Berthrong M (1953) Liver in sickle cell anemia. *Bull Johns Hopkins Hosp* 92:99–127.

Gregory KW, Smith CZ, Booth R (1972) Diurnal variations in rat liver 3-hydroxy-3-methyl-glutaryl-Coenzyme A reductase activity in relation to feeding. *Biochem J* 130:1163–1165.

Gregory DH, Vlahcevic ZR, Schatzki P, Swell L (1975) Mechanism of secretion of biliary lipids. I. Role of bile canalicular and microsomal membranes in the synthesis and transport of biliary lecithin and cholesterol. *J Clin Invest* 55:105–114.

Greiner L, Münks C, Heil W, Jakobeit C (1990) Gallbladder stone fragments in feces after biliary extracorporeal shock wave lithotripsy. *Gastroenterology* 98:1620–1624.

Grodzki M, Mazurkiewicz-Rozynska E, Czyzyk A (1968) Diabetic cholecystopathy. *Diabetologia* 4:345–348.

Groen AK, Stout JPJ, Drapers JAG, Hoek FJ, Grijm R, Tytgat GNJ (1988) Cholesterol nucleation-influencing activity in T-tube bile. *Hepatology* 8:347–352.

Groen AK, Noordam C, Drapers JAG, Egbers P, Hoek FJ, Tytgat GNJ (1989a) An appraisal of the role of biliary phospholipases in the pathogenesis of gallstone disease. *Biochim Biophys Acta* 1006:179–182.

Groen AK, Ottenhoff R, Jansen PLM, van Marle J, Tytgat GNJ (1989b) Effect of cholesterol nucleation-promoting activity on cholesterol solubilization in model bile. *J Lipid Res* 30:51–58.

Groen JN, Lock MTWT, Lameris JS, Van Blankenstein M, Terpstra OT (1989c) Removal of common duct stones by the combination of percutaneous balloon dilatation and extracorporeal shock-wave lithotripsy. *Gastroenterology* 97:202–206.

Groen AK, Noordam C, Drapers JAG, Egbers P, Jansen PLM, Tytgat GNJ (1990) Isolation of a potent cholesterol nucleation-promoting activity from human gallbladder bile: role in the pathogenesis of gallstone disease. *Hepatology* 11:525–533.

Gross DMB (1929) A statistical study of cholelithiasis. *J Pathol Bacteriol* 32:502–526.

Grosse H (1966) Die Cholelithiasis. Jena, Gustav Fischer Verlag.

Grundy SM, Metzger AL, Adler RD (1972) Mechanism of lithogenic bile formation in American Indian women with cholesterol gallstones. *J Clin Invest* 51:3026–3043.

Grundy SM, Duane WC, Adler RD, Aron JM, Metzger AL (1974) Biliary lipid outputs in young women with cholesterol gallstones. *Metabolism* 23:67–73.

Güldütuna S, Elze A, Bhatti S, Imhof M, You T, Zimmer G, Leuschner U (1993a) Ursodeoxycholate (UDC) prevents glutamate dehydrogenase (GLDH) release of isolated liver mitochondria by chenodeoxycholic acid (CDC). *Gastroenterology* 104:A361 (abstract).

Güldütuna S, Zimmer G, Imhof M, Bhatti S, You TG, Leuschner U (1993b) Molecular aspects of membrane stabilization by ursodeoxycholate. *Gastroenterology* 104:1736–1744.

Gullikson GW, Cline WS, Lorenzsonn V, Benz L, Olsen WA, Bass P (1977) Effects of anionic surfactants on hamster small intestinal membrane structure and function: relationship to surface activity. *Gastroenterology* 73:501–511.

Gurantz D, Hofmann AF (1984) Influence of bile acid structure on bile flow and biliary lipid secretion in the hamster. *Am J Physiol* 247:G736–G748.

Gurll N, Den Besten L (1978) Animal models of human cholesterol gallstone disease: a review. *Lab Animal Sci* 28:428–432.

Hada R, Mikami M, Sugiyama Y, Kikuchi A, Konn M (1993) High incidence of gallstone disease after curative gastrectomy for cancer. *Gastroenterology* 104:A362.

Haffner SM, Diehl AK, Stern MP, Hazuda HP (1989) Central adiposity and gallbladder disease in Mexican Americans. *Am J Epidemiol* 129:587–595.

Hagey LR, Crombie DL, Espinosa E, Carey MC. Igimi H, Hofmann AF (1993) Ursodeoxycholic acid in the Ursidae: biliary bile acids of bears, pandas and related carnivores. *J Lipid Res* 34:1911–1917.

Hahm JS, Ostrow JD, Mukerjee P, Celic L (1992) Ionization and self-association of unconjugated bilirubin, determined by rapid solvent partition from chloroform, with further studies of bilirubin solubility. *J Lipid Res* 33:1123–1137.

Hall RI, Ingoldby JH, Denyer ME (1990) Periampullary diverticula predispose to primary rather than secondary stones in the common bile duct. *Endoscopy* 22:127–128.

Halpern Z, Dudley MA, Kibe A, Lynn MP, Breuer AC, Holzbach RT (1986a) Rapid vesicle formation and aggregation in abnormal human biles: a time-lapse video-enhanced contrast microscopy study. *Gastroenterology* 90:875–885.

Halpern Z, Dudley MA, Lynn MP, Nader JM, Breuer AC, Holzbach RT (1986b) Vesicle aggregation in model systems of supersaturated bile: relation to crystal nucleation and lipid composition of the vesicular phase. *J Lipid Res* 27:295–306.

Hamerton AE (1932) Report on the deaths occurring in the society's gardens during the year 1931. *Proc Zool Soc Lond* 102:613–638.

Hanis CL, Ferrell RE, Tulloch BR, Schull WJ (1985) Gallbladder disease epidemiology in Mexican Americans in Starr County, Texas. *Am J Epidemiol* 22:820–829.

Hanson DS, Duane WC (1994) Effects of lovastatin and chenodiol on bile acid synthesis, bile lipid composition, and biliary lipid secretion in healthy human subjects. *J Lipid Res* 35:1462–1468.

Harber GB, Heaton KW (1979) Lipid composition of bile in diabetics and obesity-matched controls. *Gut* 20:518–522.

Hardison WGM, Rosenberg IH, Greene EA (1967) Bile salt deficiency in the steatorrhea following resection of the ileum and proximal colon. *N Engl J Med* 277:337–342.

Harrison-Levy A (1962) The biliary obstruction syndrome of the Chinese. *Br J Surg* 49:674–685.

Hartz AJ, Rupley DC, Rimm AA (1984) The association of girth measurements with disease in 32,856 women. *Am J Epidemiol* 119:71–80.

Harvald B, Hauge M (1956) A catamnestic investigation of Danish twins. *Dan Med Bull* 3:150–158.

Harvel RJ (1986) Functional activities of hepatic lipoprotein receptors. *Annu Rev Physiol* 48:119–134.

Harvey PRC, Strasberg SM (1993) Will the real cholesterol-nucleating and -antinucleating proteins please stand up? *Gastroenterology* 104:646–650.

Harvey PRC, Rupar CA, Gallinger S, Petrunka CN, Strasberg SM (1986) Quantitative and qualitative comparison of gall bladder mucus glycoprotein from patients with and without gall stones. *Gut* 27:374–381.

Harvey PRC, Somjen G, Lichtenberg MS, Petrunka P, Gilat T, Strasberg SM (1987) Nucleation of cholesterol from vesicles isolated from bile of patients with and without cholesterol gallstones. *Biochim Biophys Acta* 921:198–204.

Harvey PRC, Somjen G, Gilat T, Gallinger S, Strasberg SM (1988) Vesicular cholesterol in bile. Relationship to protein concentration and nucleation time. *Biochim Biophys Acta* 958:10–18.

Harvey PRC, Upadhya GA, Strasberg SM (1991) Immunoglobulins as nucleating proteins in the gallbladder bile of patients with cholesterol gallstones. *J Biol Chem* 266:13996–14003.

Hashimoto K (1966) Experimental studies on gallstones in hamsters. Nippon Geka Hokan (Arch Jpn Chir, Kyoto) 35:981–996.

Haslewood GAD (1955) Recent developments in our knowledge of bile salts. *Physiol Rev* 35:178–196.

Hauch E W, Moore F J (1963) Is cholelithiasis associated with a specific blood group? *Gastroenterology* 44:125–126.

Havel RJ, Hamilton RL (1988) Hepatocytic lipoprotein receptors and intracellular lipoprotein catabolism. *Hepatology* 8:1689–1704.

Hay DW, Cahalane MJ, Timofeyeva N, Carey MC (1993) Molecular species of lecithins in human gallbladder bile. *J Lipid Res* 34:759–768.

Hayward AF, Freston JW, Bouchier IAD (1968) Changes in the ultrastructure of gall bladder epithelium in rabbits with experimental gallstones. *Gut* 9:550–556.

Heaton KW (1973) The epidemiology of gallstones and suggested aetiology. *Clin Gastroenterol* 2:67–83.

Heaton KW, Read AE (1969) Gall stones in patients with disorders of the terminal ileum and disturbed bile salt metabolism. *Br Med J* 3:494–496.

Heaton KW, Emmett PM, Symes CL, Braddon FE (1993) An explanation for gallstones in normal-weight women: slow intestinal transit. (1993) *Lancet* 341:8–10.

Hegardt FG, Dam H (1971) The solubility of cholesterol in aqueous solutions of bile salts and lecithin. *Z Ernaerungswiss* 10:223–233.

Heintze K, Goetz R, Koerlings H, Wood JR (1976) Characterisation of the prostaglandin induced secretion in the isolated gallbladder of guinea pig. *Naunyn Schmiedbergs Arch Pharmacol* 293(Suppl):34.

Hellström K, Einarsson K (1977) Bile acid metabolism in hyperlipoproteinemia. *Clin Gastroenterol* 6:103–128.

Henriksson P, Einarsson K, Eriksson A, Kelter U, Angelin B (1989) Estrogen-induced gallstone formation in males. Relation to changes in serum and biliary lipids during hormonal treatment of prostatic carcinoma. *J Clin Invest* 84:811–816.

Hepatolithiasis Research Group (1983) *Annual Report 1982 of Hepatolithiasis Research Group, Ministry of Health of Japan.* Tokyo, Ministry of Health of Japan, pp 17. (In Japanese)

Hepner GW, Hofmann AF, Thomas PJ (1972) Metabolism of steroid and amino acid moieties of conjugated bile acids in man. II. Glycine-conjugated dihydroxy bile acids. *J Clin Invest* 51:1898–1905.

Hepner GW, Hofmann AF, Malagelada JR, Szczepanik PA, Klein PD (1974) Increased bacterial degradation of bile acids in cholecystectomized patients. *Gastroenterology* 66:556–564.

Herrick AL, Moore MR, Thompson GG, Ford GP, McColl KEL (1990) Cholelithiasis in patients with variegate porphyria. *J Hepatol* 12:50–53.

Hesse FG (1959) Incidence of cholecystitis and other diseases among Pima Indians of southern Arizona. *J A M A* 170:1789–1790.

Hesse FG (1964) Incidence of disease in the Navajo Indians. A necropsy study of coronary and aortic atherosclerosis, cholelithiasis and neoplastic disease. *Arch Pathol* 77:553–557.

Heubi JE, Soloway RD, Balistreri WF (1983) Biliary lipid composition in healthy and diseased infants, children, and young adults. *Gastroenterology* 82:1295–1299.

Heubi JE, O'Connell NC, Setchell KDR (1992) Ileal resection/dysfunction in childhood predisposes to lithogenic bile only after puberty. *Gastroenterology* 103:636–640.

Heuman DM (1989) Quantitative estimation of the hydrophilic-hydrophobic balance of mixed bile salt solutions. J Lipid Res 30:719–730.

Heuman R, Norrby R, Sjödahl NG, Tiselius C, Tagesson C (1980) Altered gallbladder bile composition in gallstone disease. Relation to gallbladder wall permeability. *Scand J Gastroenterol* 15:581–586.

Heuman DM, Vlahcevic ZR, Bailey M, Hylemon PB (1988) Regulation of bile acid synthesis. II. Effect of bile acid feeding on enzymes regulating hepatic cholesterol and bile acid synthesis in the rat. *Hepatology* 8:892–897.

Heuman DM, Hylemon PB, Vlahcevic ZR (1989) Regulation of bile acid synthesis. III. Correlation between biliary bile salt hydrophobicity index and the activities of enzymes regulating cholesterol and bile acid synthesis in the rat. *J Lipid Res* 30:1161–1171.

Hikasa Y, Nagase M, Tanimura H, Shioda R, Setoyama M, Kobayashi N, Mukaihara S, Kamata T, Maruyama K, Kato H, Mori K (1980) Epidemiology and etiology of gallstones. *Nippon Gekahokan* (*Arch Jpn Chir, Kyoto*) 49:555–571.

Hill MJ (1974) Bacteria and the etiology of colonic cancer. *Cancer* 34:815–818.

Hill MJ (1983) Bile, bacteria and bowel cancer. *Gut* 24:871–875.

Hill MJ (1985) Cancer of the large bowel: human carcinogenesis. *Br J Surg* 72:S37–S39.

Hill GL, Mair WSJ, Goligher JC (1975) Gallstones after ileostomy and ileal resection. *Gut* 16:932–936.

Hirota I, Chijiiwa K, Noshiro H, Nakayama F (1992) Effect of chenodeoxycholate and ursodeoxycholate on nucleation time in human gallbladder bile. *Gastroenterology* 102:1668–1674.

Hirst BH, Lund PK, Reed JD, Sanders DJ, Shaw B, Taylor W (1979) Effects of a combined oestrogen-progestin preparation on gastric acid and pepsin secretion, serum gastrin concentration and biliary secretion of bile acids, phospholipids, and cholesterol in the cat. *Br J Pharmacol* 65:87–95.

Ho YD, Ho KJ (1990) Biliary D-glucaric acid: its quantitation and preventive role in gallstone formation. *Scand J Gastroenterol* 25:631–640.

Ho KJ, Ho LHC, Kruger OR (1979) Characterization and determination of the activity of biliary $\beta$-glucuronidase in rats. *J Lab Clin Med* 93:916–925.

Ho KJ, Hsu SC, Chen JS, Ho LHC (1986) Human biliary $\beta$-glucuronidase: correlation of its activity with deconjugation of bilirubin in the bile. *Eur J Clin Invest* 16:361–367.

Ho KY, Weissberger AJ, Marbach P, Lazarus L (1990) Therapeutic efficacy of the somatostatin analog SMS 201-995 (Octreotide) in acromegaly. Effects of dose and frequency and long-term safety. *Ann Intern Med* 112:173–181.

Hoare AM (1974) Carcinoma of the colon and cholecystectomy. *Lancet* 2: 1395–1396.

Hoerr SO (1962) Stoneless gallbladder but stones in the common bile duct. Report of 10 cases. *Arch Surg* 85:821–827.

Hofmann AF (1984a) Animal models of calcium cholelithiasis. *Hepatology* 4 (Suppl):209S–211S.

Hofmann AF (1984b) Medical treatment of cholesterol gallstones by bile desaturating agents. *Hepatology* 4(Suppl):199S–208S.

Hofmann AF (1988) Pathogenesis of cholesterol gallstones. *J Clin Gastroenterol* 10(Suppl 2):S1–S11.

Hofmann AF, Hofmann NE (1974) Measurement of bile acid kinetics by isotope dilution in man. *Gastroenterology* 67:314–323.

Hofmann AF, Mekhjian HS (1973) Bile acids and the intestinal absorption of fat and electrolytes in health and disease. In Nair PP, Kritchevesky D (eds): *The Bile Acids*, Vol 2. New York, Plenum Press, pp 103–152.

Hofmann AF, Mosbach EH (1964) Identification of allodeoxycholic acid as the major component of gallstones induced in the rabbit by 5$\alpha$-cholestan-3$\beta$-ol. *J Biol Chem* 239:2813–2821.

Hofmann AF, Mysels KJ (1992) Bile acid solubility and precipitation in vitro and in vivo: the role of conjugation, pH, and $Ca^{2+}$ ions. *J Lipid Res* 33:617–626.

Hofmann AF, Bokkenheuser V, Hirsch RL, Mosbach EH (1968) Experimental cholelithiasis in the rabbit induced by cholestanol feeding: effect of neomycin treatment on bile composition and gallstone formation. *J Lipid Res* 9:244–253.

Hofmann AF, Thistle JL. Klein PD, Szczepanik PA, Yu PYS (1978) Chemotherapy for gallstone dissolution. II. Induced changes in bile composition and gallstone response. *J A M A* 2391138–1144.

Hofmann AF, Schmack B, Thistle JL, Babayan VK (1981) Clinical experience with monooctanoin for dissolution of bile duct stones. An uncontrolled multicenter trial. *Dig Dis Sci* 26:954–955.

Hofmann AF, Grundy SM, Lachin JM, Lan SP, Baum RA, Hanson RF, Hersh T, Hightower NC Jr, Marks JW, Mekhjian H, Shaefer RA, Soloway RD, Thistle JL, Thomas FB, Tyor MP, National Cooperative Gallstone Group (1982) Pretreatment biliary lipid composition in white patients with radiolucent gallstones in the National Cooperative Gallstone Study. *Gastroenterology* 83:738–752.

Holan KR, Holzbach RT, Herman RE, Cooperman AM, Claffey WJ (1979) Nucleation time: a key factor in the pathogenesis of cholesterol gallstone disease. *Gastroenterology* 77:611–617.

Holzbach RT (1983a) Pathogenesis and medical treatment of gallstones. In Sleisenger MH, Fordtran JS (eds): *Gastrointestinal disease*. 3rd ed. Philadelphia, W B Saunders, pp 1356–1373.

Holzbach RT (1983b) Gallbladder stasis: consequence of long-term parenteral hyperalimentation and risk factor for cholelithiasis. *Gastroenterology* 84:1055–1058.

Holzbach RT (1984) Animal models of cholesterol gallstone disease. Hepatology 4(Suppl):191S–198S.

Holzbach RT (1986) Recent progress in understanding cholesterol crystal nucleation as a precursor to human gallstone formation. *Hepatology* 6:1403–1406.

Holzbach RT, Busch N (1991) Nucleation and growth of cholesterol crystals. Kinetic determinants in supersaturated native bile. *Gastroenterol Clin North Am* 20:67–84.

Holzbach R T, Corbusier C (1978) Liquid crystals and cholesterol nucleation during equilibration in supersaturated bile analogs. Biochim Biophys Acta 528: 436–444.

Holzbach RT, Marsh M (1974) Transient liquid crystals in human bile analogues. *Molecular crystals and liquid crystals* 28:217–222.

Holzbach RT, Marsh ME, Hallberg MC (1971) The effect of pregnancy on lipid composition of guinea pig gallbladder bile. *Gastroenterology* 60:288–293.

Holzbach RT, Marsh ME, Olszewski M, Holan K (1973) Cholesterol solubility in bile. Evidence that supersaturated bile is frequent in healthy man. J Clin Invest 52:1467–1479.

Holzbach RT, Corbusier C, Marsh M (1976) The process of cholesterol cholelithiasis induced by diet in the prairie dog: a physicochemical characterization. *J Lab Clin Med* 87:987–998.

Holzbach RT, Kibe A, Thiel E, Howell JH, Marsh M, Hermann RE (1984) Biliary proteins. Unique inhibitors of cholesterol crystal nucleation in human gallbladder bile. *J Clin Invest* 73:35–45.

Honda A, Yoshida T, Tanaka N, Matsuzaki Y, He BF, Osuga T, Kobayashi N, Ozawa K (1992) Hepatic cholesterol and bile acid synthesis in Japanese patients with cholesterol gallstones. *Gastroenterology* 102:A823 (abstract).

Honoré LH (1980a) Cholesterol cholelithiasis in adolescent females. Its connection with obesity, parity, and oral contraceptive use – a retrospective study of 31 cases. *Arch Surg* 115:62–64.

Honoré LH (1980b) The lack of a positive association between symptomatic cholesterol cholelithiasis and clinical diabetes mellitus: a retrospective study. *J Chronic Dis* 33:465–469.

Honoré LH (1980c) Increased incidence of symptomatic cholesterol cholelithiasis in perimenopausal women receiving estrogen replacement therapy: a retrospective study. *J Reprod Med* 25:187–190.

Hood K, Gleeson D, Ruppin DC, Dowling RH (1988) Prevention of gallstone recurrence by non-steroidal anti-inflammatory drugs. *Lancet* 2:1223–1225.

Hoogerbrugge van der Linden N, de Rooy FWN, van Blankenstein M (1990) The effect of pravastatin on biliary lipid composition and bile acid synthesis in familial hypercholesterolemia. *Gut* 31:348–350.

Horn G (1956) Observations on the aetiology of cholelithiasis. *Br Med J* II:732–737.

Horwitz A, Kirson SM (1965) Cholecystitis and cholelithiasis as a sequel to gastric surgery. *Am J Surg* 109:760–762.

Huang CC (1959) Partial resection of the liver in treatment of intrahepatic stones. *Chin Med J* 79:40–45.

Huang ZQ (1976) *Biliary Tract Surgery*. Beijing, People's Health Publishing Company, pp 161. (In Chinese)

Huang ZQ (1987) Characteristics of cholelithiasis in China. Clinical study on 11,342 operated cases. *Collected Abstracts of the Third National Congress of Cholelithasis, Nanjing, China, Oct. 11–13, 1987*, pp 1–11. (In Chinese)

Huang YQ, Zhang XW, Liao YT, Luo TL, Dueng YW, Zhang CL, Kou HR, Hue WS, Su ZH, Zhang J (1987) Prevalence of gallstone cases in Tianjin. Study on 28,519 cases. *Collected Abstracts of the Third National Congress of Cholelithiasis, Nanjing, China, Oct 11–13, 1987*, pp 18–19. (In Chinese)

Hultén O (1968a) Formation of gallstones I. *Acta Chir Scand* 134: 125–130.

Hultén O (1968b) Formation of gallstones II. *Acta Chir Scand* 134: 557–561.

Hultén O (1970) Contraction of gallbladder and the formation of gallstones. III. *Acta Chir Scand* 136:53–56.

Hur KB, Rice RG, Hong SS (1963) Cholelithiasis in Koreans. *Yonsei Med J* 4:103–118.

Hussaini SH, Murphy GM, Kennedy C, Besser GM, Wass JAH, Dowling RH (1994) The role of bile composition and physical chemistry in the pathogenesis of octreotide-associated gallbladder stones. *Gastroenterology* 107:1503–1513.

Hutton SW, Sievert CE, Vennes JA, Duane WC (1981) The effect of sphincterotomy on gallstone formation in the prairie dog. *Gastroenterology* 81:663–667.

Hwang WS (1970) Cholelithiasis in Singapore. Part 1. A necropsy study. *Gut* 11:141–152.

Hylemon PB, Ericke RJ, Mosbach EH (1982) Antibacterial properties of bile acid oxazoline compounds. *Steroids* 40:347–357.

Ichimiya H, Kono S, Ikeda M, Tokudome S, Nakayama F, Kuratsune M (1986) Cancer mortality among patients undergoing cholecystectomy for benign biliary diseases. *Jpn J Cancer Res* 77:579–583.

Ihasz M, Griffith CA (1981) Gallstones after vagotomy. *Am J Surg* 141:48–50.

Ikeda S, Tanaka M, Yoshimoto H, Itoh H, Nakayama F (1981) Improved visualization of intrahepatic bile ducts by endoscopic retrograde balloon catheter cholangiography. *Ann Surg* 194:171–175.

Ilias AM, Connor WE, Cory HT, Lin DS, Daves GD Jr, Krippaehne WW (1980) Sterols of human gallstones: the recent identification of eight different digitonin precipitable sterols. *Gastroenterology* 79:539–544.

Imamoglu K, Perry JF, Wangensteen OH (1957) Experimental production of gallstones by incomplete stricture of the terminal common bile duct. *Surgery* 42:623–630.

Innis SM (1985) Hepatic transport of bile salt and bile composition following total parenteral nutrition with and without lipid emulsion in the rat. *Am J Clin Nutr* 41:1283–1288.

Inoue S, Endoh M, Itoh T, Ebina Y, Satoh S, Munakata H, Konn M (1985) Microwave lithotomy for intrahepatic gallstones. *Hirosaki Med J* 37:1029–1039.

Inoue K, Fuchigami A, Higashide S, Sumi S, Kogire M, Suzuki T, Tobe T(1992) Gallbladder sludge and stone formation in relation to contractile function after gastrectomy. *Ann Surg* 215:19–26.

Iser JH, Maton PN, Murphy GM, Dowling RH (1978) Resistance to chenodeoxycholic acid (CDCA) treatment in obese patients with gallstones. *Br Med J* 1:1509–1512.

Ivy AC, Oldberg E (1928) Hormone mechanism for gall-bladder contraction and evacuation. *Am J Physiol* 86:599–613.

Jackson CE, Gay BC (1959) Inheritance of gallbladder disease. *Surgery* 46:853–857.

Jacyna MR, Ross PE, Hopwood D, Bouchier IAD (1988a) Studies on the mechanism of non-visualisation of diseased human gallbladders during oral cholecystography. *Postgrad Med J* 64:931–934.

Jacyna MR, Ross PE, Hopwood DH, Bouchier IAD (1988b) Sodium transport in the diseased human gallbladder and the effects of indomethacin. *Clin Sci* 75:147–149.

Jandl JH (1955) The anemia of liver disease: observation on its mechanism. *J Clin Invest* 34:390–404.

Janowitz P, Swobodnik W, Wechsler JG, Zöller A, Kuhn K, Ditschuneit H (1990) Comparison of gallbladder bile and endoscopically obtained duodenal bile. *Gut* 31:1407–1410.

Janowitz P, Kratzer W, Zemmler T, Tudyka J, Wechsler JG (1994) Gallbladder sludge: spontaneous course and incidence of complications in patients without stones. *Hepatology* 20:291–294.

Janzon L, Aspelin P, Eriksson S, Hildell J, Trell E, Östberg H (1985) Ultrasonographic screening for gallstone disease in middle-aged women. Detection rate, symptoms and biochemical features. *Scand J Gastroenterol* 20:706–710.

Japanese Society of Gastroenterology, Committee for the Study of Cholelithiasis (Yamagata K, Osuga T, Kajiyama G, Kameda H, Kasugai T, Sato H, Tanimura H, Nakayama F, Hikasa Y, Miyoshi A, Matsushiro T, Suzuki N) (1986) New classification of gallstones in Japan. *Nihon Shokakibyo Gakkkai Zasshi (Jpn J Gastroenterol)* 83:309–316. (In Japanese)

Jaskiewicz K, Weight MJ, Christopher KJ, Benade AJS, Kritchevsky D (1987) A comparison of the effects of soyabean protein and casein on bile composition, cholelithiasis and serum lipoprotein lipids in the velvet monkey (*Cercopithecus aethiops*). *Br J Nutr* 58: 257–263.

Jazrawi RP, Northfield TC (1986) Effect of a pharmacological dose of cholecystokinin on bile acid kinetics and biliary cholesterol saturation in man. *Gut* 27:355–362.

Jelinek DF, Andersson S, Slaughter CA, Russell DW (1990) Cloning and regulation of cholesterol $7\alpha$-hydroxylase, the rate-limiting enzyme in bile acid synthesis. *J Biol Chem* 265:8190–8197.

Jenkins SA (1977) Hypovitaminosis C and cholelithiasis in guinea pig. Biochem Biophys Res Commun 77:1030–1035.

Jensen KH, Jørgensen T (1991) Incidence of gallstones in a Danish population. Gastroenterology 100:790–794.

Jensen J, Christiansen C, Rødbro P (1985) Cigarette smoking, serum estrogens and bone loss during hormone-replacement therapy early and after menopause. *N Engl J Med* 313:973–975.

Jivegard L, Radberg G, Wahlin T (1986) An experimental study on the role of gallbladder mucosal fluid secretion and intramural pressure in cholecystitis. *Acta Chir Scand* 152:605–610.

Johnson FE, Boyden EA (1952) The effect of double vagotomy on motor activity of human gallbladder. *Surgery* 32:591–601.

Johnston CG, Irvin JL (1947) The biliary excretion of various bile acids by patients with choledochostomy drainage and the effect of oral administration of dessicated bile of the ox and the hog. *J Clin Invest* 26:802–814.

Johnston CG, Nakayama F (1957) Solubility of cholesterol and gallstones in metabolic material. *Arch Surg* 75:436–442.

Johnston CG, Irvin JL, Walton C (1939) The free choline and phospholipid of hepatic and gallbladder bile. *J Biol Chem* 131:425–437.

Jones RS (1990) *Atlas of Liver and Biliary Surgery*. Chicago, Year Book Medical, pp 180.

Jones RS, Peric-Golia L (1962) Experimental cholelithiasis in the guinea pig. *Proc Soc Exp Biol Med* 109:991–995.

Jones PN, Weinstein IM, Ettinger RH, Capps RB (1955) Decreased red cell survival associated with liver disease. Use of radioactive sodium chromate in measurement of red cell survival. *Arch Intern Med* 95:93–102.

Jones C, Hofmann AF, Mysels KJ, Roda A (1986) The effect of calcium and sodium ion concentration on the properties of dilute aqueous solutions of glycine-conjugated bile salts. *J Colloid Interface Sci* 114:452–470.

Jones MP, Pandak WM, Heuman DM, Chiang JYL, Hylemon PB, Vlahcevic ZR (1993) Cholesterol 7$\alpha$-hydroxylase: evidence for transcriptional regulation by cholesterol or metabolic products of cholesterol in the rat. *J Lipid Res* 34:885–892.

Jonnalagadda SS, Angert R, Pronczuk A, Hayes KC (1993) Low-level dietary saturated fats (12:0, 14:0, 16:0) enhance gallstone formation relative to monos (18:1) in cholesterol-fed hamsters. *Gastroenterology* 104:A366 (abstract).

Jonnalagadda SS, Trautwein EA, Hayes KC (1995) Dietary fats rich in saturated fatty acids (12:0, 14:0, and 16:0) enhance gallstone formation relative to monounsaturated fat (18:1) in cholesterol-fed hamsters. *Lipids* 30:415–424.

Jordan RA (1957) Cholelithiasis in sickle cell disease. *Gastroenterology* 33:952–957.

Jørgensen T (1987) Prevalence of gallstones in a Danish population. *Am J Epidemiol* 126:912–921.

Jørgensen T (1988a) Gallstones in a Danish population: fertility period, pregnancies and exogenous female sex hormones. *Gut* 29:433–439.

Jørgensen T (1988b) Gallstones in a Danish population: familial occurrence and social factors. *J Biosoc Sci* 20:111–120.

Jørgensen T (1989a) Gallstones in a Danish population. Relation to weight, physical activity, smoking, coffee consumption and diabetes mellitus. *Gut* 30:528–534.

Jørgensen T (1989b) Estrogen use and gallstone disease. *Am J Public Health* 79:654.

Jørgensen T (1989c) Gallstones and plasma lipids in a Danish population. *Scand J Gastroenterol* 24:916–922.

Jørgensen T, Jørgensen L M (1989) Gallstones and diet in a Danish population. *Scand J Gastroenterol* 24:821–826.

Jüngst D, Brenner G, Pratschke E, Paumgartner G (1989) Low-dose ursodeoxycholic acid prolongs cholesterol nucleation time in gallbladder bile of patients with cholesterol gallstones. *J Hepatol* 8:1–6.

Jüngst D, Lang T, Von Ritter C, Paumgartner G (1991) Role of high total protein in gallbladder bile in the formation of cholesterol gallstones. *Gastroenterology* 100:1724–1729.

Jüngst D, Lang T, Huber P, Lange V, Paumgartner G (1993) Effect of phospholipids and bile acids on cholesterol nucleation time and vesicular/micellar cholesterol in gallbladder bile of patients with cholesterol stones. *J Lipid Res* 34:1457–1464.

Juniper K Jr, Burson EN Jr (1957) Biliary tract studies. II. The significance of biliary crystals. *Gastroenterology* 32:175–211.

Juniper K Jr, Woolf WE (1956) Biliary tract studies. l. X-ray diffraction analysis of gallstones; correlation with occurrence of microspheroliths in bile. *Am J Med* 20:383–391.

Juttijudata P, Chiemchaisri C, Palavatana C, Churuafanakul S (1984) Biliary tract disease in Thailand. *Surg Gynecol Obstet* 158:13–16.

Kajiyama G, Kubota S, Sasaki H, Kawamoto T, Miyoshi A (1981) Lipid metabolism in the development of cholesterol gallstones in hamsters. The effect of dietary cholesterol on its biliary concentration and lithogenicity. *Hiroshima J Med Sci* 30:141–143.

Kakar F, Weiss NS, Strite SA (1988) Non-contraceptive estrogen use and the risk of gallstone disease in women. *Am J Public Health* 78:564–566.

Kalk H, Schöndube W (1926) Über die Funktion der Gallenblase. Untersuchungen an normalen an Hand der Pituitrin – bezw. Hypophysinprobe. *Z Exp Med* 53:461–483.

Kameda H (1964) Gallstone disease in Japan. A report of 812 cases. *Gastroenterology* 46:109–114.

Kameda H (1991) Types of gallstones in Japan: current status. *Tan to Sui (Biliary Tract Pancreas)* 12:1179–1183. (In Japanese)

Kameda H, Ishihara F, Shibata K, Tsukie K, Tanaka M, Yamashita H, Mori W (1980) Chronological change in cholelithiasis in Japan. *Nihon Ijishinpo (Jpn J Clin Exp Med)* 2924:24–31. (In Japanese)

Kameda H, Ishihara F, Shibata K, Tsukie E, Takagi I (1981) Regional differences in cholelthiasis in Japan. *Nihon Ijishinpo (Jpn J Clin Exp Med)* 2980:26–30. (In Japanese)

Kanazawa T, Shimazaki A, Sato T, Hoshino T (1954) Synthesis of ursodeoxycholic acid and its conjugated bile acid. *Proc Jpn Acad* 30:391–392.

Karayalcin G, Hassani N, Abrams M, Lanzkowsky P (1979) Cholelithiasis in children with sickle cell disease. *Am J Dis Child* 133:306–307.

Kataruam RS, Verma GP (1967) Intra-hepatic stones in the horse. *Ind Vet J* 44:1025–1029.

Kaufman HS, Magnuson TH, Lillemoe KD, Frasca P, Pitt HA (1989) The role of bacteria in gallbladder and common duct stone formation. *Ann Surg* 209:584–591.

Kaufman HS, Magnuson TH, Pitt HA, Frasca P, Lillemoe KD (1994) The distribution of calcium salt precipitates in the core, periphery and shell of cholesterol, black pigment and brown pigment gallstones. *Hepatology* 19:1124–1132.

Kawamoto T, Akino T, Nakamura M, Mori M (1980) Metabolism of individual molecular species of phosphatidylcholine in the liver subcellular membranes and bile: origin of bile phosphatidylcholine. *Biochim Biophys Acta* 619:35–47.

Kawata S, Imai Y, Inui Y, Kakimoto H, Fukuda K, Maeda Y, Tarui S (1991) Modulation of cholesterol 7$\alpha$-hydroxylase activity by nonspecific lipid transfer protein in human liver – possibly altered regulation of its cytosolic level in patients with gallstones. *Clin Chim Acta* 197:201–208.

Keane P, Colwell D, Baer HP, Clanachan AS. Scott GW (1986) Effects of age, gender and female sex hormones upon contractility of the human gallbladder in vitro. *Surg Gynecol Obstet* 163:555–560.

Kehr H (1897) Die Behandlung der calculösen Cholangitis durch die direkte Drainage des Ductus Hepaticus. *Münch Med Wochenschr* 44:1127–1131.

Keida Y, Nakano T, Tabata M, Shimizu S, Nakayama F (1991) Significance of different conjugate forms of bilirubin in the formation of pigment gallstones. *J Gastroenterol Hepatol* 6:595–598.

Kellett MJ, Wickham JEA, Russell RCG (1988) Percutaneous cholecystolithotomy. *Br Med J* 296:453–455.

Kelley MJ, Story JA (1985) Effect of type of diet and feeding status on modulation of hepatic HMG-Co A reductase in rats. *Lipids* 20:53–55.

Kellum JM, Kuemmerle J, O'Dorisio TM, Rayford P, Martin D, Engle K, Wolf N, Sugerman HJ (1990) Gastrointestinal hormone responses to meals before and after bypass and vertical banded gastroplasty. *Ann Surg* 211:763–771.

Kennedy RH, Thompson MH (1988) Are duodenal diverticula associated with choledocholithiasis? *Gut* 29:1003–1006.

Ker CG, Huang TJ, Sheen PC (1981) Intrahepatic stones. I. Etiological study. *J Formosan Med Assoc* 80:698–711. (In Chinese with an English summary)

Kerlan RK, LaBerge JM, Ring EJ (1985) Percutaneous cholecystolithotomy: preliminary experience. *Radiology* 157:653–656.

Kern F Jr, Everson GT (1987) Contraceptive steroids increase cholesterol in bile: mechanism of action. *J Lipid Res* 28:828–839.

Kern F Jr, Eriksson H, Curstedt T, Sjövall J (1977) Effect of ethinylestradiol on biliary excretion of bile acids, phosphatidylcholines, and cholesterol in the bile fistula rat. *J Lipid Res* 18:623–634.

Kern F Jr, Everson GT, DeMark B, McKinley C, Showalter R, Erfling W, Braverman DZ, Szczepanik-Van Leeuwen P, Klein PD (1981) Biliary lipids, bile acids, and gallbladder function in the human female. *J Clin Invest* 68:1229–1242.

Kervinen K, Savolainen MJ, Heikkilä JI, Kesäniemi YA (1993) Lovastatin enhances hepatic uptake of low density lipoprotein in humans. *J Lipid Res* 34:1975–1982.

Kessler MJ (1982) Calcium bilirubinate gallstones in an aged rhesus monkey (*Macaca mulatta*). *Am J Primatol* 2:291–294.

Key PH, Bonorris GG, Marks JW, Chung A, Schoenfield LJ (1980) Biliary lipid synthesis and secretion in gallstone patients before and during treatment with chenodeoxycholic acid. *J Lab Clin Med* 95:816–826.

Khail T, Walker JP, Wiener I, Fagan CJ, Townsend CM, Greeley GH Jr, Thompson JC (1985) Effect of aging on gallbladder contraction and release of cholecystokinin-33 in humans. *Surgery* 98:423–429.

Khuroo MS, Zargar SA (1985) Biliary ascariasis: a common cause of biliary and pancreatic disease in an endemic area. *Gastroenterology* 88:418–423.

Khuroo MS, Mahajan R, Zargar SA, Javid G, Sapru S (1989) Prevalence of biliary tract disease in India: a sonographic study in adult population in Kashmir. *Gut* 30:201–205.

Kibe A, Holzbach RT, LaRusso NF, Mao SJT (1984) Inhibition of cholesterol crystal formation by apolipoproteins in supersaturated model bile. *Science* 225:514–516.

Kibe A, Dudley MA, Halpern Z, Lynn MP, Breuer AC, Holzbach RT (1985) Factors affecting cholesterol monohydrate crystal nucleation time in model systems of supersaturated bile. *J Lipid Res* 26:1102–1111.

Kimura T, Yoshida M, Umehara Y, Sakuramachi S, Matsuda S, Takabayashi N, Harada Y (1991) Operative procedure of laparoscopic cholecystectomy. *Geka Shinryo (Surg Diagn Treat)* 33:967–975. (In Japanese)

King MS (1971) Biliary tract disease in Malaya. *Br J Surg* 58:829–832.

King DR, Ginn-Pease ME, Lloyd TV, Hoffman J, Hohenbrink K (1987) Parenteral nutrition with associated cholelithiasis: another iatrogenic disease of infants and children. *J Pediatr Surg* 22:593–596.

Kjølbye JE, Nielsen EL (1959) ABO blood groups in cholelithiasis. *Acta Genet Basel* 9:213–220.

Kleeberg J (1960) Etiology of gallstone formation in human beings. In *Rudolf Virchow Medical Society in the City of New York. Jubilee Volume, 100th anniversary (1860–1960)*, Basel, Karger, pp 224–257.

Kleeberg J (1961) The incidence of cholelithiasis among the different ethnic groups in Israel. *Harefuah* (J Med Assoc Isr) 59:381–382. (In Hebrew and English)

Klingensmith WC, Cioffi-Ragan DT (1988) Fetal gallstones. *Radiology* 167:143–144.

Knyrim K, Vakil N (1992) Bile composition, microspheroliths, antinucleating activity, and gallstone calcification. *Gastroenterology* 103:552–559.

Koga A, Todo S (1977) Structure study of so-called black gallstones. *Nihon Shokakibyo Gakkai Zasshi (Jpn J Gastroenterol)* 74:1154–1159. (In Japanese with an English abstract)

Koga A, Miyazaki K, Ichimiya H, Nakayama F (1984) Choice of treatment for hepatolithiasis based on pathological findings. *World J Surg* 8:36–40.

Koga A, Ichimiya H, Yamaguchi K, Miyazaki K, Nakayama F (1985) Hepatolithiasis associated with cholangiocarcinoma. Possible etiological significance. *Cancer* 55:2826–2829.

Koga A, Watanabe K, Takiguchi S, Miyazaki K, Nakayama F (1987) Etiological significance of anatomic variations in the main intrahepatic ducts in hepatolithiasis. *Acta Pathol* 28:285–288.

Kohse KP, Stehle P, Walker S (1992) N-acetylcysteine is useless for oral gallstone dissolution. *Gastroenterology* 103:351.

Konikoff FM, Chung DS, Donovan JM, Small DM, Carey MC (1992) Filamentous, helical, and tubular microstructures during cholesterol crystallization from bile. Evidence that cholesterol does not nucleate classic monohydrate plates. *J Clin Invest* 90:1155–1160.

Konikoff FM, Cohen DE, Carey MC (1994) Phospholipid molecular species influence crystal habits and transition sequences of metastable intermediates during cholesterol crystallization from bile salt-rich model bile. *J Lipid Res* 35:60–70.

Kono S, Kochi S, Ohyama S, Wakisaka A (1988) Gallstones, serum lipids, and glucose intolerance among male officials of self-defense forces in Japan. *Dig Dis Sci* 33:839–844.

Kozoll DD, Dwyer G, Meyer KA (1959) Pathologic correlation of gallstones. A review of 1,874 autopsies of patients with gallstones. *Arch Surg* 79:514–536.

Kravetz RE (1964) Etiology of biliary tract disease in southwest American Indians. Analysis of 105 consecutive cholecystectomies. *Gastroenterology* 46:392–398.

Kritchevsky D, Klurfeld DM (1983) Gallstone formation in hamsters: effect of varying animal and vegetable protein levels. *Am J Clin Nutr* 37:802–804.

Kubota K, Itoh T, Shibayama K, Shimada K, Nomura Y, Idezuki Y (1989) Papillary function of patients with juxtapapillary duodenal diverticulum. Consideration of pathogenesis of common bile duct stones. *Scand J Gastroenterol* 24:140–144.

Kümmell H (1890) Zur Chirurgie der Gallenblase. *Dtsch Med Wochenschr* 12:237–239.

Kuroki S, Muramoto S, Kuramoto T, Hoshita T (1983) Sex differences in gallbladder bile acid composition and hepatic steroid 12$\alpha$-hydroxylase activity in hamsters. *J Lipid Res* 24:1543–1549.

Kuroki S, Cohen BI, Carey MC, Mosbach EH (1986) Rapid computation with the personal computer of the percent cholesterol saturation of bile samples. *J Lipid Res* 27:442–446.

Kuroki S, Mosbach EH, Cohen BI, McSherry CK (1987a) Metabolism of the bile acid analogues, 7$\beta$-methyl-cholic acid and 7$\alpha$-methyl-ursocholic acid. *Gastroenterology* 92:876–884.

Kuroki S, Mosbach EH, Cohen BI, Stenger RJ, McSherry CK (1987b) 7-Methyl bile acids: 7$\beta$-Methyl-cholic acid inhibits bacterial 7-dehydroxylation of cholic acid and chenodeoxycholic acid in the hamster. *J Lipid Res* 28:856–863.

Kwon OJ, Park YH, Kim JP (1982) A clinical study of cholelithiasis in Korean. *J Korean Surg Soc* 24:1052–1058. (In Korean with an English abstract)

Kyd PA, Bouchier IAD (1971) Absorption of water, unconjugated bilirubin, and sodium glycodeoxycholate by the rabbit gallbladder with dietary-induced gallstones. *Gastroenterology* 61:723–732.

Kyd PA, Bouchier IAD (1972) Experimental oleic acid-induced cholelithiasis in the rabbit associated with increased biliary 5$\alpha$-deoxycholic acid. *Biochem J* 128:169–172.

Lachman BS, Lazerson J, Starshak RJ, Vaughters FM, Werlin SL (1979) The prevalence of cholelithiasis in sickle cell disease as diagnosed by ultrasound and cholecystography. *Pediatrics* 64:601–603.

Lafont H, Nalbone G, Lairon D, Dagorn J C, Domingo N, Amic J, Hauton JC (1977) Zone electrophoresis study of the bile lipoprotein complex. *Biochemie (Paris)* 59:445–452.

Lafont H, Halpern Z, Domingo N, Peled Y, Grosclaude J, Gilat T (1993) Anionic polypeptide fraction (APF/CBP) in normal and abnormal human biles; its distribution between cholesterol carriers in bile and its effect on nucleation. *Gastroenterology* 104:A367 (abstract).

Lam RC (1954) Gallbladder diseases among the American Indians. *J Lancet* 74:305–309.

LaMont JT, Turner BS, Bernstein SE, Trotman BW (1983a) Gallbladder glycoprotein secretion in mice with hemolytic anemia and pigment gallstones. *Hepatology* 3:198–200.

LaMont JT, Turner BS, DiBenedetto D, Handin R, Schafer AI (1983b) Arachidonic acid stimulates mucin secretion in prairie dog gallbladder. *Am J Physiol* 245:G92–G98.

LaMont JT, Smith BF, Moore JRL (1984) Role of gallbladder mucin in the pathophysiology of gallstones. *Hepatology* 4(Suppl): 51Sf–56S

LaMorte WW, Schoetz DJ, Birkett DH, Williams LF Jr (1979) The role of the gallbladder in the pathogenesis of cholesterol gallstones. *Gastroenterology* 77:580–592.

LaMorte WW, Booker ML, Scott TE, Williams LF Jr (1985a) Increases in gallbladder prostaglandin synthesis before the formation of cholesterol gallstones. *Surgery* 98:445–451.

La Morte WW, Brotschi EA, Scott TE, Williams LF Jr (1985b) Pigment gallstone formation in the cholesterol-fed guinea pig. *Hepatology* 5:21–27.

LaMorte WW, LaMont JT, Hale W, Booker ML, Scott TE, Turner B (1986) Gallbladder prostaglandins and lysophospholipids as mediators of mucin secretion during cholelithiasis. *Am J Physiol* 251:G701–G709.

LaMorte WW, O'Leary D, Booker M, Scott T (1993) High dietary fat accelerates cholesterol (CHL) gallstone formation in th prairie dog. *Gastroenterology* 104:A368 (abstract).

Langenbuch C (1882) Ein Fall von Exstirpation der Gallenblase wegen chronischer Cholelithiasis. Heilung. *Berl Klin Wochenschr* 90:725–727.

Lanzini A, Northfield TC (1990) Hepatic biliary lipid secretion and gall bladder biliary lipid mass in gall stone patients: effect of ursodeoxycholic acid. *Gut* 31: 226–230.

Lanzini A, Jazrawi RP, Northfield TC (1987) Simultaneous quantitative measurements of absolute gallbladder storage and emptying during fasting and eating in humans. *Gastroenterology* 92:852–861.

Lapin BA, Krilova RI, Cherkovich GM, Asanov NS (1979) Observations from Sukhumi. In Bowden DM (ed): *Aging in nonhuman primates.* New York, Van Nostrand Reinhold, pp 26–27.

Lapin BA, Yakovleva LA (1963) *Comparative Pathology in Monkeys.* Springfield, IL, C C Thomas, pp 236–237.

Lauffer GL, Jazrawi RJ, Ahmed H, Grundy A, Northfield TC (1993) In-vivo comparison for gallstone dissolution (using MTBE) with computerized pump and hand syringe at two temperatures. *Gastroenterology* 104:A368 (abstract).

Lawson M, Everson GT, Klingensmith W, Kern F Jr (1983) Coordination of gastric and gallbladder emptying after ingestion of a regular meal. *Gastroenterology* 85:866–870.

Layde PM, Vessey MP, Yeates D (1982) Risk factors for gall-bladder disease: a cohort study of young women attending family planning clinics. *J Epidemiol Commun Health* 36:274–278.

LeBlanc GA, Waxman DJ (1990) Regulation and ligand-binding specificities of two sex-specific bile acid-binding proteins of rat liver cytosol. *J Biol Chem* 265:5654–5661.

Lee SP (1978) Enhanced fluid transport across gallbladder mucosa in experimental cholelithiasis. *Am J Physiol* 234:E575–E578.

Lee SP (1990) Pathogenesis of biliary sludge. *Hepatology* 12:200S–205S.

Lee SP, Nicholls JF (1986) Nature and composition of biliary sludge. *Gastroenterology* 90:677–686.

Lee SP, Scott AJ (1982) The evolution of morphologic changes in the gallbladder before stone formation in mice fed a cholesterol-cholic acid diet. *Am J Pathol* 108:1–8.

Lee TJ, Smith BF (1989) Bovine gallbladder mucin promotes cholesterol crystal nucleation from cholesterol-transporting vesicles in supersaturated model bile. *J Lipid Res* 30:491–498.

Lee SP, Thomsen LL (1982) Toxin-induced cell membrane injury in guinea pigs given lincomycin. *Pathology*

14:317–322.

Lee SP, Lim TH, Scott AJ (1979) Carbohydrate moieties of glycoproteins in human hepatic and gall-bladder bile, gall-bladder mucosa and gall stones. *Clin Sci* 56:533–538.

Lee SP, Carey MC, LaMont JT (1981a) Aspirin prevention of cholesterol gallstone formation in prairie dogs. *Science* 211:1429–1431.

Lee SP, LaMont JT, Carey MC (1981b) The role of gallbladder mucus hypersecretion in the evolution of cholesterol gallstones. Studies in the prairie dog. *J Clin Invest* 67:1712–1723.

Lee SP, Tasman-Jones C, Carlisle V (1986) Oleic acid-induced cholelithiasis in rabbits. Changes in bile composition and gallbladder morphology. *Am J Pathol* 124:18–24.

Lee SP, Park HZ, Madani H, Kaler EW (1987a) Partial characterization of a nonmicellar system of cholesterol solubilization in bile. *Am J Physiol* 252:G374–G383.

Lee SP, Tasman-Jones C, Carlisle V (1987b) Oleic acid-induced cholelithiasis in the rabbit: conversion of dietary oleic acid to cholestanol as a cause of calcium-bile salt gallstones. *Hepatology* 7:529–534.

Lee SP, Maher K, Nicholls JF (1988) Origin and fate of biliary sludge. *Gastroenterology* 94:170–176.

Lee VS, Paulson EK, Libby E, Flannery JE, Meyers WC (1993) Cholelithoptysis and cholelithorrhea: rare complications of laparoscopic cholecystectomy. *Gastroenterology* 105:1877–1881.

Leinkram C, Roberts-Thomson IC, Kune GA (1980) Juxtapapillary duodenal diverticula. Association with gallstones and pancreatitis. *Med J Aust* 1:209–210.

Lembcke B, Creutzfeldt W, Schleser S, Ebert R, Shaw C, Koop I (1987) Effect of the somatostatin analogue sandostatin (SMS 201-995) on gastrointestinal, pancreatic and biliary function and hormone release in normal men. *Digestion* 36:108–124.

Lemmel G (1934) Die klinische Bedeutung der Duodenaldivertikel. *Arch Verdauungskr* 56:59–70.

Leo H (1914) Die Gallensteinlösende Wirkung des Karlsbaderwassers. *Dtsch Med Wochenschr* 40:786–788.

Leslie BR, Sander NW, Gerwin LE (1985) Runner's hemolysis and pigment gallstones. *N Engl J Med* 7:1230.

Levy PF, Smith BF, LaMont JT (1984) Human gallbladder mucin accelerates nucleation of cholesterol in artificial bile. *Gastroenterology* 87:270–275.

Leyssac P, Bukhave K, Frederiksen O (1974) Inhibitory effect of prostaglandins on isoosmotic fluid transport by rabbit gallbladder in vitro, and its modification by blockade of endogenous PGE-biosynthesis by indomethacin. *Acta Physiol Scand* 92:496–507.

Li J, Stahlgren LH (1995) Glutamine prevents the biliary lithogenic effect of total parenteral nutrition in rats. *J Surg Res* 58:491–495.

Li Y, Luo GZ (1990a) Qualitative and quantitative comparison of gallbladder proteins from patients with and without cholesterol gallstones. *Dig Dis Sci* 35:47–49.

Li YC, Wang DP, Chang JYL (1990b) Regulation of cholesterol $7\alpha$-hydroxylase in the liver. Cloning, sequencing, and regulation of cholesterol $7\alpha$-hydroxylase mRNA. *J Biol Chem* 265:12012–12019.

Li YF, Russell DH, Myers SI, Weisbrodt NW, Moody FG (1994) Gallbladder contractility in aspirin- and cholesterol-fed prairie dogs. *Gastroenterology* 106:1662–1667.

Lichtenberg D, Ragimova S, Peled Y, Halpern Z (1988) Phospholipid peroxidation as a factor in gallstone pathogenesis. *FEBS Lett* 228:179–181.

Liddle RA, Goldstein RB, Saxton J (1989) Gallstone formation during weight-reduction dieting. *Arch Intern Med* 149:1750–1753.

Lieber MM (1952) The incidence of gallstones and their correlation with other diseases. *Ann Surg* 135:394–405.

Lilja P, Fagan CJ, Wiener I, Inoue K, Watson LC, Rayford PL, Thompson JC (1982) Infusion of pure cholecystokinin in humans. Correlation between plasma concentration of cholecystokinin and gallbladder size. *Gastroenterology* 83:256–261.

Lillemoe KD, Magnuson TH, Webb TH, Kaufman HS, Watt PC, D'Souza MP, Pitt HA (1988) Bilirubin monoglucuronide promotes cholesterol gallstone formation. Hepatology 8:1373 (abstract).

Lin SD, Conner WE, Phillipson BE (1984) Sterol composition of normal human bile. Effects of feeding shellfish (marina) sterols. *Gastroenterology* 86:611–617.

Lindner HH, Green RB (1964) Embryology and surgical anatomy of the extrahepatic biliary tract. *Surg Clin North Am* 44:1273–1285.

Lindström CG (1977) Frequency of gallstone disease in a well-defined Swedish population: a prospective necropsy study in Malmö. *Scand J Gastroenterol* 12:341–346.

Linos DA, Beard CM, O'Fallon WM, Dockerty MB, Beart RW Jr, Kurland LT (1981) Cholecystectomy and carcinoma of the large bowel. *Lancet* 2:379–381.

Lipsett PA, Burrow CR, Fox-Talbot MK, Pitt HA, Lillemoe KD (1993) Identification of a ubiquitous $CaCO_3$ inhibitory factor in human bile. *Gastroenterology* 104:A369 (abstract).

Little TE, Madani H, Lee SP, Kaler EW (1993) Lipid vesicle fusion induced by phospholipase C activity in model bile. *J Lipid Res* 34:211–217.

Loefler IJP (1988) Gallstones and glaciers: hypothesis meeting at the equator. *Lancet* 2:683.

Lofland H B (1976) Cholelithiasis, Model No. 74. *Handbook: Animal Models of Human Disease*. In Jones TC, Hackel DB, Migaki G (eds): *Registry of Comparative Pathology*. Washington, DC: Armed Forces Institute of Pathology (AFIP).

Logan GM, Duane WC (1990) Lovastatin added to ursodeoxycholic acid further reduces biliary cholesterol saturation. *Gastroenterology* 98:1572–1576.

Lointier PH, Kauffmann P, Francannet P, Pezet D, Chipponi J (1990) Management of intrahepatic calculi in Caroli's disease by extracorporeal shock wave lithotripsy. *Br J Surg* 77:987–988.

Lorentz TG (1966) Observations on the pathogenesis of gall-stones. *Br J Surg* 53:503–509.

Lorusso D, Misciagna G, Noviello MR, Tarantino S (1988) Cholelithiasis after Billroth II gastric resection. *Surgery* 103:579–583.

Løtveit T (1982) The composition of biliary calculi in patients with juxtapapillary duodenal diverticula. *Scand J Gastroenterol* 17:653–656.

Løtveit T, Osnes M, Aune S (1978) Bacteriological studies of common bile duct bile in patients with gallstone disease and juxta-papillary duodenal diverticula. *Scand J Gastroenterol* 13:93–95.

Løtveit T, Osnes M, Aune S, Larsen S (1980) Studies of the choledochoduodenal sphincter in patients with and without juxta-papillary duodenal diverticula. *Scand J Gastroenterol* 15:875–880.

Løtveit T, Osnes, Larsen S (1982) Recurrent biliary calculi. Duodenal diverticula as a predisposing factor. *Ann Surg* 196:30–32.

Low-Beer TS, Nutter S (1978) Colonic bacterial activity, biliary cholesterol saturation and pathogenesis of gallstones. *Lancet* 2:1063–1065.

Low-Beer TS, Pomare EW (1973) Regulation of bile salt pool size in man. *Br Med J* 2:338–340.

Low-Beer TS, Pomare EW (1975) Can colonic bacterial metabolites predispose to cholesterol gallstones? *Br Med J* 1:438–440.

Lowenfels AB (1980) Gallstones and the risk of cancer. *Gut* 21:1090–1092.

Lowenfels AB (1988) Gallstones and glaciers: the stone that came from the cold. *Lancet* I:1385–1386.

Lowenfels AB (1991) Smoking and the risk of gallstones. *Arch Intern Med* 151:398.

Lowenfels AB, Domellöf L, Lindström CG, Bergman F, Monk MA, Sternby NH (1982) Cholelithiasis, cholecystectomy and cancer: a case-control study in Sweden. *Gastroenterology* 83:672–676.

Lowenfels AB, Walker AM, Althaus DP, Townsend G, Domellöff L (1989) Gallstone growth, size and risk of gallbladder cancer: an interracial study. *Int J Epidemiol* 18:50–54.

Ludlow AI (1930) Cholelithiasis in the Korean. *Surg Gynecol Obstet* 50:51–58.

Lund J (1960) Surgical indication in cholelithiasis. Prophylactic cholecystectomy elucidated on the basis of long-term follow-up on 526 nonoperated cases. *Ann Surg* 151:153–162.

Lundgren O, Svanvik J, Jivegåd L (1989) Enteric nervous system II. Physiology and pathophysiology of the gallbladder. *Dig Dis Sci* 34:284–288.

Lutton RG, Large AM (1957) Gallstones: solubility studies. *Surgery* 42:488–492.

Lynn J, Williams L, O'Brien J, Wittenberg J, Egdahl RH (1973) Effects of estrogen upon bile: Implications with respect to gallstone formation. *Ann Surg* 178:514–524.

Ma L (1968) The formation of biliary mud in Chinese liver fluke infections. *Clin Chim Acta* 19:7–10.

Ma Y (1989) *China's Minority Nationalities*. Beijing, Foreign Language Press.

Mabee TM, Meyer P, DenBesten L, Mason EE (1976) The mechanism of increased gallstone formation in obese human subjects. *Surgery* 79:460–468.

Maclure KM, Hayes KG, Colditz GA, Stampfer MJ, Speizer FE, Willet WC (1989) Weight, diet and the risk of symptomatic gallstones in middle-aged women. *N Engl J Med* 321:563–569.

Maclure KM, Hayes KC, Colditz GA, Stampfer MJ, Willett WC (1990) Dietary predictors of symptom-associated gallstones in middle-aged women. *Am J Clin Nutr* 52:916–922.

MacPharson BR, Pemsingh RS, Scott GW (1987) Experimental cholelithiasis in the ground squirrel. *Lab Invest* 56:138–145.

Magnus IA, Jarrett A, Prankerd TAJ, Rimington C (1961) Erythropoietic protoporphyria. A new porphyria syndrome with solar urticaria due to protoporphyrinaemia. *Lancet* 2:448–451.

Magnuson TH, Lillemoe KD, High RC, Pitt HA (1989a) Fish oil prevents cholesterol crystal nucleation and gallstone formation. *Gastroenterology* 96:A625 (abstract).

Magnuson TH, Lillemoe KD, Peoples GE, Pitt HA (1989b) Oral calcium promotes pigment calcium formation. *J Surg Res* 46:286–291.

Magnuson TH, Lillemoe KD, Scheeres DE, Pitt HA (1990) Altered bile composition during cholesterol gallstone formation: cause or effect? *J Surg Res* 48:584–589.

Mahfouz-Cercone S, Johnson JE, Liepa GU (1984) Effects of animal and vegetable protein on gallstone formation and biliary constituents in the hamster. *Lipids* 19:5–10.

Mahmoud H, Schell M, Pui CH (1991) Cholelithiasis after treatment of childhood cancer. *Cancer* 67:1439–1442.

Maingot R (1974) Congenital anomalies of the gallbladder, the bile ducts, and the hepatic and cystic arteries. In Maingot R (ed): *Abdominal Operations*, 6th ed., New York, Appleton-Century-Crofts, pp 928–948.

Majoor CLH, Suren TJJ (1947) Gallbladder complications following resection of stomach for peptic ulcer. *Br Med J* 2:8–11.

Maki T (1961) Cholelithiasis in the Japanese. *Arch Surg* 82:599–612.

Maki T (1966) Pathogenesis of calcium bilirubinate gallstone: role of *E. coli*, $\beta$-glucuronidase and coagulation by inorganic ions, polyelectrolytes and agitation. *Ann Surg* 164:90–100.

Maki T, Sato T, Yamaguchi I, Saito Y (1964) Autopsy incidence of gallstones in Japan. *Tohoku J Exp Med* 84:37–45.

Maki T, Matsushiro T, Suzuki N, Nakamura N (1971) Role of sulfated glycoproteins in gallstone formation. *Surg Gynecol Obstet* 132:846–851.

Maki T, Matsushiro T, Suzuki N (1982) Clarification of the nomenclature of pigment gallstones. Am J Surg 144: 302–305.

Makino I, Shinozaki K, Yoshino K, Nakagawa S (1975) Cases of cholesterol gallstone dissolution after prolonged administration of ursodeoxycholic acid. *Nihon Shokakibyo Gakkai Zasshi (Jpn J Gastroenterol)* 72:690–702. (In Japanese)

Makino I, Chijiiwa K, Higashijima H, Nakahara S, Kishinaka M, Mibu R (1994) Rapid cholesterol nucleation time and cholesterol gall stone formation after subtotal or total colectomy in humans. *Gut* 35:1760–1764.

Malagelada JR, Go VLW, Summerskill WHJ, Gamble WS (1973) Bile acid secretion and biliary bile acid composition altered by cholecystectomy. *Am J Dig Dis* 18:455–459.

Malagelada JR, Go VLW, Summerskill WHJ (1974) Altered pancreatic and biliary function after vagotomy and pyloroplasty. *Gastroenterology* 66:22–27.

Malavolti M, Fromm H, Ceryak S, Roberts IM (1987) Modulation of low density lipoprotein receptor activity by bile acids: differential effects of chenodeoxycholic and ursodeoxycholic acids in the hamster. *J Lipid Res* 28:1281–1295.

Malet PF (1985) Animal models of gallstone formation. In Cohen S, Soloway RD (eds): *Gallstones.* New York, Churchill Livingstone, pp 309–333.

Malet PF, Takabayashi A, Trotman BW, Soloway RD, Weston NE (1984) Black and brown pigment gallstones differ in microstructure and microcomposition. *Hepatology* 4:227–234.

Malet PF, Locke C L, Trotman BW, Soloway RD (1986a) The calcium ionophore A23187 stimulates glycoprotein secretion by the guinea pig gallbladder. *Hepatology* 6:569–573.

Malet PF, Williamson CE, Trotman BW, Soloway RD (1986b) Composition of pigmented centers of cholesterol gallstones. *Hepatology* 6:477–481.

Malet PF, Dabezies MA, Huang GG, Long WB, Gadacz TR, Soloway R D (1988) Quantitative infrared spectroscopy of common bile duct gallstones. *Gastroenterology* 94:1217–1221.

Malet PF, Deng SQ, Soloway RD (1989) Gallbladder mucin and cholesterol and pigment gallstone formation in hamsters. *Scand J Gastroenterol* 24:1055–1060.

Malhotra SI (1968) Epidemiological study of cholelithiasis among railroad workers in India with a special reference to causation. *Gut* 9:290–295.

Malone BS, Werlin SL (1988) Cholecystectomy and cholelithiasis in sickle cell anemia. *Am J Dis Child* 142:799–800.

Mann GV (1970) Quoted by Portman et al., (1975). In Harris RS (ed): *Feeding and Nutrition of Nonhuman Primates.* New York, Academic Press, pp. 143–158.

Marcus SN, Heaton KW (1986a) Intestinal transit, deoxycholic acid and the cholesterol saturation of bile – three inter-related factors. *Gut* 27:550–558.

Marcus SN, Heaton KW (1986b) Effects of a new, concentrated wheat fibre preparation on intestinal transit, deoxycholic acid metabolism and the composition of bile. *Gut* 27:893–900.

Marcus SN, Heaton KW (1988) Deoxycholic acid and the pathogenesis of gall stones. *Gut* 29:522–533.

Maringhini A, Marceno MP, Lanzarone F, Caltagirone M, Fusco G, Di Cuonzo G, Cittadini E, Pagliaro L (1987) Sludge and stones in gallbladder after pregnancy. Prevalence and risk factors. *J Hepatol* 5:218–223.

Maringhini A, Clambra M, Baccelliere P, Raimondo M, Pagliaro L (1988) Sludge, stones and pregnancy. *Gastroenterology* 95:1160–1161.

Maringhini A, Ciambra M, Baccelliere P, Raimondo M, Orlando A, Tiné F, Grasso R, Randazzo MA, Barresi L, Gullo D, Musico M, Pagliaro L (1993) Biliary sludge and gallstones in pregnancy: incidence, risk factors, and natural history. *Ann Intern Med* 119:116–120.

Marks JW, Conley DR, Capretta TL, Bonorris GG, Chung A, Coyne MJ, Schoenfield LJ (1977) Gallstone prevalence and biliary lipid composition in inflammatory bowel disease. *Dig Dis Sci* 22:1097–1100.

Marks JW, Sue SO, Pearlman BJ, Bonorris GG, Varady P, Lachin JM, Schoenfield LJ (1981) Sulfation of lithocholate as a possible modifier of chenodeoxycholic acid-induced elevations of serum transaminase in patients with gallstones. *J Clin Invest* 68:1190–1196.

Marks JW, Bonorris GG, Schoenfield LJ (1991) Roles of deoxycholate and arachidonate in pathogenesis of cholesterol gallstones in obese patients during rapid loss of weight. *Dig Dis Sci* 36:957–960.

Marks JW, Bonorris GG, Albers G, Schoenfield LJ (1992) The sequence of biliary events preceding the formation of gallstones in humans. *Gastroenterology* 103:566–570.

Marks JW, Stein T, Schoenfield LJ (1994) Natural history and treatment with ursodiol of gallstone formed during rapid loss of weight in man. *Dig Dis Sci* 39:1981–1984.

Marteau P, Chretien Y, Calmus Y, Parc R, Poupon R (1989) Pharmacological effect of somatostatin on bile secretion in man. *Digestion* 42:16–21.

Marteau C, Sastre B, Iconomidis N, Portugal H, Pauli AM, Gerolami A (1990) pH regulation in human gallbladder bile: study in patients with and without gallstones. *Hepatology* 11:997–1002.

Mårtensson KM (1937) The incidence of gallstones in Sweden. The correlation of gallstones with various diseases and pathologic changes. *Ann Surg* 34:650–669.

Martigne M, Domingo N, Lechene de la Porte P, Lafont H, Hauton J (1988) Identification and localization of the apoprotein fraction of the bile lipoprotein complex in human gallstones. *Scand J Gastroenterol* 23:731–737.

Martin DE, Wolf RC, Houser WD (1973) Naturally occurring cholelithiasis in a rhesus monkey and its effects on plasma and biliary lipid concentration. *Am J Vet Res* 34:971–974.

Martin DE, Wolf RC, Meyer RK (1972) The effects of pregnancy on biliary lipids in rhesus monkeys. *Proc Soc Exp Biol Med* 139:115–117.

Martin KO, Budai K, Javitt NB (1993) Cholesterol and 27-hydroxycholesterol $7\alpha$-hydroxylation: evidence for two different enzymes. *J Lipid Res* 34:581–588.

Marzolo MP, Rigotti A, Nervi F (1990) Secretion of biliary lipids from the hepatocyte. *Hepatology* 12:135S–142S.

Masclee AAM, Jansen JBM, Driessen WMM, Geuskens LM, Lamers CBHW (1990) Effect of truncal vagotomy on cholecystokinin release, gallbladder contraction and gallbladder sensitivity to cholecystokinin in humans. *Gastroenterology* 98:1338–1344.

Massarrat S, Klingemann HG, Kappert J, Jaspersen D, Schmitz-Moormann P (1982) Die Häfigkeit der Cholelithiasis im autoptischen Material und ambulaten Krankengut aus Deutschland. *Z Gastroenterol* 20:341–345.

Masuda H, Nakayama F (1979) Composition of bile pigment in gallstones and bile and their etiological significance. *J Lab Clin Med* 73:353–360.

Matoba N, Une M, Hoshita T (1986) Identification of unconjugated bile acids in human bile. *J Lipid Res* 27:1154–1162.

Matoba N, Cohen BI, Mosbach EH, Stenger RJ, Kuroki S, Une M, McSherry CK (1989a) 7-Methyl bile acids: effects of chenodeoxycholic acid, cholic acid, and their $7\beta$-methyl analogues on the formation of cholesterol gallstones in the prairie dog. *Gastroenterology* 96:178–185.

Matoba N, Mosbach EH, Cohen BI, Une M, McSherry CK (1989b) Synthesis of new bile acid analogues and their metabolism in the hamster: $3\alpha,6\alpha$-dihydroxy-$6\beta$-methyl-$5\beta$-cholanoic acid and $3\alpha,6\beta$-dihydroxy-$6\alpha$-methyl-$5\beta$-cholanoic acid. *J Lipid Res* 30:1005–1014.

Maton PN, Murphy GM, Dowling RH (1977) Ursodeoxycholic acid treatment of gallstones. *Lancet* 2: 1297–1301.

Maton PN, Ellis HJ, Higgins MJP, Dowling RH (1980) Hepatic HMG-CoA reductase in human cholelithiasis: effect of chenodeoxycholic and ursodeoxycholic acids. *Eur J Clin Invest* 10:325–332.

Maton PN, Iser JH, Reuben A, Saxton HM, Murphy GM, Dowling RH (1982) Outcome of chenodeoxycholic acid (CDCA) treatment in 125 patients with radiolucent gallstones. Factors influencing efficacy, withdrawal, symptoms and side effects and post-dissolution recurrence. *Medicine* 61:86–96.

Matsumoto S, Tanaka M, Yoshimoto H, Miyazaki K, Ikeda S, Nakayama F (1987) Electrohydraulic lithotripsy of intrahepatic stones during choledochoscopy. *Surgery* 102:852–856.

Matsushiro T (1965) Identification of glucaro-l,4-lactone in bile as a factor responsible for inhibitory effect of bile on bacterial $\beta$-glucuronidase. *Tohoku J Exp Med* 85:330–339.

Matsushiro T, Suzuki N, Sato H, Maki T (1977) Effects of diet on glucaric acid concentration in bile and the formation of calcium bilirubinate gallstones. *Gastroenterology* 72:630–633.

Maugdal DP, Kupfer RM, Zentler-Munro PL, Northfield TC (1980) Postprandial gall-bladder emptying in patients with gallstones. *Br Med J* 280:141–143.

Maurer KR, Everhart JE, Knowler WC, Shawker TH, Roth HP (1990) Risk factors for gallstone disease in the Hispanic populations of the United States. *Am J Epidemiol* 131:836–844.

Mauret F (1987) Personal communication. Quoted by Cuschieri et al (1991) The European experience with laparoscopic cholecystectomy. *Am J Surg* 161:385–387.

Mayo WJ (1911) "Innocent" gall-stones a myth. *J A M A* 56:1021–1024.

Mazer NA, Carey MC (1983) Quasi-elastic light-scatter studies of aqueous biliary lipid systems. Cholesterol solubilization and precipitation in model bile solutions. *Biochemistry* 22:426–442.

Mazer NA, Carey MC, Kwasnick RF, Benedek GB (1979) Quasi-elastic light scattering studies of aqueous biliary lipid systems. Size, shape and thermodynamics of bile salt micelles. *Biochemistry* 18:3064–3075.

Mazer NA, Benedek GB, Carey MC (1980) Quasielastic light-scattering studies of aqueous biliary lipid systems. Mixed micelle formation in bile salt-lecithin solutons. *Biochemistry* 19:601–615.

Mazer NA, Schurtenberger P. Carey MC, Preisig R, Weigand K, Känzig W (1984) Quasi-elastic light scattering studies of native hepatic bile from the dog: comparison with aggregative behavior of model biliary lipid systems. *Biochemistry* 23:1994–2005.

Mazzella G, Bazzoli F, Festi D, Ronchi M, Aldini R, Roda A, Grigolo B, Simoni P, Villanova N, Roda E (1991) Comparable evaluation of chenodeoxycholic and ursodeoxycholic acids in obese patients. Effects on biliary lipid metabolism during weight maintenance and weight reduction. *Gastroenterology* 101:490–496.

McCall IW, Desai P, Serjeant BE, Serjeant GR (1977) Cholelithiasis in Jamaican patients with homozygous sickle cell disease. *Am J Hematol* 3:15–21.

McClure HM (1974) Observations in a necropsy series of 1,512 nonhuman primates. *Annual Proceedings of the American Association of Zoo Veterinarians, Philadelphia*

McDole M (1980) Cholelithiasis in a horse. *Equine Pract* 2:37–39.

McDougall RM, Walker K, Thurston OG (1976) Bile acid alterations in patients with cholesterol gallstones. *J Surg Res* 21:233–237.

McLean LR, Philips MC (1982) Cholesterol desorption from clusters of phosphatidylcholine and cholesterol in unilamellar vesicle bilayers during lipid transfer or exchange. *Biochemistry* 21:4053–4059.

McMaster P, Herbertson BM, Cusick C, Calne RY, Syrakos T, Marni A (1979) The development of biliary 'sludge' following liver transplantation. *Transplant Proc* 11:262–266.

McPherson K, Strong PM, Jones L, Britton BJ (1985) Do cholecystectomy rates correlate with geographic variations in the prevalence of gallstones? *J Epidemiol Commu Health* 39:179–182.

McSherry CK (1989) Cholecystectomy: the gold standard. *Am J Surg* 158:174–178.

McSherry CK, Javitt NB, de Carvalho JM, Glenn F (1971) Cholesterol gallstones and the chemical composition of bile in baboons. *Ann Surg* 173:569–577.

McSherry CK, Deitrick JE, May PS, Niemann W, Morrissey KP, Palmer RH, Glenn F (1977) Biliary lipid metabolism in pregnant baboon. *Surg Gynecol Obstet* 144:727–733.

McSherry CK, Ferstenberg H, Calhoun WF, Lahman E, Virshup M (1985) The natural history of diagnosed gallstone disease in symptomatic and asymptomatic patients. *Ann Surg* 202:59–63.

McSherry CK, Cohen BI, Bokkenheuser VD, Mosbach EH, Winter J, Matoba N, Scholes J (1989) Effects of calcium and bile acid feeding on colon tumors in the rat. *Cancer Res* 49:6039–6043.

Mellström D, Asztely M, Svanvik J (1988) Gallstones and previous cholecystectomy in 77- to 78-year-old women in an urban population in Sweden. *Scand J Gastroenterol* 23:1241–1244.

Mentzer SH (1926) A clinical and pathologic study of cholecystitis and cholelithiasis. *Surg Gynecol Obstet* 42:782–793.

Mentzer SH (1934) Cholecystic disease in pigs, sheep and cattle. *Calif West Med* 40:333–336.

Messing B, DeOliveira F, Bernier JJ (1981) Cholestasis during total parenteral nutrition (TPN): demonstration of facilitating factors and association with gallbladder lithiasis. *Gastroenterology* 80:1231 (abstract).

Messing B, Bories C, Kunstlinger F, Bernier JJ (1983) Does total parenteral nutrition induce gallbladder sludge formation and lithiasis? *Gastroenterology* 84:1012–1019.

Messing B, Aprahamian M, Rautureau M, Bories C, Bisalli A, Stock-Damge S (1984) Gallstone formation during total parenteral nutrition: a prospective study in man. *Gastroenterology* 86:1183 (abstract).

Metzger AL, Alder R, Heymsfield S, Grundy SM (1973) Diurnal variation in biliary lipid composition. Possible role in cholesterol gallstone formation. N Engl J Med 288:333–336.

Meyer WW, Hottenrott C (1986) Lithotripsie intrahepatischer Gallensteine. Dtsch Med Wochenschr lll: 1280–1282.

Miettinen TA (1971) Cholesterol production in obesity. *Circulation* 44:842–850.

Miettinen M, Turpeinen O, Karvonen MJ, Paavilainen E, Elosuo R (1976) Prevalence of cholelithiasis in men and women ingesting a serum-cholesterol-lowering diet. *Ann Clin Res* 8:111–116.

Miettinen TA, Kesäniemi YA, Järvinen H, Hästbacka J (1986) Cholesterol precursor sterols, plant sterols and cholestanol in human bile and gallstones. *Gastroenterology* 90:858–864.

Miki S, Mosbach EH, Cohen BI, Yoshii M, Ayyard N, McSherry CK (1992) Sulfonate analogues of chenodeoxycholic acid: Metabolism of sodium $3\alpha,7\alpha$-dihydroxy-25-homo-$5\beta$-cholane-25-sulfonate and sodium $3\alpha,7\alpha$-dihydroxy-24-nor-$5\beta$-cholane-23-sulfonate in the hamster. *J Lipid Res* 33:1629–1637.

Min PC, Cho MH, Im HM, Kim JH, Chin BH, Hahn SS (1966) Biliary tract diseases among Koreans. Analysis of 100 consecutive cases. *J Korean Surg Soc* 8:1–11. (In Korean with an English abstract)

Mingrone G, Greco AV, Finotti E, Passi S (1988) Free fatty acids: a stimulus for mucin hypersecretion in cholesterol gallstone biles. *Biochim Biophys Acta* 958:52–59.

Miquel J F, Nunez L, Rigotti A, Amigo L, Brandan E, Nervi F (1993) Isolation and partial characterization of cholesterol pronucleating hydrophobic glycoproteins associated with native biliary vesicles. *FEBS Lett* 318:45–49.

Mirizzi PL (1937) Operative cholangiography. *Surg Gynecol Obstet* 65:702–710.

Mirizzi PL (1948) Sindrome del conducto hepatico. *J Int Chir* 8:731–777.

Mitchell JC, Logan GM, Stone BG, Duane WC (1991a) Effects of lovastatin on biliary lipid secretion and bile acid metabolism in humans. *J Lipid Res* 32:71–78.

Mitchell JC, Stone BG, Logan GM, Duane WC (1991b) Role of cholesterol synthesis in regulation of bile acid synthesis and biliary cholesterol secretion in humans. *J Lipid Res* 32:1143–1149.

Miyake H Sr (1913) Statistische, klinische und chemische Studien zur Aetiologie der Gallensteine, mit besonderer Berücksichtigung der japanischen und deutschen Verhältnisse. *Arch Klin Chir* 101:54–117.

Miyake H Jr (1962) Gallstones in Kyushu. *Arch Surg* 85:425–429.

Miyake H Jr (1970) *Cholelithiasis*. Tokyo, Kanehara Shuppan Publishing Co. (In Japanese)

Miyake H Sr, Ishiyama F (1930) Statistische und klinische Studien auf Grund von 754 Fällen von Cholelithiasisoperationen bei Japanern. *Dtsch Z Chir* 225: 187–214.

Miyake H Jr, Johnston CG (1968) Gallstones: ethnological studies. *Digestion* 1:219–228.

Miyake H Jr, Kuwatsuka T, Tamesue N, Nakayama H, Izumi K, Yamamoto H, Onishi N, Aono K, Hara A, Johnston CG, Watanabe N, Ong GB (1963) Comparative studies on the chemical composition of gallstones in Japan, China and the United States. *Fukuoka Igakukai Zasshi (Fukuoka Acta Med)* 54: 781–826. (In Japanese with an English summary)

Miyazaki K, Nakayama F, Koga A (1984) Effect of chenodeoxycholic and ursodeoxycholic acids on isolated adult human hepatocytes. *Dig Dis Sci* 29:1123–1130.

Moesch C, Sautereau D, Letard JC, Daudon M, Leymarie J, Cessot F, Pillegand B (1993) Biliary drug lithiasis due to glaphenine: three cases identified by Fournier transform infrared spectrometery. *Gastroenterology* 104:A371 (abstract).

Mok HYI, Von Bergmann K, Grundy SM (1977) Regulation of pool size of bile acids in man. *Gastroenterology* 73:684–690.

Mok HYI, Von Bergmann K, Crouse JR, Grundy SM (1979) Biliary lipid metabolism in obesity. Effects of bile acid feeding before and during weight reduction. *Gastroenterology* 76:556–567.

Mok HYI, Von Bergman K, Grundy SM (1980) Kinetics of the enterohepatic circulation during fasting: biliary lipid secretion and gallbladder storage. Gastroenterology 78:1023–1033.

Mok HYI, Druffel ERM, Rampone WM (1986) Chronology of cholelithiasis. Dating gallstones from atmospheric radiocarbon produced by nuclear bomb explosions. *N Engl J Med* 314:1075–1077.

Mok K, Out T, deBruijn M, Goldhoorn B, Tytgat GNJ (1992) An evaluation of the quantitative importance of individual pronucleating proteins in the biliary concanavalin A-binding protein fraction. *Gastroenterology* 102:A323 (abstract).

Moody FG, Amerson JR, Berci G, Bland KL, Cotton PB, Graham JB, Jones RS, Maher JW, Munson JL, Pennell TC, Way LW (1989a) Lithotripsy for bile duct stones. *Am J Surg* 158:241–247.

Moody FG, Haley-Russell D, Li YF, Husband KJ Weisbrodt NW, Dewey RB (1989b) The effects of lithogenic bile on gallbladder epithelium. *Ann Surg* 210:406–416.

Moore EW (1984) The role of calcium in the pathogenesis of gallstones: $Ca^{++}$ electrode studies of model bile salt solutions and other biologic systems. With a hypothesis on the structural requirements for $Ca^{++}$ binding to proteins and bile acids. *Hepatology* 4:228S–243S.

Moore EW (1990) Biliary calcium and gallstone formation. *Hepatology* 12:206S–218S.

Moore EW, Celic L, Ostrow JD (1982) Interactions between ionized calcium and sodium taurocholate: bile salts are important buffers for prevention of calcium-containing gallstones. *Gastroenterology* 83:1079–1089.

Moore EW, Verine HJ (1985) Pathogenesis of pancreatic and biliary $CaCO_3$ lithiasis: the solubility product [K'sp] of calcite determined with the $Ca^{++}$ electrode. *J Lab Clin Med* 106:611–618.

Moorehead RJ, Kernohan RM, Patterson CC, McKelvey STD, Parks TG (1986) Does cholecystectomy predispose to colorectal cancer? A case control study. *Dis Colon Rectum* 29:36–38.

Moran S, Guevara L, Ramos M, Vargas F, Lizardi J, Cruzgonzalez I, Mendez N, De la Mora G, Uribe M (1993) Asymptomatic gallstone disease: prevalence and associated risk factors. *Gastroenterology* 104:A372 (abstract).

Morrissey K, Panveliwalla D, McSherry C, Deitrick J, Niemann W, Gupta G (1977) Effects of contraceptive steroids and pregnancy on bile composition and kinetics in the baboon. *J Surg Res* 22:598–604.

Mosbach EH, Bevans M (1960) Early pathologic and biochemical changes in rabbits fed dihydrocholesterol. *Am J Pathol* 37:631–639.

Mukaihara S (1981) Chemical analysis of gallstones II. Classification and composition of human gallstones. *Nippon Geka Hokan (Arch Jpn Chir, Kyoto)* 50:476–500. (In Japanese with an English abstract)

Mundth ED (1962) Cholecystitis and diabetes mellitus. *N Engl J Med* 267:642–646.

Munizaga J, Allison MJ, Paredes C (1978) Cholelithiasis and cholecystitis in pre-Columbian Chileans. *Am J Phys Anthrop* 48:209–212.

Munoz-Ortiz PE, Calvo C, Taxonera C, Abreu L, Marin PE (1993a) Adverse effects of shock-wave therapy in 200 patients. *Gastroenterology* 104:A360 (abstract).

Munoz-Ortiz PE, Calvo C, Taxonera C, Abreu L, Marin PE (1993b) Gallstone recurrence rate after successful shock-wave therapy. *Gastroenterology* 104: A360 (abstract).

Murai N, Nakata N (1988) Rounded spikes of Kompeitoh and scaling relations. *Am J Physics* 56:459–462.

Murray FE, Logan RFA, Hannaford PC, Kay CR (1994) Cigarette smoking and parity as risk factors for the development of symptomatic gall bladder disease in women: results of the Royal College of General Practitioners' oral contraception study. *Gut* 35:107–111.

Myers SI, Li YF, Weisbrodt NW, Russell DH, Moody FG (1989) Endogenous gallbladder prostaglandin biosynthesis is not related to gallstone formation in the prairie dog fed a high-cholesterol diet. *Surg Forum* 40:157–158.

Nagakawa T (1989) Indications and limitations of nonlaparotomized cholecystolithotomy with mucoklase. *Geka Shinryo (Surg Diagn Treat)* 61:739–742. (In Japanese)

Nagakawa T, Konishi I, Oyama S, Kayahara M, Kanno M, Ota I, Noto K, Miyazaki I (1985) Nonlaparotomized cholecystolithotomy with mucoklase. *Nippon Ijishinpo (Jpn J Clin Exp Med)* 134:387–388. (In Japanese)

Nagase M, Tanimura H, Setoyama M, Hikasa Y (1978) Present features of gallstones in Japan. A collective review of 2,144 cases. *Am J Surg* 135:788–790.

Nagashima H, Suzuki N, Yosizawa S (1974) Coagulating effect of calcium carbonate on sulfated glycoproteins isolated from pathological human bile. *Tohoku J Exp Med* 113:159–168.

Nahrwold DL, Rose RC, Ward SP (1976) Abnormalities in gallbladder morphology and function in patients with cholecystitis. *Ann Surg* 184:415–421.

Nakagawa S, Makino I, Ishizaki T, Dohi I (1977) Dissolution of cholesterol gallstones by ursodeoxycholic acid. *Lancet* 2:367–369.

Nakagawa Y, Abram V, Rarks JH, Lau HSH, Kawooya JK, Coe FL (1985) Urine glycoprotein crystal growth inhibitors. Evidence for a molecular abnormality in calcium oxalate nephrolithiasis. *J Clin Invest* 76:1455–1461.

Nakanishi M, Goldstein JL, Brown MS (1988) Multivalent control of 3-hydroxy-3-methylglutaryl coenzyme A reductase. *J Biol Chem* 263:8929–8937.

Nakano T, Tabata M, Nakayama F (1988a) Unconjugated bilirubin in hepatic bile with brown pigment gallstones and cholangitis. *Dig Dis Sci* 33:1116–1120.

Nakano T, Yanagisawa J, Nakayama F (1988b) Phospholipase activity in human bile. *Hepatology* 8:1560–1564.

Nakanuma Y, Terada T, Tanaka Y, Ohta G (1985) Are hepatolithiasis and cholangiocarcinoma aetiologically related? A morphological study of 12 cases of hepatolithiasis associated with cholangiocarcinoma. *Virchows Arch* (A) 406:45–58.

Nakanuma Y, Yamaguchi K, Ohta G, Terada T, Japanese Hepatolithiasis Study Group (1988) Pathologic features of hepatolithiasis in Japan. *Hum Pathol* 19:1181–1186.

Nakayama F (1967) Composition of gallstone and bile: species difference. *J Lab Clin Med* 73:623–630.

Nakayama F (1968) Quantitative microanalysis of gallstone. *J Lab Clin Med* 72:602–611.

Nakayama F (1971) Studies on calculus versus milieu: gallstone and bile. *J Lab Clin Med* 77:366–377.

Nakayama F (1980) Oral cholelitholysis – Cheno versus urso. Japanese experience. *Dig Dis Sci* 25:129–134.

Nakayama F (1981) Classification of gallstones (Kyushu). *Tan to Sui ( Biliary tract Pancreas)* 2:9–12. (In Japanese)

Nakayama F (1982) Intrahepatic calculi: a special problem in East Asia. *World J Surg* 6:802–804.

Nakayama F (1994) Intrahepatic stones. In Blumgart LH (ed): Surgery of the Liver and Biliary Tract, Second edition, Vol l. Edinburgh, Churchill Livingstone, pp 765–774.

Nakayama F, Blomstrand R (1960) Occurrence of cephalin, sphingomyelin and lysolecithin in bile. *Acta Chem Scand* 14:1211–1212.

Nakayama F, Blomstrand R (1961) Neutron activation paper chromatographic analysis of phospholipids in human liver and bile. *Acta Chem Scand* 15:1595–1603.

Nakayama F, Johnston CG (1960) Solubility of human gallstones in primate gallbladder. *Proc Soc Exp Biol Med* 104:73–75.

Nakayama F, Johnston CG (1962) Fractionation of bile lipids with silicic acid chromatography. *J Lab Clin Med* 59:364–370.

Nakayama F, Miyake H Jr (1965) Cholesterol complexing macromolecular fractions in human gallbladder bile. *J Lab Clin Med* 65:638–648.

Nakayama F, Miyake H Jr (1966) Species difference in cholesterol complexing macromolecular fractions in bile. *J Lab Clin Med* 67:78–86.

Nakayama F, Miyake H Jr (1970) Changing state of gallstone disease in Japan. Composition of the stones and treatment of the condition. *Am J Surg* 120: 794–799.

Nakayama F, Van der Linden W (1970) Bile from gallbladder harbouring gallstone: can it indicate stone formation? *Acta Chir Scand* 136:605–610.

Nakayama F, Van der Linden W (1971) Bile composition: Sweden versus Japan. Possible significance in the difference in gallstone incidence. *Am J Surg* 122:8–12.

Nakayama F, Van der Linden W (1974) Role of gallbladder in gallstone formation. *Acta Chir Scand* 139:45–49.

Nakayama F, Van der Linden W (1975) Stratification of bile in gallbladder and gallstone formation. *Surg Gynecol Obstet* 141:587–590.

Nakayama F, Furusawa T, Nakama T (1980) Hepatolithiasis in Japan: present status. *Am J Surg* 139:216–220.

Nakayama F, Soloway RD, Nakama T, Miyazaki K, Ichimiya H, Sheen PC, Ker CG, Ong GB, Choi TK, Boey J, Foong WC, Tan EC, Tung KH, Lee CN (1986) Hepatolithiasis in East Asia. Retrospective study. *Dig Dis Sci* 31:21–26.

Nakayama F, Ichimiya H, Keida Y, Koga A, Ikeda M (1987) Epidemiological survey of hepatolithiasis in Japan. In *Annual Report, 1986, of the Research Group for the Study of Hepatolithiasis*. Tokyo, Ministry of Health of Japan, pp11–48. (In Japanese)

Nakayama F, Koga A, Ichimiya H, Todo S, Shen K, Guo RX, Zeng XJ, Zhang ZH (1991) Hepatolithiasis in East Asia: Comparison between Japan and China. *J Gastroenterol Hepatol* 6:155–158.

Narisawa T, Magadia NE, Weisburger JH, Wynder EL (1974) Promoting effect of sodium deoxycholate on colon carcinogenesis after intrarectal instillation of N-methyl-N'-nitro-N-nitroguanidine in rats. *J Natl Cancer Inst* 53:1093–1097.

Naunyn B (1892) *Klinik der Cholelithiasis*. Leipzig, F C Vogel.

Naus MJ, Jones BR (1978) Cholelithiasis and choledocholithiasis in a cat. *N Z Vet J* 26:160–161.

Neiderhiser DH, Roth HP (1970) Effect of phospholipase A on cholesterol solubilization in a bile salt solution. *Gastroenterology* 58:26–31.

Neiderhiser DH, Roth HP (1972a) The effect of modifications of lecithin and cholesterol on the micellar solubilization of cholesterol. *Biochim Biophys Acta* 270:407–413.

Neiderhiser DH, Roth HP (1972b) Absorption of lecithin by the gallbladder. *Gastroenterology* 62:190 (abstract).

Neiderhiser DH, Roth HP, Webster LT Jr (1966) Studies on the importance of lecithin for cholesterol solubilization in bile. *J Lab Clin Med* 68:90–102.

Neiderhiser DH, Morgenstar WA, Roth HP (1973) Absorption of cholesterol by the gallbladder. *Clin Res* 21: 828.

Neiderhiser DH, Harmon CK, Roth PH (1976) Absorption of cholesterol by the gallbladder. *J Lipid Res* 17:117–124.

Neiderhiser DH, Thornell E, Björck S, Svanvik J (1983) The effect of lysophosphatidylcholine on gallbladder function in the cat. *J Lab Clin Med* 101:699–707.

Neithercut WD (1989) Effect of calcium, magnesium and sodium ions on in vitro nucleation of human gallbladder bile. *Gut* 30:665–670.

Nelson NC, Piker JP, Welsh RR (1968) Cholelithiasis in a dog. *J Am Vet Med Assoc* 152:47–50.

Nelson PE, Moyer TP, Thistle JL (1990) Gallstone dissolution in vitro using methyl tert-butyl ether: radiologic selection criteria. *Gastroenterology* 98:1280–1283.

Nervi FO, Covarrubias CF, Valdivieso VD, Rouco BO, Solari A, Tocornal J (1981) Hepatic cholesterogenesis in Chileans with cholesterol gallstone disease. Evidence for sex differences in the regulation of hepatic cholesterol metabolism. *Gastroenterology* 80:539–545.

Nervi FO, Del Pozo R, Covarrrubias CF, Ronco BO (1983) The effect of progesterone on the regulatory mechanisms of biliary cholesterol secretion in the rat. *Hepatology* 3:360–367.

Nervi F, Bronfman M, Allalon W, Depiereux E, Del Pozo R (1984) Regulation of biliary cholesterol secretion in the rat. Role of hepatic cholesterol esterification. *J Clin Invest* 74:2226–2237.

Nervi F, Marinovic I, Rigotti A, Ulioa N (1988) Regulation of biliary cholesterol secretion. Functional relationship between the canalicular and sinusoidal cholesterol secretory pathways in the rat. *J Clin Invest* 82:1818–1825.

Nervi F, Covarrubias C, Bravo P, Velasco N, Ulloa N, Cruz F, Fava M, Severin C, Del Pozo R, Antezana C, Valdivieso V, Arteaga A (1989) Influence of legume intake on biliary lipids and cholesterol saturation in young Chilean men. Identification of a dietary risk factor for cholesterol gallstone formation in a highly prevalent area. *Gastroenterology* 96:825–830.

Ness GC, Keller RK, Pendleton LC (1991) Feedback regulation of hepatic 3-hydroxy-3-methylglutaryl-CoA reductase activity by dietary cholesterol is not due to altered mRNA levels. *J Biol Chem* 266:14854–14857.

Nestel PJ, Monger EA (1967) Turnover of plasma esterified cholesterol in normocholesterolemic and hypercholesterolic subjects and its relation to body build. *J Clin Invest* 46:967–974.

Nestel PJ, Whyte HM, Goodman DS (1969) Distributon and turnover of cholesterol in humans. *J Clin Invest* 48:982–991.

Nestel PJ, Schreibman PH, Ahrens EH Jr (1973) Cholesterol metabolism in human obesity. *J Clin Invest* 52:2389–2397.

Neubrand M, Sauerbruch T, Stellaard F, Paumgartner G (1986) In vitro cholesterol gallstone dissolution after fragmentation with shock waves. *Digestion* 34:51–59.

Newman DE (1973) Gallstones in children. *Pediatr Radiol* 1:100–104.

Newman HF, Northup JD (1959) The autopsy incidence of gallstones. *Int Abst Surg* 109:1–13.

Nicholas P, Rinaudo PA, Conn HO (1972) Increased incidence of cholelithiasis in Laennec's cirrhosis. A postmortem evaluation of pathogenesis. *Gastroenterology* 63:112–121.

Nichols JW (1988) Phospholipid transfer between phosphatidylcholine-taurocholate mixed micelles. *Biochemistry* 27:3925–3931.

Nicolau G, Shefer S, Salen G, Mosbach EH (1974) Determination of hepatic 3-hydroxy-3-methylglutaryl CoA reductase activity in man. *J Lipid Res* 15:94–98.

Nilsell K, Angelin B, Leijd B, Einarsson K (1983) Comparative effects of ursodeoxycholic acid and chenodeoxycholic acid on bile acid kinetics and biliary lipid secretion in humans. Evidence for different modes of action on bile acid synthesis. *Gastroenterology* 85:1248–1256.

Nilsell K, Angelin B, Liljeqvist L, Einarsson K (1985) Biliary lipid output and bile acid kinetics in cholesterol gallstone disease. Evidence for an increased hepatic secretion of cholesterol in Swedish patients. *Gastroenterology* 89:287–293.

Nilsson S (1966) Gallbladder disease and sex hormones. Statistical study. *Acta Chir Scand* 132:275–279.

Nilsson S, Scherstén T (1969) Importance of bile acids for phospholipid secretion into human hepatic bile. *Gastroenterology* 57:525–532.

Nilsson S, Scherstén T (1970) Influence of bile acids on the synthesis of biliary phospholipids in man. *Eur J Clin Invest* 1:109–111.

Nilsson S, Statin S (1967) Gallbladder emptying during the normal menstrual cycle. A cholecystographic study. *Acta Chir Scand* 133:648–652.

Nimura Y, Shionoya S, Hayakawa N, Kamiya J, Kondo S, Yasui A (1988) Value of percutaneous transhepatic cholangioscopy (PTCS). Surg Endosc 2: 213–219.

Nishimura M (1938) Über die chemische Zusammensetzung der Gallensteine. *J Biochem* 28:265–292.

Niu N, Gourdin T, Smith BF (1989) Calcium ($Ca^{++}$) augments hydrophobic binding properties of bovine gallbladder mucin (BGM). *Gastroenterology* 98: A615 (abstract).

Niu N, Smith BF (1990) Addition of N-acetylcysteine to aqueous model bile systems accelerates dissolution of cholesterol gallstones. *Gastroenterology* 98:454–463.

Nobles ER Jr (1966) Vagotomy and gastroenterostomy: 15-year follow-up of 175 patients. *Am Surg* 32:177–182.

Nomura H, Kashiwagi S, Hayashi J, Kajiyama W, Ikematsu H, Noguchi A, Tani S, Goto M (1988) Prevalence of gallstone disease in a general population in Okinawa, Japan. *Am J Epidemiol* 128:598–605.

Norman A (1954) On conjugation of bile acids in rat. Bile acid and steroids. *Acta Physiol Scand* 32:1–10.

Norrby S, Fagerberg G, Sjödahl R (1986) Decreasing incidence of gallstone disease in a defined Swedish population. *Scand J Gastroenterol* 21:158–162.

Northfield TC, Hofmann AF (1973) Biliary lipid secretion in gallstone patients. Lancet 1:747–748.

Northfield TC, Hofmann AF (1975) Biliary lipid output during three meals and an overnight fast. I. Relationship to bile acid pool size and cholesterol saturation of bile in gallstone and control subjects. *Gut* 16:1–17.

Northfield TC, Kupfer RM, Maudgal DP, Zentlee-Munro PL, Meller ST, Garvie NW, McCready R (1980) Gall-bladder sensitivity to cholecystokinin in patients with gall stones. *Br Med J* 280:143–144.

Norton JJ, Smith LR, Hamper E (1968) Diabetes mellitus and gallstones with special reference to insulin assay. *Am J Gastroenterol* 50:214–220.

Noshiro M, Okuda K (1990) Molecular cloning and sequence analysis of cDNA encoding human cholesterol $7\alpha$-hydroxylase. *FEBS Lett* 268:137–140.

Nürnberg D, Berndt H, Pannwitz H (1989) Familiäre Häufung von Gallensteinen. *Dtsch Med Wochenschr* 114:1059–1063.

Nuutinen H, Abei M, Schwarzendrube J, Kawczak P, Holzbach RT (1992) Biliary $\alpha_1$-acid glycoprotein is higher in cholesterol gallstone patients than in gallstone-free controls. *Hepatology* 16:154A (abstract).

O'Brien TR, Mitchum GD (1970) Cholelithiasis in a cat. *J Am Vet Med Assoc* 156:1015–1017.

Oda H, Yamashita H, Kosahara K, Kuroki S, Nakayama F (1990) Esterified and total $7\alpha$-hydroxycholesterol in human serum as an indicator for hepatic bile acid synthesis. *J Lipid Res* 31:2209–2218.

Odom FC, Oliver DD, Kline M, Rogers W (1976) Gallbaldder disease in patients 20 years of age and under. *Southern Med J* 69:1299–1300.

O'Donnell LDJ, Heaton KW (1988) Recurrence and re-recurrence of gall stones after medical dissolution: a long-term follow-up. *Gut* 29:655–658.

Ohkubo H, Ostrow JD, Carr SH, Rege RV (1984) Polymer networks in pigment and cholesterol gallstones assessed by equilibrium swelling and infrared spectroscopy. *Gastroenterology* 87:805–814.

Ohya F, Schwarzendrube J, Busch N, Gresky S, Chandler K, Takabayashi A, Igimi H, Egami K, Holzbach RT (1993) Isolation of a human biliary glycoprotein inhibitor of cholesterol crystallization. *Gastroenterology* 104:527–538.

Okamoto S, Fukushima K, Higashijima H, Makino I, Kishinaka M, Oda H, Yamashita H, Ichimiya H, Chijiiwa K, Kuroki S (1994) Serum $7\alpha$-hydroxycholesterol reflects hepatic bile acid synthesis in patients with obstructive jaundice after external biliary drainage. *Hepatology* 20:95–100.

Okey R (1942) Gallstone formation and intake of B vitamins in cholesterol-fed guinea pig. *Proc Soc Exp Biol Med* 51:349–350.

Okey R, Greaves VD (1939) Anemia caused by feeding cholesterol to guinea pigs. *J Biol Chem* 129:111–123.

Okido M, Shimizu S, Ostrow JD, Nakayama F (1992) Isolation of a calcium regulatory protein from black pigment gallstones: similarity with a protein from cholesterol gallstones. *Hepatology* 15:1079–1085.

Okido M, Soloway RD, Crowther RS (1993) Inhibition of vaterite ($CaCO_3$) formation by a calcium binding protein from black pigment gallstones. Gastroenterology 104:A968 (abstract).

Okuda K, Nakayama F, Wong J (1984) *Intrahepatic Calculi*. New York, Alan R Liss.

O'Leary DP (1994) Artificial bile inhibits bile salt-induced gallbladder glycoprotein release *in vitro*. *Hepatology* 19:771–774.

O'Leary DP, LaMorte WW, Scott TE, Booker ML, Stevenson J (1991a) Inhibition of prostaglandin synthesis fails to prevent gallbladder mucin hypersecretion in the cholesterol-fed prairie dog. *Gastroenterology* 101:812–820.

O'Leary DP, Murray FE, Turner BS, LaMont JT (1991b) Bile salts stimulate glycoprotein release by guinea pig gallbladder in vitro. *Hepatology* 13:957–961.

Olszewski MF, Holzbach RT, Saupe A, Brown GH (1973) Liquid crystals in human bile. *Nature* 242:336–337.

Ong GB (1962) A study of recurrent pyogenic cholangitis. *Arch Surg* 84:199–225.

Ong GB (1979) Helminthic disease of the liver and biliary tract. In Wright R, Alberti KGMM, Karran S, Millward-Sadler GH (eds): Liver and Biliary Disease. Pathophysiology, Diagnosis, Management. London, W B Saunders, pp 1267–1303.

Onodera H, Sugawara H, Hirata T, Imai N, Nagasaki A, Yoda B, Toyota T, Goto Y (1983) Diurnal profile of gallbladder size in diabetic patients: ultrasonographic evaluation of diabetic neurogenic gallbladder. *Tohoku J Exp Med*

139:179–186.

Onuigbo WIB (1977) A biopsy study of gallstones in Nigerian Igbos. *Digestion* 15:353–355.

Orii K, Ozaki A, Takase Y (1983) Lithotomy of intrahepatic and choledochal stones with Yag laser. *Surg Gynecol Obstet* 156:485–488.

Osborne TF, Gill G, Brown MS, Kowal RC, Goldstein JL (1987) Identification of promotor elements required for in vitro transcription of hamster 3-hydroxy-3-methylglutaryl coenzyme A reductase gene. *Proc Natl Acad Sci USA* 84:3614–3618.

Osnes M, Løtveit T, Larsen S, Aune S (1981) Duodenal diverticula and their relationship to age, sex and biliary calculi. *Scand J Gastroenterol* 16:103–107.

Ostrow JD (1967) Absorption of bile pigments by the gall bladder. *Clin Invest* 46:2035–2052.

Ostrow JD (1969) Absorption by the gallbladder of bile salts, sulfobromophthalein and iodipamide. *J Lab Clin Med* 74:482–494.

Ostrow JD (1971) Absorption of organic compounds by the injured gallbladder. *J Lab Clin Med* 78:255–264.

Ostrow JD (1984) The etiology of pigment gallstones. *Hepatology* 4(Suppl):215S–222S.

Ostrow JD (1990) Unconjugated bilirubin and cholesterol gallstone formation. *Hepatology* 12(Suppl):219S–226S.

Ostrow JD, Murphy NH (1970) Isolation and properties of conjugated bilirubin from bile. *Biochem* J 120:311–327.

Ostrow JD, Celic L, Mukerjee P (1988) Molecular and micellar associations in the pH-dependent stable and metastable dissolution of unconjugated bilirubin by bile salts. *J Lipid Res* 29:335–348.

Ostrow JD, Mukerjee P, Tiribelli C (1994) Structure and binding of unconjugated bilirubin: relevence for physiological and pathophysiological function. *J Lipid Res* 35:1715–1737.

Osuga T, Portman OW (1971) Experimental formation of gallstones in the squirrel monkey. *Proc Soc Exp Biol Med* 136:722–726.

Osuga T, Portman OW (1972) Relationship between bile composition and gallstone formation in the squirrel monkeys. *Gastroenterology* 63:122–133.

Osuga T, Portman OW, Mitamura K, Alexander M (1974) A morphologic study of gallstone development in the squirrel monkey. *Lab Invest* 30:486–493.

Osuga T, Portman OW, Tanaka N, Alexander M, Ochsner J III (1976) The effect of diet on hepatic bile formation and bile acid metabolism in squirrel monkeys with and without cholesterol gallstones. *J Lab Clin Med* 88:649–661.

Owor R (1964) Gallstones in the autopsy population at Mulago hospital, Kampala. *East Afr Med* J 41:251–253.

Owor R (1971) Study of gallstones in Ugandan Africans. *East Afr Med J* 48:193–195.

Oyabu H, Tabata M, Nakayama F (1987) Nonbacterial transformation of bilirubin in bile. *Dig Dis Sci* 32:809–816.

Palmer RH (1965) Gallstones produced experimentally by lithocholic acid in rats. *Science* 148:1339–1340.

Palmer RH 1972) Bile acids, liver injury, and liver disease. *Arch Int Med* 130:606–617.

Palmer RH, Hruban Z (1966) Production of bile duct hyperplasia and gallstones by lithocholic acid. *J Clin Invest* 45:1255–1267.

Pandak WM, Li YC, Chiang YL, Studer EJ, Gurley EC, Heuman DM, Vlahcevic ZR, Hylemon PB (1991) Regulation of cholesterol $7\alpha$-hydroxylase mRNA and transcriptional activity by taurocholate and cholesterol in the chronic biliary diverted rat. *J Biol Chem* 266:3416–3421.

Pandak WM, Vlahcevic ZR, Chiang JYL, Heuman DM, Hylemon PB (1992) Bile acid synthesis. VI. Regulation of cholesterol $7\alpha$-hydroxylase by taurocholate and mevalonate. *J Lipid Res* 33:659–668.

Papasteriades C, Al-Mahmoud I, Papageorgakis N, Romania S, Katsas A, Ollier W, Economidou I (1990) HLA antigens in Greek patients with cholelithiasis. *Dis Markers* 8:17–21.

Park YH, Igimi H, Carey MC (1984) Dissolution of human cholesterol gallstones in simulated chenodeoxycholate-rich and ursodeoxycholate-rich biles. An in vitro study of dissolution rates and mechanisms. *Gastroenterology* 87:150–158.

Parkin GJS, Smith RB, Johnston D (1973) Gallbladder volume and contractility after truncal, selective, and highly selective (parietal-cell) vagotomy in man. *Ann Surg* 178:581–586.

Parnis RO (1964) Gall bladder disease in Nigeria. A five-year review. *Trans R Soc Trop Med* 58:437–440.

Pastides H, Tzonou A, Tichopoulos D, Katsouyanni K, Trichopoulou A, Kefalogiannis N, Manousos O (1990) A case-control study of the relationship between smoking, diet, and gallbladder disease. *Arch Intern Med* 150:1409–1412.

Pathak RK, Yokode M, Hammer RE, Hofmann SL, Brown MS, Goldstein JL, Anderson RGW (1990) Tissue-specific sorting of the human LDL receptor in polarized epithelia of transgenic mice. *J Cell Biol* 111:347–359.

Pattinson NR (1985) Solubilization of cholesterol in human bile. *FEBS Lett* 181:339–342.

Pattinson NR (1988) Identification of a phosphatidylcholine active phospholipase C in human gallbladder bile. *Biochem Biophys Res Commun* 150:890–896.

Pattinson NR, Chapman BA (1986) Distribution of biliary cholesterol between mixed micelles and nonmicelles in relation to fasting and feeding in humans. *Gastroenterology* 91:697–702.

Pattinson NR, Willis KE (1990) Phospholipase C and diacylglycerol lipase in human gallbladder and hepatic bile. *Gastroenterology* 99:1798–1806.

Pattinson NR, Willis KE (1991a) Nucleation of cholesterol crystals from native bile and the effect of protein hydrolysis. *J Lipid Res* 32:215–221.

Pattinson NR, Willis KE (1991b) Efffect of phospholipase C on cholesterol solubilization in model bile. A concanavalin A-binding nucleation-promoting factor from human gallbladder bile. *Gastroenterology* 101:1339–1344.

Pattinson NR, Willis KE, Frampton CM (1991) Comparative analysis of cholesterol transport in bile from patients with and without cholesterol gallstones. *J Lipid Res* 32:205–214.

Patton DE, Plotner K, Cox GE, Taylor CB (1961) Biliary cholesterol deposits in ground squirrels and prairie dogs. *Fed Proc* 20:248 (abstract)

Patton GM, Fasulo JM, Robins SJ (1994) Hepatic phosphatidylcholines: evidence for synthesis in the rat by extensive reutilization of endogenous acylglycerides. *J Lipid Res* 35:1211–1221.

Paul O, Lepper MJ, Phelan WH, Dupertuis GW, MacMillan A, McKean H, Park H (1983) A longitudinal study of coronary heart disease. *Circulation* 28:20–31.

Pauletzki J, Sailer C, Klüppelberg U, Ritter CV, Neubrand M, Holl J, Sauerbruch T, Sackmann M, Paumgartner G (1994) Gallbladder emptying determines early gallstone clearance after shock-wave lithotripsy. *Gastroenterology* 107:1496–1502.

Pausawasdi A, Pausawasdi S, Mahaweero W (1979) Clinical study of gallstones in Thai patients. *J Med Assoc Thailand* 62:227–234.

Peled Y, Halpern Z, Baruch R, Goldman G, Gilat T (1988) Cholesterol nucleation from its carriers in human bile. *Hepatology* 8:914–918.

Pellerin D, Bertin P, Nihoul-Fekete C, Ricour C (1975) Cholelithiasis and ileal pathology in childhood. *J Pediatr Surg* 10:35–41.

Pemsingh RS, MacPharson BR, Scott GW (1987) Mucus hypersecretion in the gallbladder epithelium of ground squirrels fed a lithogenic diet for the induction of cholesterol gallstones. *Hepatology* 7:1267–1271.

Peric-Golia L, Jones RS (1962) Ornithocholanic acids – abnormal conjugates of bile acids. *Proc Soc Exp. Biol Med* 110:327–331.

Peric-Golia L, Jones RS (1963) Ornithocholanic acids and cholelithiasis in man. *Science* 142:245–246.

Percy-Robb IW, Jalan KN, McManus JPA, Sircus W (1971) Effect of ileal resection on bile salt metabolism in patients with ileostomy following proctocolectomy. *Clin Sci* 41:371–382.

Perrine RP (1973) Cholelithiasis in sickle cell anemia in a Caucasian population. *Am J Med* 54:327-332.

Pertsemlidis D, Panveliwalla D, Ahrens EH Jr (1974) Effects of clofibrate and of an estrogen-progestin combination on fasting biliary lipids and cholic acid kinetics in man. *Gastroenterology* 66:565–573.

Peters JH, Ellison EC, Innes JT, Liss JL, Nichols KE, Lomano JM, Roby SR. Front ME, Carey LC (1991) Safety and efficacy of laparoscopic cholecystectomy. A prospective analysis of 100 initial patients. *Ann Surg* 213:3–12.

Petersen SR, Sheldon GF (1979) Acute acalculous cholecystitis: a complication of hyperalimentation. *Am J Surg* 138:814–817.

Petersen BT, Segura JW, Thistle JL (1988) Gallstone lithotripsy: in vitro comparison of four different shock wave generators. Gastroenterology 96:A581 (abstract)

Petitti DB, Friedman GD, Klatsky AL (1981) Association of a history of gallbladder disease with a reduced concentration of high-density-lipoprotein cholesterol. *N Engl J Med* 304:1396–1398.

Petitti DB, Sidney S, Perlman JA (1988) Increased risk of cholecystectomy in users of supplemental estrogen. *Gastroenterology* 94:91–95.

Phemister DB, Rewbridge AG, Rudisill H Jr (1931) Calcium carbonate gallstones and calcification of the gallbladder following cystic duct obstruction. *Ann Surg* 94:493–516.

Phemister DB, Day L, Hastings AB (1932) Calcium carbonate gall-stones and their experimental production. *Ann Surg* 96:595–614.

Phemister DB, Aronsohn HG, Pepinsky R (1939) Variation in the cholesterol, bile pigment and calcium salt contents of gallstones formed in gallbladder and in bile ducts with the degree of associated obstruction. *Ann Surg* 109:161–186.

Philips GB (1960) The lipid composition of human bile. *Biochim Biophys Acta* 41:361–363.

Phillips MC (1990) Cholesterol packing, crystallization and exchange properties in phosphatidylcholine vesicle systems. *Hepatology* 12(Suppl):75S–82S.

Phinney PR, Austin GE, Kadell BM (198l) Cholangiocarcinoma arising in Caroli's disease. *Arch Pathol Lab Med* 105:194–197.

Piehler JM, Crichlow RW (1978) Primary carcinoma of the gallbladder. *Surg Gynecol Obstet* 147:929–942.

Pitchumoni CS, Viswanathan KV, Moore EW (1987) Analysis and localization of elements in human cholesterol gallstones: calcium and other elements are present in the central (nidus) region. *Gastroenterology* 92:1764 (abstract)

Pitt HA, Roslyn JJ, Kuchenbecker SL, Doty JE, DenBesten L (1981) The role of cystic duct resistance in the pathogenesis of cholesterol gallstones. *J Surg Res* 30:508–514.

Pitt HA, Berquist WE, Mann LL, Porter-Fink V, Fonkalsrud EW, Ament ME, DenBesten L (1983a) Parenteral nutrition induces calcium bilirubinate gallstones. *Gastroenterology* 84:1274 (abstract)

Pitt HA, King W III, Mann LL , Roslyn JJ, Berqvist WE, Ament ME, DenBesten L (1983b) Increased risk of cholelithiasis with prolonged total parenteral nutrition. *Am J Surg* 145:106–112.

Pitt HA, Lewinski MA, Muller EL, Porter-Fink V, DenBesten L (1984) Ileal resection-induced gallstones: altered bilirubin or cholesterol metabolism? *Surgery* 96:154–162.

Pixley F, Mann J (1988) Dietary factors in the aetiology of gall stones: a case control study. *Gut* 29:1511–1515.

Pixley F, Wilson D, McPherson K, Mann J (1985) Effect of vegetarianism on development of gall stones in women. *Br Med* J 291:11–12.

Pomare EW, Heaton KW (1973a) Bile salt metabolism in patients with gallstones in functioning gallbladders. *Gut* 14:885–890.

Pomare EW, Heaton KW (1973b) The effect of cholecystectomy on bile salt metabolism. *Gut* 14:753–762.

Pomare EW, Low-Beer TS (1975) The selective inhibition of chenodeoxycholate synthesis by cholate metabolites in man. *Clin Sci* 48:315–321.

Pomare EW, Heaton KW, Low-Beer TS, Espiner HJ (1976) The effect of wheat bran upon bile salt metabolism and upon lipid composition of bile in gallstone patients. *Am J Dig Dis* 21:521–526.

Pomeranz IS, Shaffer EA (1985) Abnormal gallbladder emptying in a subgroup of patients with gallstones. *Gastroenterology* 88:787–791.

Pomeranz IS, Davison JS, Shaffer EA (1986) The effects of prosthetic gallstones on gallbladder function and bile composition. *J Surg Res* 41:47–52.

Ponchon T, Martin X, Barkun A, Mestas JL, Chavaillon A, Boustiere C (1990) Extracorporeal lithotripsy of bile duct stones using ultrasonography for stone localization. *Gastroenterology* 98:726–732.

Ponchon T, Gagnon P, Valette PJ, Henry L, Chavaillon A, Thieulin F (1991) Pulsed dye laser lithotripsy of bile duct stones. *Gastroenterology* 100:1730–1736.

Portman OW, Osuga T (1975) Biliary lipids and cholesterol gallstone formation. *Adv Lipid Res* 13:136–194.

Portman OW, Alexander M, Tanaka N, Osuga T (1980) Relationships between cholesterol gallstones, biliary function and plasma lipoproteins in squirrel monkeys. *J Lab Clin Med* 96:90–101.

Poston GJ, Draviam EJ, Yao CZ, Townsend CM, Thompson JC (1990) Effect of age and sensitivity to cholecystokinin on gallstone formation in the guinea pig. *Gastroenterology* 98:993–999.

Potter MG (1936) Observations of the gallbladder and bile during pregnancy at term. *J A M A* 106:1070–1074.

Praderi RC (1982) One hundred years of biliary surgery. *Surg Gastroenterol* 1:269–287.

Prange I, Christensen F, Dam H (1962) Alimentary production of gallstones in hamsters. II. Relation between diet and composition of the bladder bile. *Z Ernährungswiss* 3:59–78.

Quigley EMM, Marsh MN, Shaffer JL, Markin RS (1993) Hepatobiliary complications of total parenteral nutrition. *Gastroenterology* 104:286–301.

Qureshi A, Browne A, Leahy A, Courtney G, Grace P, Osborne H, Bouchier-Hayes D (1993a) The use of ERCP in patients having laparoscopic cholecystectomy (LC). *Gastroenterology* 104:A376 (abstract).

Qureshi A, Sheehan S, Burke P, Leahy A, Grace P, Broe P, Lane B, Lynch G, Deasy J, Osborne H, Bouchier-Hayes D (1993b) Laparoscopic cholecystectomy and the acute gallbladder. Gastroenterology 104:A377 (abstract).

Rådberg G, Svanvik J (1986) Influence of pregnancy, oophorectomy and contraceptive steroids on gallbladder concentrating function and hepatic bile flow in the cat. *Gut* 27:10–14.

Rådberg G, Jivegard L, Friman S, Zettergren L, Svanvik J (1988) Relationship between gallbladder histopathology and ability to concentrate biliary lipids and bilirubin. A study on gallstone patients with functioning gallbladder. *Acta Chir Scand* 154:581–584.

Rådberg G, Friman S, Svanvik J (1989) The influence of pregnancy and contraceptive steroids on the biliary tract and its reference to cholesterol gallstone formation. *Scand J Gastroenterol* 25:97–102.

Rains AJH (1964) *Gallstones. Cause and Treatment*. London, W Heinemann Medical Books.

Rajagopalan N, Lindenbaum S (1982) The binding of $Ca^{2+}$ to taurine- and glycine-conjugated bile salt micelles. *Biochim Biophys Acta* 711:66–74.

Rajagopalan SU, Keightley A, Bills P, Walters JPF, Murphy GM, Dowling RH (1989) Predictive value of pre-treatment CT scanning vs. conventional radiology in determining composition, dissolvability and fragmentability of gallbladder stones (GBS). *J Hepatol* 9:S211 (abstract).

Ratner J, Lisbona A, Rosenbloom M, Palayew M, Szabolcsi S, Tupaz T (1991) The prevalence of gallstone disease in very old institutionalized persons. *JAMA* 265:902–903.

Ravussin E, Lillioja S, Knowler WC, Christin L, Freymond D, Abbott WGH, Boyce V, Howard BV, Bogardus C (1988) Reduced rate of energy expenditure as a factor for body-weight gain. *N Engl J Med* 318:467–472.

Reddy BS, Watanabe K (1979) Effect of cancer metabolites and promoting effect of lithocholic acid in colon carcinogenesis in germ-free and conventional F344 rats. *Cancer Res* 39:1521–1524.

Reddy BS, Wynder EL (1977) Metabolic epidemiology of colon cancer. Fecal bile acids and neutral sterols in colon cancer patients and patients with adenomatous polyps. *Cancer* 39:2533–2539.

Reddy BS, Narisawa T, Weisburger JH, Wynder EL (1976) Promoting effect of sodium deoxycholate on colonic adenocarcinoma in germ-free rats. *J Natl Cancer Inst* 56:441–442.

Redinger RN, Small DM (1972) Bile composition, bile salt metabolism and gallstones. *Arch Intern Med* 130:618–630.

Redinger RN, Herman AH, Small DM (1971) Effect of diet on bile composition in the rhesus monkey. *Gastroenterology* 60:A198 (abstract).

Rege RV, Moore EW (1986) Pathogenesis of calcium-containing gallstones. Canine ductular bile, but not gallbladder bile, is supersaturated with calcium carbonate. *J Clin Invest* 77:21–26.

Rege RV, Moore EW (1987) Evidence for $H^+$ secretion by the in vivo canine gallbladder. *Gastroenterology* 92:281–289.

Rege RV, Nahrwold DL (1987) Animal models of pigment gallstone disease. *J Surg Res* 43:196–203.

Rege RV, Nahrwold DL, Moore EW (1987) Absorption of biliary calcium from the canine gallbladder: protection against the formation of calcium-containing gallstones. *J Lab Clin Med* 110:381–386.

Rege RV, Dawes LG, Moore EW (1989) Canine common duct and gallbladder bile contain antinucleating factors that inhibit CaCO3 precipitation. *J Lab Clin Med* 113:642–650.

Reichenbach DD (1967) Autopsy incidence of diseases among Southwestern American Indians. *Arch Pathol* 84:81–86.

Reihnér E, Björkhem I, Angelin B, Ewerth S, Einarsson K (1989) Bile acid synthesis in humans: Regulation of hepatic microsomal cholesterol 7$\alpha$-hydroxylase activity. *Gastroenterology* 97:1498–1505.

Reihnér E, Angelin B, Rudling M, Ewerth S, Björkhem I, Einarsson K (1990a) Regulation of hepatic cholesterol metabolism in humans – stimulatory effects of cholestyramine on HMG-CoA reductase activity and low density lipoprotein receptor expression in gallstone patients. *J Lipid Res* 31:2219–2226.

Reihnér E, Rudling M, Ståhlberg D, Berglund L, Ewerth S, Björkhem I, Einarsson K, Angelin B (1990b) Influence of pravastatin, a specific inhibitor of HMG-CoA reductase, on hepatic metabolism of cholesterol. *N Engl J Med* 323:224–228.

Reihnér E, Angelin B, Björkhem I, Einarsson K (1991) Hepatic cholesterol metabolism in gallstone disease. *J Lipid Res* 32:469–475.

Rennels MB, Dunne MG, Grossman NJ, Schwartz AD (1984) Cholelithiasis in patients with major sickle hemoglobinopathies. *Am J Dis Child* 138:66–67.

Renshaw PF, Janoff AS, Miller KW (1983) On the nature of dilute aqueous cholesterol suspensions. *J Lipid Res* 24:47–51.

Reuben A, Dowling RH (1978) Does obesity complicate chenodeoxycholic acid (CDCA) treatment of gallstones? *Gut* 19:A452 (abstract).

Rewbridge AG (1937) The disappearance of gallstone shadows following the prolonged administration of bile salts. *Surgery* 1:395–400.

Riegel C, Ravdin IS, Johnston CG (1931) Studies of gallbladder function. VI. The absorption of bile salts and cholesterol from the bile-free gallbladder. *Am J Physiol* 99:656–665.

Riegel C, Johnston CG, Ravdin IS (1932) Studies of gallbladder function. VIII. The fate of bile pigment and cholesterol in hepatic bile subjected to gallbladder activity. *J Exp Med* 56:1–11.

Riemann JF, Seuberth K, Demling L (1982) Clinical application of a new mechanical lithotripter for smashing common duct stones. *Endoscopy* 14:226–230.

Rigotti A, Nunez L, Amigo L, Puglielli L, Garrido J, Santos M, Gonzalez S, Mingrone G, Greco A, Nervi F (1993) Biliary lipid secretion: immunolocalization and identification of a protein associated with lamellar cholesterol carriers in supersaturated rat and human bile. *J Lipid Res* 34:1883–1894.

Rinaldo JA, Baltz JI (1957) Familial cholelithiasis with special reference to its relation to familial pancreatitis. *Am J Med* 23:880–885.

Ringsted J (1963) A Korean autospy material. *Dan Med Bull* 10:90–96.

Robertson HE (1945) The preponderance of gallstones in women. An etiological study. *Int Abst Surg* 80:1–23.

Robertson HE, Dochat GR (1944) Pregnancy and gallstones: collective review. *Int Abst Surg* 78:193–204.

Robins SJ, Armstrong MJ (1976) Biliary lecithin secretion. II. Effects of dietary choline and biliary lecithin synthesis. *Gastroenterology* 70:397–402.

Robins SJ, Brunengraber H (1982) Origin of biliary cholesterol and lecithin in the rat: contribution of new synthesis and preformed hepatic stores. *J Lipid Res* 23:604–608.

Robins SJ, Fasulo JM, Patton GM (1982) Lipids of pigment gallstones. *Biochim Biophys Acta* 712:21–25.

Robins SJ, Fasulo JM, Lessard PD, Patton GM (1993a) Hepatic cholesterol synthesis and the secretion of newly synthesized cholesterol in bile. *Biochem J* 289:41–44.

Robins SJ, Fasulo JM, Lessard PD, Patton GM (1993b) Changes in biliary lipid secretion during normal development and diurnal cycling in the rat. *J Lipid Res* 34:1445–1450.

Robins SJ, Fasulo JM, Collins MA, Patton GM (1985) Evidence for separate pathways of transport of newly synthesized and preformed cholesterol into bile. *J Biol Chem* 260:6511–6513.

Roda E, Bazzoli F, Labata AMM, Mazzella G, Roda A, Sama C, Festi D, Aldini R, Taroni F, Barbara L (1982) Ursodeoxycholic acid vs. chenodeoxycholic acid as cholesterol gallstone-dissolving agents: a comparative randomized study. *Hepatology* 2:804–810.

Rogers L (1925) Quoted by Malhotra (1968).

Rolleston H, McNee JW (1929) *Diseases of the Liver, Gallbladder and Bile Ducts*. London, Macmillan

Rome Group for Epidemiology and Prevention of cholelithiasis (GREPCO) (1984) Prevalence of gallstone disease in an Italian adult female population. *Am J Epidemiol* 119:796–805.

Rome Group for Epidemiology and Prevention of Cholelithiasis (GREPCO) (1987) Radiologic appearance of gallstones and its relationship with biliary symptoms and awareness of having gallstones. Observations during epidemiological studies. *Dig Dis Sci* 32:349–353.

Rome Group for Epidemiology and Prevention of Cholelithiasis (GREPCO) (1988a) The epidemiology of gallstone disease in Rome, Italy. Part I. Prevalence data in men. *Hepatology* 8:904–906.

Rome Group for Epidemiology and Prevention of Cholelithiasis (GREPCO) (1988b) The epidemiology of gallstone disease in Rome, Italy. Part II. Factors associated with the disease. *Hepatology* 8:907–913.

Ros E, Navarro S, Bru C, Gilabert R, Bianchi L, Bruguera M (1993) Ursodeoxycholic acid treatment of primary hepatolithiasis in Caroli's syndrome. *Lancet* 342:404–406.

Roslyn JJ, DenBesten L, Thompson JE (1979) Effects of periodic emptying of the gallbladder on gallbladder function and formation of cholesterol gallstone. *Surg Forum* 30:403–404.

Roslyn JJ, DenBesten L, Thompson JE, Cohen K (1980) Chronic cholelithiasis and cholesterol bile salt pool size. Cause or effect? *Am J Surg* 139:119–124.

Roslyn JJ, DenBesten L, Pitt HA, Kuchenbecker S, Polarek JW (1981a) Effects of cholecystokinin on gallbladder stasis and cholesterol gallstone formation. *J Surg Res* 30:200–204.

Roslyn JJ, Pitt HA, Mann LL, Ament ME, DenBesten L (1981b) Long-term total parenteral nutrition induces gallbladder disease. *Gastroenterology* 80:1264 (abstract)

Roslyn JJ, Berquist WE, Pitt HA, Mann LL, Kangarloo H, DenBesten L, Ament M E (1983a) Increased risk of gallstones in children receiving total parenteral nutrition. *Pediatrics* 71:784–789.

Roslyn JJ, Pitt HA, Mann LL, Ament ME, DenBesten L (1983b) Gallbladder disease in patients on long-term parenteral nutrition. *Gastroenterology* 84:148–154.

Roslyn JJ, Conter RL, DenBesten L (1987a) Altered gallbladder concentration of biliary lipids during early cholesterol gallstone formation. *Dig Dis Sci* 32:609–614.

Roslyn JJ, Conter RL, Julian E, Abedin MZ (1987b) The role of dietary iron in pigment gallstone formation. *Surgery* 102:327–333.

Roslyn JL, Abedin MZ, Strichartz SD, Abdou MS, Palant CE (1989) Regulation of gallbladder ion transport: role of biliary lipids. Surgery 105:207–212.

Roy CC, Weber AM, Morin CL Combes JC, Nusslé D, Mégevand A, Lasalle R (1977) Abnormal biliary lipid composition in cystic fibrosis. Effect of pancreatic enzymes. *N Engl J Med* 297:1301–1305.

Royal College of General Practitioners' Oral Contraceptive Study (1982) Oral contraceptives and gallbladder disease. *Lancet* 2:957–959.

Ruch TC (1959) *Diseases of Laboratory Primates*. Philadelphia, WB Saunders.

Rudel L, Deckelman C, Wilson M, Scobey M, Anderson R (1994) Dietary cholesterol and downregulation of cholesterol 7$\alpha$-hydroxylase and cholesterol absorption in African green monkeys. *J Clin Invest* 93:2463–2472.

Rudick J, Hutchison JSF (1965) Evaluation of vagotomy and biliary function by combined oral cholecystography and intravenous cholangiography. *Ann Surg* 162:234–240.

Ruetz S, Fricker G, Hugantobler G, Winterhalter K, Kurz G, Meier PJ (1987) Isolation and characterization of the putative canalicular bile salt transport system of rat liver. *J Biol Chem* 262:11324–11330.

Russell PW, Brown CH (1950) Primary carcinoma of gallbladder. Report of 29 cases. *Ann Surg* 132:121–128.

Russel DW, Setchell KDR (1992) Bile acid biosynthesis. *Biochemistry* 31:4737–4749.

Sackmann M, Delius M, Sauerbruch T, Holl J, Weber W, Ippisch E, Hagelauer U, Wess O, Hepp W, Brendel W, Paumgartner G (1988) Shock-wave lithotripsy of gallbladder stones. The first 175 patients. *N Engl J Med* 318:393–397.

Sackmann M, Ippisch E, Sauerbruch T, Holl J, Brendel W, Paumgartner G (1990) Early gallstone recurrence rate after successful shock-wave therapy. *Gastroenterology* 98:392–396.

Sackmann M, Pauletzki J, Sauerbruch T. Holl J, Schelling G, Paumgartner G (1991) The Munich gallbladder lithotripsy study. Results of the first 5 years with 711 patients. *Ann Intern Med* 114:290–296.

Sackmann M, Pauletzki J, Delius M, Holl J, Neubrand M, Sauerbruch T, Paumgartner G (1992) Noninvasive therapy of gallbladder calculi with a radiopaque rim. *Gastroenterology* 102:988–993.

Sackmann M, Niller H, Klüppelberg U, Von Ritter C, Pauletzki J, Holl J, Berr F, Neubrand M, Sauerbruch T, Paumgartner G (1994) Gallstone recurrence after shock-wave therapy. *Gastroenterology* 106:225–230.

Sacquet E, Parquet M, Riottot M, Raizman A, Jarrige P, Huguet C, Infante R (1983) Intestinal absorption, excretion, and biotransformation of hyodeoxycholic acid in man. *J Lipid Res* 24:604–613.

Sahlin S, Danielsson Å, Angelin B, Reihnér E, Henriksson R, Einarsson K (1988) Mucin in gall bladder bile of gall stone patients: influence of treatment with chenodeoxycholic acid and ursodeoxycholic acid. *Gut* 29:1506–1510.

Sahlin S, Ahlberg J, Einarsson K, Henriksson R, Danielsson Å (1990) Quantitative ultrastructural studies of gall bladder epithelium in gall stone free subjects and patients with gall stones. *Gut* 31:100–105.

Sahlin S, Ahlberg J, Reihnér E, Ståhlberg D, Einarsson K (1992) Cholesterol metabolism in human gallbladder mucosa: Relationship to cholesterol gallstone disease and effects of chenodeoxycholic acid and ursodeoxycholic acid treatment. *Hepatology* 16:320–326

Sahlin S, Granström U, Gustafsson U, Ståhlberg D, Backman L, Einarsson K (1994) Hepatic esterification rate of cholesterol and biliary lipids in human obesity. *J Lipid Res* 35:484–490.

Saisho H, Sodeki H, Tsuyuguchi T, Yamaguchi T, Ohto M (1990) Peroral cholangioscopic lithotripsy for intrahepatic calculi. *Tan to Sui (J Biliary Tract Pancreas)* ll:825–830. (In Japanese)

Sakata R, Aoki T, Minetoma T, Kimura Y, Torimura T, Inuzuka S, Ueno T, Sata M, Tanikawa K (1993) Morphological observation on extrahepatic bile duct of golden hamsters fed with a lithogenic diet: histochemical, ultrastructural and cell kinetic studies. *Gastroenterology* 104:A377 (abstract).

Salen G, Nicolau G, Shefer S, Mosbach EH (1975) Hepatic cholesterol metabolism in patients with gallstones. *Gastroenterology* 69:676–684.

Salen G, Colalillo A, Verga D, Bagan E, Tint GS, Shefer S (1980) Effect of high and low doses of ursodeoxycholic acid on gallstone dissolution in humans. *Gastroenterology* 78:1412–1418.

Salisbury CG (1947) Incidence of certain diseases among the Navajos. *Arizona Med* 4:29–31.

Salky BA, Bauer JJ, Kreel I, Gelernt IM, Gorfine SR (1991) Laparoscopic cholecystectomy: an initial report. *Gastrointest Endosc* 37:1–4.

Salvioli G, Salati R, Bondi K, Fratalocchi A, Sala BM, Gibertini A (1982) Bile acid transformation by the intestinal flora and cholesterol saturation in bile. Effects of *Streptococcus faecium* administration. *Digestion* 23:80–88.

Salvioli G, Igimi H, Carey MC (1983) Cholesterol gallstone dissolution in bile. Dissolution kinetics of crystalline cholesterol monohydrate by conjugated chenodeoxycholate-lecithin and conjugated ursodeoxycholate-lecithin mixtures: dissimilar phase equilibria and dissolution mechanisms. *J Lipid Res* 24:701–720.

Salvioli G, Romani M, Loria P, Caruli N, Pradelli JM (1985) Effect of acute administration of bile acids on fatty acid composition of biliary phosphatidylcholine in man. *J Hepatol* 1:291–300.

Sampliner RE, Bennett PH, Comess LJ, Rose FA, Burch TA (1970) Gallbladder disease in Pima Indians. Demonstration of high prevalence and early onset by cholecystography. *N Engl J Med* 283:1358–1364.

Sanchez NM, Esquivel MU (1991) Mucolytic agents and cholesterol gallstones. *Gastroenterology* 100:581.

Sandler RS (1993) Cholecystectomy and colorectal cancer. *Gastroenterology* 105:286–288.

Sandstad O, Osnes T, Skar V, Urdal P, Osnes M (1994) Common bile duct stones are mainly brown and associated with duodenal diverticula. *Gut* 35:1464–1467.

Sanghvi A, Grassi E, Warty V, Diven W, Wight C, Lester R ( 1981) Reversible activation-inactivation of cholesterol $7\alpha$–hydroxylase possibly due to phosphorylation-dephosphorylation. *Biochem Biophys Res Commun* 103:886–892.

Sanjo T (1970) Biochemical and histochemical study on fatty acid-calcium gallstones. *Tohoku J Exp Med* 101:237–249.

Sapala MA, Sapala JA, Resto Soto AD, Bouwman DL (1979) Cholelithiasis following subtotal gastric resection with truncal vagotomy. *Surg Gynecol Obstet* 148:36–38.

Sarin SK, Kapur BML, Tandon RK (1986) Cholesterol and pigment gallstones in northern India: a prospective analysis. *Dig Dis Sci* 31:1041–1045.

Sarles H, Chabert C, Pommeau Y (1969) Diet and cholesterol gallstones. A study of 101 patients with cholelithiasis compared to 101 matched controls. *Am J Dig Dis* 14:531–537.

Sarles H, Hauton J, Planche NE, Lafont H, Gerolami A (1970) Diet, cholesterol gallstones and composition of the bile. *Am J Dig Dis* 15:251–260.

Sarles H, Crotte C, Gerolami A, Mule A, Domingo N, Hauton J (1971) The influence of calorie intake and of dietary protein on the bile lipids. *Scand J Gastroenterol* 6:189–191.

Sarles H, Gerolami A, Cros RC (1978) Diet and cholesterol gallstones. A multicenter study. *Digestion* 17:121–127.

Sarnaik S, Slovis TL, Corbett DP, Emami A, Whitten CF (1980) Incidence of cholelithiasis in sickle cell anemia using the ultrasonic gray-scale technique. *J Pediatr* 96:1005–1008.

Sastry M R (1945) A case of biliary disease in a horse. *Ind Vet J* 21:350–353.

Sauerbruch T, Delius M, Paumgartner G, Holl J, Wess O, Weber W, Hepp W, Brendel W (1986) Fragmentation of gallstones by extracorporeal shock waves. *N Engl J Med* 314:818–822.

Sauerbruch T, Stern M, The Study Group for Shock-Wave Lithotripsy of Bile Duct Stones (1989) Fragmentation of bile duct stones by extracorporeal shock-waves. A new approach to biliary calculi after failure of routine endoscopic measures. *Gastroenterology* 96:146–152.

Saunders DR, Hedge JR, Sillery J, Matsumura EK, Rubin CE (1975) Morphological and functional effects of bile salts on rat colon. *Gastroenterology* 68:1236–1245.

Schall WD, Chapman WL Jr, Finco DR, Greiner TP, Mather GW, Rosin E, Welser JR (1973) Cholelithiasis in dogs. *J Am Vet Med Ass* 163:469–472.

Schattenkerk ME, Li AKC, Jeppsson BW, Eggink WF, Jamieson CG, Ross JS, Malt RA (1980) Chloecystectomy has no influence on frequency of chemically induced colonic cancer in mice. *Br J Cancer* 42:791–793.

Scheibner J, Fuchs M, Hörmann E, Tauber G, Stange E (1994) Biliary cholesterol secretion and bile acid formation in the hamster: the role of newly synthesized cholesterol. J Lipid Res 35: 690–697.

Schein CJ, Gliedman ML (1970) The influence of vagotomy on the normal and diseased gallbladder. *Digestion* 3:243–250.

Schmassmann A, Fehr HF, Locher J, Lillienau J, Schteingart CD, Rossi SS, Hofmann AF (1993) Cholylsarcosine, a new bile acid analogue: metabolism and effect on biliary secretion in humans. *Gastroenterology* 104:1171–1181.

Schmid R (1978) Bilirubin metabolism: state of the art. *Gastroenterology* 74:1307–1312.

Schmidt JH, Hocking MP, Rout WR, Woodward ER (1988) The case for prophylactic cholecystectomy concomitant with gastric restriction for morbid obesity. *Am Surg* 54:269–272.

Schneider MU, Matek W, Bauer R, Domschke W (1988) Mechanical lithotripsy of bile duct stones in 209 patients – effect of technical advances. *Endoscopy* 20:248–253.

Schoenfield LJ (1972) Animal models of gallstone formation. *Gastroenterology* 63:189–191.

Schoenfield LJ, Sjövall J (1966) Bile acids and cholesterol in guinea pigs with induced gallstones. Am J Physiol 211:1069–1074.

Schoenfield LJ, Sjövall J, Sjövall K (1966) Bile acid composition of gallstones from man. *J Lab Clin Med* 68:186–194.

Schoenfield LJ, Lachin JM, The NCGS Steering Committee and the National Cooperative Gallstone Study Group (NCGS) (1981) Chenodiol (chenodeoxycholic acid) for dissolution of gallstones: the National Cooperative Gallstone Study. A controlled trial of efficacy and safety. *Ann Intern Med* 95:257–282.

Schoenfield LJ, Grundy SM, Hofmann AF, Lachin JM, Thistle JL, Tyor MP (1983) The National Cooperative Gallstone Study viewed by its investigators. *Gastroenterology* 84:644–648.

Schoenheimer R, Breusch F (1933) Synthesis and destruction of cholesterol in the organism. *J Biol Chem* 103:439–448.

Schoenheimer R, Johnston CG (1937) Lithocholic acid gallstones from hog bile. *J Biol Chem* 120:499–501.

Schriever CE, Jüngst D (1989) Association between cholesterol-phospholipid vesicles and cholesterol crystals in human gallbladder. *Hepatology* 9:541–546.

Schwaier A (1979) Tupaia (tree shrews) – A new animal model for gallstone research. I. First observations of gallstones. *Res Exp Med* 176:15–24.

Schwaier A, Weis HJ, Van der Linden J (1979) Tupaia (tree shrews) – a new animal model for gallstone research. II. Influence of fat, sugar, and cholesterol on bile composition. *Res Exp* Med 176:157–172.

Schwartz CC, Vlahcevic ZR, Halloran LG, Gregory DH, Meek JB, Swell L (1975) Evidence for the existence of definitive hepatic cholesterol precursor compartments for bile acids and biliary cholesterol in man. *Gastroenterology* 69:1379–1382.

Schwartz CC, Berman M, Vlahcevic ZR, Halloran LG, Gregory DH, Swell L (1978a) Multicompartmental analysis of cholesterol metabolism in man. Characterization of the hepatic bile acid and biliary cholesterol precursor sites. *J Clin Invest* 61:408–423.

Schwartz CC, Halloran LG, Vlahcevic ZR, Gregory DH, Swell L (1978b) Preferential utilization of free cholesterol from high-density lipoproteins for biliary cholesterol secretion in man. *Science* 200:62–64.

Schwartz CC, Berman M, Vlahcevic ZR, Swell L (1982) Multicompartmental analysis of cholesterol metabolism in man: A quantitative kinetic evaluation of precursor sources and turnover of high density lipoprotein cholesterol esters. *J Clin Invest* 70:864–876.

Schwarzendrube J, Nuutinen H, Abei M, Chandler K, Williams C, Holzbach RT (1992) Amino acid sequence and immunological localization of unique human 120 kD dimeric crystal growth-inhibiting biliary glycoprotein. Gastroenterology 102:A882 (abstract).

Schwesinger WE, Kurtin WE, Johnson R (1988) Alcohol protects aginst cholesterol gallstone formation. *Ann Surg* 207:641–647.

Sciarretta G, Ligabue A, Garuti G, Pieromaldi S, Verri A, Giacobazzi G, Malaguti P (1984) Inhibitory activity of gallbladder bile on calcium carbonate crystallization in vitro. A comparison between normal subjects and gallstone patients. *Scand J Gastroenterol* 19:626–630.

Scobey MW, Johnson FL, Parks JS, Rudel LL (1988) Dietary fish oil reduces bile lithogenicity in the African green monkey. *Gastroenterology* 94:A588 (abstract).

Scopinaro N, Gianetta HE, Civalleri D, Bonalumi U, Friedman D, Bachi V (1981) Partial and total biliopancreatic bypass in the surgical treatment of obesity. *Int J Obesity* 5:421–429.

Scoppola A, Maher VMG, Thompson GR, Rendell NB, Taylor GW (1991) Quantitation of plasma mevalonic acid using gas chromatography-electron capture mass spectrometry. *J Lipid Res* 32:1057–1060.

Scott MB (1976) Lincomycin-induced cholecystitis and gallstones in guinea pigs. *Gastroenterology* 71:814–820.

Scott AJ (1978) Epithelial cell proliferation of diverse models of experimental cholelithiasis. *Gut* 19:558–562.

Scott WJ, Block GE (1989) Biliary stone disease in adults with cystic fibrosis. *Surgery* 105:671–673.

Scott DW, Hoffer RE, Amand WB, Roenigk WJ (1973) Cholelithiasis in a dog. *J Am Vet Med Assoc* 163:254–257.

Scragg RKR, Calvert GD, Oliver JR (1984a) Plasma lipids and insulin in gall stone disease: a case-control study. *Br Med J* 289:521–525.

Scragg RKR, McMichael AJ, Baghurst PA (1984b) Diet, alcohol and relative weight in gall stone disease: a case-control study. *Br Med J* 288:1113-1119.

Scragg RKR, McMichael AJ, Seamark RF (1984c) Oral contraceptives, pregnancy, and endogenous oestrogen in gall stone disease – a case-control study. *Br Med J* 288:1795–1799.

Sedaghat A, Grundy SM (1980) Cholesterol crystals and the formation of cholesterol gallstones. *N Engl J Med* 302:1274–1277.

Selle JG, Altmeier WA, Fullen WD, Goldsmith RE (1972) Cholelithiasis in hyperparathyroidism. *Arch Surg* 105:369–374.

Senaati S, Gumruk FU, Delbakhsh P, Balkanci P, Altay C (1993) Gallbladder pathology in pediatric beta-thalassemic patients. A prospective ultrasonographic study. *Pediatr Radiol* 23:357–359.

Sewell RB, Mao SJT, Kawamoto T, LaRusso NF (1983) Apolipoproteins of high, low and very low density lipoproteins in human bile. *J Lipid Res* 24:391–401.

Shaffer EA (1982) The effect of vagotomy on gallbladder function and bile composition in man. *Ann Surg* 195:413–418.

Shaffer EA (1992) Abnormalities in gallbladder function in cholesterol gallstone disease: bile and blood, mucosa and muscle – the list lengthens. *Gastroenterology* 102:1808–1812.

Shaffer EA, Small DM (1977) Biliary lipid secretion in cholesterol gallstone disease. The effect of cholecystectomy and obesity. *J Clin Invest* 59:828–840.

Shaffer EA, Braasch JW, Small DM (1972) Bile composition at and after surgery in normal persons and patients with gallstones. Influence of cholecystectomy. *N Engl J Med* 287:1317–1322.

Shafffer EA, McOrmond P, Duggan H (1980) Quantitative cholescintigraphy: assessment of gallbladder filling and emptying and duodenographic reflux. *Gastroenterology* 79:899–906.

Shaffer EA, Taylor PJ, Logan K, Gadomski S, Corenblum B (1984) The effect of a progestin on gallbladder function in young women. *Am J Obstet Gynecol* 148:504–507.

Shaheb S (1990) Cholelithiasis among American Indians. Gastroenterology 98: 251–252

Shamburek RD, Schwartz CC (1993) Selective composition of biliary phosphatidylcholines is affected by secretion rate but not by bile acid hydrophobicity. *J Lipid Res* 34:1833–1842.

Shaper AG, Patel KM (1964) Diseases of the biliary tract in Africans in Uganda. *East Afr Med J* 41:246–250.

Sheen PC (1971) Risk of developing cholelithiasis after vagotomy. *Jpn J Surg* 1:19–31.

Sheen IS, Liaw YF (1989) The prevalence and incidence of cholelithiasis in patients with chronic liver disease: a prospective study. *Hepatology* 9:538–540.

Shefer S, Hauser S, Lapar V, Mosbach EH (1973) Regulatory effects of sterols and bile acids on hepatic 3-hydroxy-3-methylglutaryl CoA-reductase and cholesterol 7$\alpha$-hydroxylase in the rat. *J Lipid Res* 14:573–580.

Shefer S, Nguyen LB, Salen G, Ness GC, Tint S, Batta AK, Hauser S, Rani I (1991) Regulation of cholesterol 7$\alpha$-hydroxylase by hepatic 7$\alpha$-hydroxylated bile acid flux and newly synthesized cholesterol supply. *J Biol Chem* 266:2693–1696.

Shefer S, Nguyen LB, Salen G, Ness GC, Chowdhary IR, Lerner S, Batta AK, Tint GS (1992) Differing effects of cholesterol and taurocholate on steady state hepatic HMG-CoA reductase and cholesterol 7$\alpha$-hydroxylase activities and mRNA levels in the rat. *J Lipid Res* 33:1193–1200.

Shi WJ, Jiang GS, Xie MS, Ji F, Wu JH, Fang GF (1987) Prevalence of cholelithiasis in Shanghai. *Collected Abstracts of the Third National Congress of Choleltihiasis, Nanjing, China, Oct 11–13, 1987*, pp 28. (In Chinese)

Shiffman ML, Moore EW (1987) Bile is supersaturated with calcium in most patients with cholesterol and mixed gallstones . *Gastroenterology* 92:1775 (abstract)

Shiffman ML, Moore EW (1988a) Acidification of gallbladder bile is defective in patients with all types of gallstones: A selective defect. *Gastroenterology* 94:A591 (abstract).

Shiffman ML, Moore EW (1988b) Defective acidification leads to $CaCO_3$ supersaturation of gallbladder bile in patients with all types of gallstones. *Gastroenterology* 94: A591 (abstract).

Shiffman ML, Sugerman HJ, Moore EW (1990) Human gallbladder mucosal function. Effect of concentration and acidification of bile on cholesterol and calcium solubility. *Gastroenterology* 99:1452–1459.

Shiffman ML, Sugerman HJ, Kellum JM, Brewer WH, Moore EW (1991) Gallstone formation following rapid weight loss: a prospective study in patients undergoing gastric bypass surgery for treatment of morbid obesity. *Am J Gastroenterol* 86:1000–1005.

Shiffman ML, Sugerman HJ, Kellum JM, Moore EW (1992a) Changes in gallbladder bile composition following gallstone formation and weight reduction. *Gastroenterology* 103:214–221.

Shiffman ML,Sugerman HJ, Kellum JM, Moore EW (1992b) Calcium in human gallbladder bile. *J Lab Clin Med* 120:875–884.

Shiffman ML, Shamburek RD, Schwartz CC, Sugerman HJ, Kellum JM, Moore EW (1993a) Gallbladder mucin, arachidonic acid, and bile lipids in patients who develop gallstones during weight reduction. *Gastroenterology* 105:1200–1208.

Shiffman ML, Sugerman HJ, Kellum JM, Brewer WH, Moore EW (1993b) Gallstones in patients with severe obesity. Relationship to body weight, weight loss and gallbladder bile cholesterol solubility. *Int J Obesity* 17:153–158.

Shimizu S, Sabsay B, Ostrow JD, Rege RV, Dawes LG (1989) Isolation of an acidic protein from cholesterol gallstones, which inhibits the precipitation of calcium carbonate in vitro. *J Clin Invest* 84:1990–1906.

Shioda R (1965) Experimental studies on gallstone formation. *Nippon Geka Hokan (Arch Jpn Chir, Kyoto)* 34:571–585.

Shoda J, Tanaka N, Matsuzaki Y, Honda A, Osuga T, Shigematsu S, Miyazaki H (1991) Microanalysis of bile acid composition in intrahepatic calculi and its etiological significance, *Gastroenterology* 101:821–830.

Shoda J, Tanaka N, He BF, Matsuzaki Y, Osuga T, Miyazaki H (1993a) Alterations of bile acid composition in gallstones, bile and liver of patients with hepatolithiasis and their etiological significance. *Dig Dis Sci* 38:2130–2141.

Shoda J, Toll A, Axelson M, Pieper F, Wikval K, Sjövall J (1993b) Formation of 7$\alpha$-hydroxylated bile acid precursors from 27-hydroxycholesterol in human liver microsomes and mitochondria. *Gastroenterology* 104:A994 (abstract).

Shoda J, He BF, Tanaka N, Matsuzaki Y, Osuga T (1994) Plasma levels of mevalonate and 7$\alpha$-hydroxy-4-cholestene-3-one in cholesterol gallstone disease and their etiological significance. *J Gastroenterol* 29:94 (rapid communication).

Short RV, Eton B (1959) Progesterone in blood. III. Progesterone in the peripheral blood of pregnant women. *J Endocrinol* 18:418–425.

Shull SD, Wagner CI, Trotman BW, Soloway RD ( 1977) Factors affecting bilirubin excretion in patients with cholesterol or pigment gallstones. *Gastroenterology* 72:625–629.

Sichieri R, Everhart JE, Roth HP (1990) Low incidence of hospitalization with gallbladder disease among blacks in the United States. *Am J Epidemiol* 131:826–835.

Sievers ML, Marquis JR (1962) The Southwestern American Indian's burden: biliary disease. *JAMA* 182:570–572.

Silverman A, Roy C (1983) Acute and chronic biliary tract disease. In Silverman A, Roy C (eds): *Pediatric Clinical Gastroenterology*, 3rd ed. St Louis, Mosby, pp 798–805.

Simi M, Loriga P, Basoli A, Leardi S, Speranza V (1979) Intrahepatic lithiasis. Study of thirty-six cases and review of the literature. *Am J Surg* 137:317–322.

Simonet WS, Ness GC (1988) Transcriptional and post-transcriptional regulation of rat hepatic 3-hydroxy-3-methylglutaryl-coenzyme A reductase by thyroid hormones. *J Biol Chem* 263:12448–12453.

Singhal AK, Cohen BI, Finver-Sadowsky J, McSherry CK, Mosbach EH (1984a) Role of hydrophilic bile acids and of sterols on cholelithiasis in the hamster. *J Lipid Res* 25:564–570.

Singhal AK, Cohen BI, Mosbach EH, Une M, Stenger RJ, McSherry CK, Donath P, May-Palaia T (1984b) Prevention of cholesterol-induced gallstones by hyodeoxycholic acid in the prairie dog. *J Lipid Res* 25:539–549.

Singletary BK, Van Thiel DH, Eagon PK (1986) Estrogen and progesterone receptors in human gallbladder. *Hepatology* 6:574–578.

Sitzmann JV, Pitt HA, Steinborn PA, Pasha ZR, Sanders RC (1990) Cholecystokinin prevents parenteral nutrition induced biliary sludge in humans. *Surg Gynecol Obstet* 170:25–31.

Sjövall J (1959) Dietary glycine and taurine on bile acid conjugation in man. Bile acid and steroids. *Proc Soc Exp Biol Med* 100:676–678.

Skar V, Lotveit T, Osnes M (1989a) Juxtapapillary duodenal diverticula predispose to common bile duct gallstones. *Scand J Gastroenterol* 24:202–204.

Skar V, Skar AG, Bratlie J, Osnes M (1989b) Beta-glucuronidase activity in the bile of gallstone patients both with and without duodenal diverticula. *Scand J Gastroenterol* 24:205–212.

Skornick YG, Klausner JM, Lelcuk S, Merhav A, Ratan J, Rozin RR (1983) Cholelithiasis in Dubin-Johnson syndrome. *Surg Gynecol Obstet* 157:447–449.

Skrede S, Björkhem I, Buchmann MS, Midtvedt T (1985) Biosynthesis of cholestanol from bile acid intermediates in the rabbit and the rat. *J Biol Chem* 260:77–81.

Small DM (1970) The formation of gallstones. *Adv Intern Med* 16:243–264.

Small DM (1982) The formation and treatment of gallstones. In Schiff L, Shiff ER (eds): *Disease of the Liver*. 5th ed. Philadelphia, JB Lippincott, pp 151–161.

Smit JWA, Van Erpecum KJ, Stolk MFJ, Geerdink RA, Cluysenaer OJJ, Erkelens DW, Van Berge Henegouwen GP (1992) Successful dissolution of cholesterol gallstone during treatment with pravastatin. *Gastroenterology* 103:1068–1070.

Smit MJ Verkade HJ, Havinga R, Vonk RJ, Scherphof GL, Veld GI, Kuipers F (1994) Dietary fish oil potentiates bile acid-induced cholesterol secretion into bile in rats. *J Lipid Res* 35:301–310.

Smith BF (1987) Human gallbladder mucin binds biliary lipids and promotes cholesterol crystal nucleation in model bile. *J Lipid Res* 28:1088–1097.

Smith DA, Gee MI (1979) A dietary survey to determine the relationship between diet and cholelithiasis. *Am J Clin Nutr* 32:1519–1526.

Smith BF, LaMont JT (1983) Bovine gallbladder mucin binds bilirubin in vitro. *Gastroenterology* 85:707–712.

Smith BF, LaMont JT (1984) Hydrophobic binding properties of bovine gallbladder mucin. *J Biol Chem* 259:12170–12177.

Smith BF, LaMont JT (1985) Identification of gallbladder mucin-bilirubin complex in human cholesterol gallstone matrix. Effects of reducing agents on in vitro dissolution of matrix and intact gallstones. *J Clin Invest* 76:439–445.

Smith JJ, Pomaranc MM, Ivy AC (1941) Influence of pregnancy and sex hormones on gall bladder motility in guinea pig. *Am J Physiol* 132:129–140.

Smith LC, Pownall HJ, Gotto AM Jr (1978) The plasma lipoproteins: structure and metabolism. *Annu Rev Biochem* 47:751–777.

Smith BF, LaMont JT, Small DM (1987) The sequence of events in gallstone formation. *Lab Invest* 56:125–126.

Smith BF, Peetermans JA, Tanaka T, LaMont JT (1989) Subunit interactions and physical properties of bovine gallbladder mucin. *Gastroenterology* 97:179–187.

Smith JL, Hardie IR, Pillay SP, de Jersey J (1990) Hepatic acyl-coenzyme A : cholesterol acyltransferase activity is decreased in patients with cholesterol gallstones. *J Lipid Res* 31:1993–2000.

Soehendra N, Nam VC, Bihnacker S, Schreiber HW (1994) Pulverisation of calcified and non-calcified gallbladder stones: extracorporeal shock wave lithotripsy used alone. *Gut* 35:417–422.

Soloway RD, Wu JG (1994) Analysis of gallstones. In Muraca M (ed): *Methods in biliary research.* Boca Raton CRC Press, Boca Raton, Florida pp 168–190.

Soloway RD, Trotman BW, Ostrow JD (1977) Pigment gallstones. *Gastroenterology* 72:167–182.

Soloway RD, Trotman BW, Maddrey WC, Nakayama F (1986) Pigment gallstone composition in patients with hemolysis or infection/stasis. *Dig Dis Sci* 31:454–460.

Sömjen GJ, Gilat T (1983) A non-micellar mode of cholesterol transport in human bile. *FEBS Lett* 156:265–268.

Sömjen GJ, Gilat T (1985) Contribution of vesicular and micellar carriers to cholesterol transport in human bile. *J Lipid Res* 26:699–704.

Sömjen GJ, Gilat T (1986) Changing concepts of cholesterol solubility in bile. *Gastroenterology* 91:772–775.

Sömjen GJ, Marikovsky Y, Wachtel E, Harvey RC, Rosenberg R, Strasberg SM, Gilat T (1990) Phospholipid lamellae are cholesterol carriers in human bile. *Biochim Biophys Acta* 1042:28–35.

Spady DK, Cuthbert JA (1991) Regulation of hepatic sterol metabolism in the rat. Parallel regulation of activity and mRNA for $7\alpha$-hydroxylase but not 3-hydroxyl-3-methylglutaryl-coenzyme A reductase or low density lipoprotein receptor. *J Biol Chem* 267:5584–5591.

Spady DK, Turley SD, Dietschy JM (1985a) Receptor-independent low density lipoprotein transport in the rat in vivo. Quantitation, characterization and metabolic consequences. *J Clin Invest* 76:1113–1122.

Spady DK, Turley SD, Dietschy JM (1985b) Rates of low density lipoprotein uptake and cholesterol synthesis are regulated independently. *J Lipid Res* 26:465–472.

Spengler U, Sackmann M, Sauerbruch T, Holl J, Paumgartner G (1989) Gallbladder motility before and after extracorporeal shockwave lithotripsy. Gastroenterology 96:860–863.

Spinapolice RX, Colmorgen GHC, Spisso K (1982) Hemoglobin SD disease associated with cholecystitis and cholelithiasis in pregnancy. *Obstet Gynecol* 60:388–390.

Spivak W, Carey M C (1985) Reverse-phase h.p.l.c. separation, quantification and preparation of bilirubin and its conjugates from native bile. Quantitative analysis of the intact tetrapyrroles based on h.p.l.c. of their ethyl anthranilate azo derivatives. *Biochem J* 225:787–805.

Spivak W, Yuey W (1986) Application of a rapid and efficient h.p.l.c. method to measure bilirubin and its conjugates from native bile and in model bile system. Potential use as a tool for kinetic reactions and as an aid in diagnosis of hepatobiliary disease. *Biochem J* 234:101–109.

Spivak W, DiVenuto D, Yuey W (1987) Non-enzymatic hydrolysis of bilirubin mono- and diglucuronide to unconjugated bilirubin in model and native bile systems. Potential role in the formation of gallstones. *Biochem J* 242:323–329.

Splitter G A (1972) Cholelithiasis in a pig. *Vet Rec* 90:73.

Sporea I, Goldis A, Mateoc A (1993) Echographic screening concerning the incidence of gallstones in a general population. *Gastroenterology* 104:A379 (abstract).

St Claire RW, Henderson GR, Heaster V, Wagner WD, Bond MG, McMahan MR (1980) Influence of dietary fats and an oral contraceptive on plasma lipids, high density lipoproteins, gallstones and atherosclerosis in African green monkeys. *Atherosclerosis* 37:103–121.

Stahlberg D, Reihnér E, Angelin B, Einarsson K (1991) Interruption of the enterohepatic circulation of bile acids stimulates the esterification rate of cholesterol in human liver. *J Lipid Res* 32:1409–1415.

Staritz M, Rambow A, Grosse A, Hurst A, Floth A, Mildenberger P, Goebel M, Junginger T, Hohenfellner R, Thelen M, Meyer zum Büschenfelde K and H (1990) Electromagnetically generated extracorporeal shockwaves for fragmentation of extra- and intrahepatic bile duct stones: Indications, success and problems during a 15 month clinical experience. *Gut* 31: 222–225.

Stark RE, Gosselin GJ, Donovan JM, Carey MC, Roberts MF (1985) Influence of dilution on the physical state of model bile systems: NMR and quasi-elastic light-scattering investigations. *Biochemistry* 24:5599–5605.

Starzl TE, Putnam CW, Hansbrough JF, Porter KA, Reid HAS (1977) Biliary complications after liver transplantation: with special reference to the biliary cast syndrome and techniques of secondary duct repair. *Surgery* 81:212–221.

Stavney LS, Kato T, Griffith CA, Nyhus LM, Harkins HN (1963) A physiologic study of motility changes following selective gastric vagotomy. *J Surg Res* 3:390–394.

Steinberg HV, Beckett WW, Chezmar JL, Torres WE, Murphy FB, Bernardino ME (1988) Incidence of cholelithiasis among patients with cirrhosis and portal hypertension. *Gastrointest Radiol* 13:347–350.

Stempel JM, Duane WC (1978) Biliary lipids and bile acid pool size after vagotomy in man. Evidence against a predisposition to gallstones. *Gastroenterology* 75:608–611.

Stephens GS. Scott RB (1980) Cholelithiasis in sickle cell anemia. Surgical or medical management. *Arch Intern Med* 140:648–651.

Stephenson TJ, Johnson AG, Ross B (1989) Piezoelectric shock wave fragmentation of biliary calculi. *Gut* 30:1435–1436.

Stevens RD, Lack L, Killenberg PG (1991) Calcium binding by monosulfate esters of taurochenodeoxycholate. *J Lipid Res* 32:621–627.

Stewart L, Smith AL, Pellegrini CA, Motson RW, Way LW (1987) Pigment gallstones form as a composite of bacterial microcolonies and pigment solids. *Ann Surg* 206:242–250.

Stitnimankarn T (1960) The necropsy incidence of gallstones in Thailand. *Am J Med Sci* 240:349–352.

Stölzel U, Koszka C, Wölfer B, Kleine U, Pommerien W, Riecken EO (1994) Relief of heterogeneous symptoms after successful gall bladder stone lithotripsy and complete stone disappearance. *Gut* 35:819–821.

Stone BG, Evans CD (1992) Evidence for a common biliary cholesterol and VLDL cholesterol precursor pool in rat liver. *J Lipid Res* 33:1665–1675.

Stone B G, Erickson S K, Craig W Y, Cooper A D (1985) Regulation of rat biliary cholesterol secretion by agents that alter intrahepatic cholesterol metabolism. Evidence for a distinct biliary precursor pool. J Clin Invest 76: 1773–1781

Stone BG, Gavaler JS, Belle SH, Shreiner DP, Peleman RR, Sarva RP, Yingvorapant N, Van Thiel DH (1988) Impairment of gallbladder emptying in diabetes mellitus. *Gastroenterology* 95:170–176.

Strasberg SM, Harvey PRC (1990) Biliary cholesterol transport and precipitation: introduction and overview of conference. *Hepatology* 12(Suppl): 1S–5S.

Strasberg SM, Toth JL, Harvey PRC (1988) High total protein (TPC) and total lipid concentration (TLC) are associated with reduced metastability in an early stage of cholesterol gallstone (CGS). *Hepatology* 8:1257 (abstract).

Strasberg SM, Toth JL, Gallinger S, Harvey PRC (1990) High protein and total lipid concentraton are associated with reduced metastability of bile in an early stage of cholesterol gallstone formation. *Gastroenterology* 98:739–746.

Strichartz SD, Abedin MZ, Abdou S, Roslyn JJ (1988) Increased biliary calcium in cholesterol gallstone formation. *Am J Surg* 155:131–137.

Strichartz SD, Abedin MZ, Abdou MS, Roslyn JJ (1989a) The effects of amiloride on biliary calcium and cholesterol gallstone formation. *Ann Surg* 209:152–156.

Strichartz SD, Abedin MZ, Ippoliti AF, Derezin M, Roslyn JJ (1991) Intrahepatic cholesterol stones: a rationale for dissolution therapy. *Gastroenterology* 100:228–232.

Strichartz SD, Abedin MZ, Safarian EK, Roslyn JJ (1989b) Pigment gallstone formation and altered ion transport.

*Am J Surg* 157:163–167.

Strom BL, West SL (1985) The epidemiology of gallstone disease. In Cohen S, Soloway RD (eds): *Gallstones*. New York, Churchill Livingstone, pp 1–26.

Strom BL, Tamragouli RN, Morse ML, Lazar EL, West SL, Stolley PD, Jones JK (1986) Oral contraceptives and other risk factors for gallbladder disease. *Clin Pharmacol Ther* 39:335–341.

Studevant RAL, Pearce ML, Dayton S (1973) Increased prevalence of cholelithiasis in men ingesting a serum-cholesterol-lowering diet. *N Engl J Med* 288:24–27.

Suckling KE, Stange EF (1985) Role of acyl-CoA:cholesterol acyltransferase in cellular cholesterol metabolism. *J Lipid Res* 26:647–671.

Sudjana-Sugiaman E, Eggertsen G, Björkhem I (1994) Stimulation of HMG-CoA reductase as a consequence of phenobarbital-induced primary stimulation of 7$\alpha$-hydroxylase in rat liver. *J Lipid Res* 35:319–327.

Sugata F, Shimizu M (1974) Reevaluation of cases with disappearing gallstone shadows. *Nihon Shokakibyo Gakkai Zasshi (Jpn J Gastroenterol)* 71:75–80. (In Japanese)

Sugerman HJ, Brewer WH, Shiffman ML, Brolin RE, Fobi MA, Linner JH, MacDonald KG, MacGregor AM, Martin LF, Oram-Smith JC, Popoola D, Schirmer BD, Vockers FF (1995) A multicenter, placebo-controlled, randomized, double-blind, prospective trial of prophylactic ursodiol for the prevention of gallstone formation following gastric-bypass-induced rapid weight loss. *Am J Surg* 169:91–96.

Sullivan MA, Duffy A, Dimarco N, Liepa G (1985) Effects of various dietary animal and vegetable proteins on serum and biliary lipids and on gallstone formation in the hamster. *Lipids* 20:1–6.

Summerskill WHJ, Davidson CS, Dible JH, Mallory GK, Sherlock S, Turner MD, Wolfe SJ (1960) Cirrhosis of the liver. A study of alcoholic and non-alcoholic patients in Boston and London. *N Engl J Med* 262:1–9.

Sutor DJ (1970) Calcium palmitate and $\alpha$-palmitic acid in gallstones. *Gut* 11:618–619.

Sutor DJ, Percival JM (1976) Presence or absence of inhibitors of crystal growth in bile. 1. Effect of bile on the formation of calcium phosphate, a constituent of gallstones. *Gut* 17:506–510.

Sutor DJ, Percival JM (1978) The effect of bile on the crystallisation of calcium carbonate, a constituent of gallstones. *Clin Chim Acta* 89:479–484.

Sutor DJ, Wilkie LI (1977a) Calcium in bile and calcium salts in gallstones. *Clin Chim Acta* 79:119–127.

Sutor DJ, Wilkie LI (1977b) The crystalline salts of calcium bilirubinate in human gallstones. *Clin Sci Mol Med* 53:101–103.

Sutor DJ, Wilkie LI (1978) Calcium carbonate in human gallstones and total $CO_2$ in bile. *Gut* 19:220–224.

Sutor DJ, Wooley SE (1971) A statistical survey of the composition of gallstones in eight countries. *Gut* 12:55–64.

Sutor DJ, Wooley S E (1973) The nature and incidence of gallstones containing calcium. *Gut* 14:215–220.

Sutor DJ, Wooley SE (1974a) The organic matrix of gallstones. *Gut* 15:487–491.

Sutor DJ, Wooley SE (1974b) The sequential deposition of crystalline material in gallstones: evidence for changing gallbladder bile composition during the growth of some stones. *Gut* 15:130–131.

Sutor DJ, Wilkie LI, Jackson MJ (1980) Ionised calcium in pathological human bile. *J Clin Pathol* 33:86–88.

Suzuki N, Yamauchi H, Takahashi W, Sato T (1984) Peripapillary duodenal diverticulum and biliary tract diseases. *Jpn J Surg* 14:479–485.

Svanvik J, Thornell E, Zettergren L (1981) Gallbladder function in experimental cholecystitis. Reversal of the inflammatory net fluid 'secretion' into the gallbladder by indomethacin. *Surgery* 89:500–506.

Svanvik J, Pellegrini CA, Allen B, Bernhoft R, Way LW (1986) Transport of fluid and biliary lipids in the canine gallbladder in experimental cholecystitis. *J Surg Res* 41:425–431.

Swell L, Bell CC Jr, Entenman C (1968) Bile acids and lipid metabolism. III. Influence of bile acids on phospholipids in liver and bile of the isolated perfused dog liver. *Biochim Biophys Acta* 164:278–284.

Swell L, Bell CC Jr, Vlahcevic ZR (1971) Relationship of bile acid pool size to biliary lipid excretion and the formation of lithogenic bile in man. *Gastroenterology* 61:716–722.

Swobodnik W, Ditschuneit H, Soloway RD (1990) *Gallstone Disease. Pathophysiology and Therapeutic Approaches.* Berlin, Springer-Verlag.

Sylwestrowicz TA, Shaffer EA (1988) Gallbladder function during gallstone dissolution: effect of bile acid therapy in patients with gallstones. *Gastroenterology* 95:740–748.

Tabata M, Nakayama F (1981) Bacteria and gallstones. Etiological significance. *Dig Dis Sci* 26:218–224.

Tabata M, Nakayama F (1984) Bacteriology of hepatolithiasis. In Okuda K, Nakayama F, Wong J (eds): *Intrahepatic Calculi.* New York, Alan R Liss, pp 163–174.

Tait L (1879) Cholecystotomy for dropsy of gall-bladder due to the impaction of gall-stone. – gastrotomy in extra-uterine pregnancy. Lancet 2: 729–732.

Tait L (1885) Cholecystotomy v. cholecystectomy. *Br Med J* I: 1224.

Takahashi I, Suzuki T, Aizawa I, Itoh Z (1982) Comparison of gallbladder contractions induced by motilin and cholecystokinin in dogs. *Gastroenterology* 82:419–424.

Takayama K, Kitayama O (1988) Extracorporeal shock wave lithotripsy: physical background. *Tan to Sui (Biliary Tract Pancreas)* 9:1081–1089. (in Japanese)

Tall AR (1990) Plasma high density lipoproteins. Metabolism and relationship to atherogenesis. *J Clin Invest* 86:379–384.

Tall AR, Small DM (1978) Plasma high-density lipoproteins. *N Engl J Med* 299:1232–1236.

Tamura K (1942) Crystallographic studies on gallstones in Japan by X-ray diffraction analysis. Nihon Gekagakukai Zasshi (J Jpn Surg Soc) 43:1556–1567. (In Japanese)

Tanaka N, Portman OW, Osuga T (1976) Effect of type of dietary fat, cholesterol, and chenodeoxycholic acid on gallstone formation, bile acid kinetics, and plasma lipids in squirrel monkeys. *J Nutr* 106:1123–1134.

Tanno N, Koizumi M, Goto Y (1988) The relationship between cholelithiasis and diabetes mellitus: discussion of age, obesity, hyperlipidemia and neuropathy. *Tohoku J Exp Med* 154:11–20.

Taylor DR, Sharrock P, Cozart J, Wu JG, Crowther RS, Soloway RD (1993) Microcomposition of gallstones reveals that different $CaCO_3$ polymorphs can be precipitated in separate pigmented areas in cholesterol gallstones. *Gastroenterology* 104:A379 (abstract).

Tazuma S, Sasaki H, Mizuno S, Sagawa H, Hashiba S, Horiuchi I, Kajiyama G (1989) Effect of ursodeoxycholic acid administration on nucleation time in human gallbladder bile. *Gastroenterology* 97:173–178.

Tedstrom MK, Bond RC, Olmstead WH, Moore S (1926) Cholecystography in diabetes mellitus. *JAMA* 87:1603–1605.

Teefey SA, Hollister MS, Lee SP, Jacobson AF, Higano CS, Bianco JA, Colacurcio CJ (1994) Gallbladder sludge formation after bone marrow transplant. *Abdom Imaging* 19:57–60.

Teilum D (1989) The prevalence of gallstones in autopsies from a Danish urban area. Frederiksberg 1914–1955. *Acta Chir Scand* 155:103–106.

Teilum D, Olsen B (1988) The prevalence of gallstones in autopsies from a Danish urban area, Frederiksberg 1959–1985. *Scand J Gastroenterol* 23:813–816.

Teoh T B (1963) A study of gall-stones and included worms in recurrent pyogenic cholangitis. *J Pathol Bacteriol* 86:123–129.

Tepperman J (1965) Experimental formation of gallstones. *Gastroenterology* 48:261–262.

Tepperman J, Caldwell FT, Tepperman HM (1964) Induction of gallstones in mice by feeding a cholesterol-cholic acid containing diet. *Am J Physiol* 206:628–634.

Tera H (1960) Stratification of human gallbladder bile in vivo. Acta Chir Scand 256 (Suppl): pp 1–85.

Tera H (1961) The passage of calcium into the gallbladder through its wall. A study in the rabbit with the isotope $Ca^{45}$. *Acta Chir Scand* 120:358–365.

Tesler J (1946) Cholecystitis and cholelithiasis in identical twins. *Gastroenterology* 7:685–686.

Thijs C, Knipschild P, Brombacher P (1990) Serum lipids and gallstones: a case-control study. *Gastroenterology*

99:843–849.

Thistle JL, Schoenfield LJ (1971) Induced alterations in composition of bile of persons having cholelithiasis. *Gastroenterology* 61:488–496.

Thistle JL, Eckhart KL, Nensel RE, Nobrega FT, Poehling GG, Schoenfield LJ (1971) Prevalence of gallbladder disease among Chippewa Indians. *Mayo Clin Proc* 46:603–608.

Thistle JL, Hofmann AF, Yu PYS, Ott BJ (1977) Effect of varying doses of chenodeoxycholic acid on bile lipid and biliary bile acid composition in gallstone patients: dose response study. *Am J Dig Dis* 22:1–6.

Thistle JL, Hofmann AF, Ott BJ, Stephens DH (1978) Chenotherapy for gallstone dissolution. I. Efficacy and safety. *JAMA* 239:1041–1046.

Thistle JL, Cleary P, Lachin JM, Tyor MP, Hersh T, the Steering Committee and the National Cooperative Gallstone Study (NCGS) Group (1984) The natual history of cholelithiasis: the National Cooperative Gallstone Study. *Ann Intern Med* 101:171–175.

Thistle JL, May GR, Bender CE, Williams HJ, LeRoy AJ, Nelson PE, Peine CJ, Petersen BT, McCullough JE (1989) Dissolution of cholesterol gallbladder stones by methyl tert-butyl ether administered by percutaneous transhepatic catheter. *N Engl J Med* 320:633–639.

Thomas PJ, Hofmann AF (1973) A simple calculation of the lithogenic index of bile: expressing biliary lipid composition on rectangular coordinate. *Gastroenterology* 65:698–700.

Thomas PJ, Hsia SL, Matschiner JT, Doisy EA Jr, Elliot WH, Thayer SA, Doisy EA (1964) Bile acids. XIX. Metabolism of lithocholic acid-24-$^{14}$C in the rat. *J Biol Chem* 239:102–105.

Thompson JC, Fried GM, Ogden WD, Fagan CJ, Inoue K, Wiener I, Watson LC (1982) Correlation between release of cholecystokinin and contraction of the gallbladder in patients with gallstones. *Ann Surg* 195:670–676.

Thompson D, Wild R, Merrick MV, Brydon G, Macintyre IM, Eastwood MA (1994) Cholelithiasis and bile acid absorption after truncal vagotomy and gastroenterostomy. *Br J Surg* 81:1037–1039.

Thornell E, Svanvik J, Wood JR (1981) Effects of intra-arterial prostaglandin $E_2$ on gallbladder fluid transport, motility and hepatic bile flow in the cat. *Scand J Gastroenterol* 16:1083–1088.

Thornell E, Jivegård L, Bukhave K, Rask-Madsen J, Svanvik J (1986) Prostaglandin $E_2$ formation by the gallbladder in experimental cholecystitis. *Gut* 27:370–373.

Thornton JR, Heaton KW (1981) Do colonic bacteria contribute to cholesterol gall-stone formation? Effects of lactulose on bile. *Br Med J* 282:1018–1020.

Thornton JR, Heaton KW, MacFarlane DG (1981) A relation between high-density-lipoprotein cholesterol and bile cholesterol saturation. *Br Med J* 283:1352–1354.

Thornton JR, Emmett PM, Heaton KW (1983) Diet and gall stones: effect of refined and unrefined carbohydrate diets on bile cholesterol saturation and bile acid metabolism. *Gut* 24:2–6.

Thudichum JLW (1863) A *Treatise on Gallstones: Their Chemistry, Pathology and Treatment*. London, John Churchill and Sons.

Thureborn E (1963) A water-soluble lipid complex obtained in the macromolecular phase by gel-filtration of human bile. *Nature* 197:1301–1302.

Tierney S, Ahrendt SA, Fox K, Talbot IC, Booker ML, Pitt HA, LaMorte WW, Lillemoe KD (1993) Fish oil reduces biliary cholesterol and prolongs nucleation of human gallbladder bile. *Gastroenterology* 104:A380 (abstract).

Tinker J, Cox AG (1969) Gall-bladder function after vagotomy. *Br J Surg* 56:779–782.

Tint GS, Dyrszka H, Sanghavi B, Patel G, Patel S, Shefer S, Salen G (1992) Lithotripsy plus ursodiol is superior to ursodiol alone for cholesterol gallstones. *Gastroenterology* 102:2042–2049.

Tipping E, Ketterer B, Christodoulides L (1979) Interactions of small molecules with phospholipid bilayers. Binding to egg phosphatidylcholine of some organic anions (bromosulphophthalein, oestrone sulphate, haem and bilirubin) that bind to ligandin and aminoazo-dye-binding protein A. *Biochem* J 180:327–337.

Tokyo Cooperative Gallstone Study Group (1980) Efficacy and indications of ursodeoxycholic acid treatment for dissolving gallstones. *Gastroenterology* 78:542–548.

Tominaga K, Chen YK, Kurata JH, Miyagawa S, Fujimoto E (1993) Prevalence of fatty liver and gallstone disease in children: relationship to childhood obesity. *Gastroenterology* 104:A26 (abstract).

Tompkins RK, Kraft AR, Zimmerman E, Lichtenstein JE, Zollinger RM (1972) Clinical and biochemical evidence of increased gallstone formation after complete vagotomy. *Surgery* 71:196–200.

Toor EW, Evans DF, Cussler EL (1978) Cholesterol monohydrate growth in model bile solutions. *Proc Natl Acad Sci USA* 75:6230–6234.

Torvik A, Høivik B (1960) Gallstones in an autopsy series. Incidence, complications and correlations with carcinoma of the gallbladder. *Acta Chir Scand* 120:168–174.

Traub JL, Rantanen N, Reed S, Schecter L (1982) Cholelithiasis in four horses. *J Am Vet Med Assoc* 181:59–62.

Trautwein EA, Liang J, Hayes KC (1993) Cholesterol gallstone induction in hamsters reflects strain differences in plasma lipoproteins and bile acid profiles. *Lipids* 28:305–312.

Tritapepe R, Di Padova C, Zuin M, Bellomi M, Podda M (1972) Lithogenic bile after conjugated estrogen. *N Engl J Med* 295:961–962.

Trock B, Lanza E, Greenwald P (1990) Dietary fiber, vegetables, and colon cancer: critical review and meta-analyses of the epidemiologic evidence. *J Natl Cancer Inst* 82:650–661.

Trotman BW, Soloway RD (1975) Pigment vs. cholesterol cholelithiasis: clinical and epidemiological aspects. *Am J Dig Dis* 20:735–740.

Trotman BW, Soloway RD (1982) Pigment gallstone disease: summary of the National Institutes of Health International Workshop. *Hepatology* 2:879–884.

Trotman BW, Morris TA III, Sanchez HM, Soloway RD, Ostrow JD (1977) Pigment versus cholesterol cholelithiasis: Identification and quantification by infrared spectroscopy. *Gastroenterology* 72:495–498.

Trotman BW, Bernstein SE, Bove KE, Wirt GD (1980) Studies on the pathogenesis of pigment gallstones in hemolytic anemia. Description and characteristics of a mouse model. *J Clin Invest* 65:1301–1308.

Trotman BW, Bernstein SE, Balistreri WF, Wirt GD, Martin RA (1981) Hemolysis-induced gallstones in mice: increased unconjugated bilirubin in hepatic bile predisposes to gallstone formation. *Gastroenterology* 81:232–236.

Trotman BW, Bongiovanni MB, Kahn MJ, Bernstein SE (1982) A morphological study of the liver and gallbladder in hemolysis-induced gallstone disease in mice. *Hepatology* 2:863–869.

Tudyka J, Kratzer W, Maier C, Mason R, Wechsler JG (1994) The relation between biliary lipids, nucleation time, and number of gallbladder stones after percutaneous gallbladder puncture. *Scand J Gastroenterol* 29:844–848.

Turley SD, Dietschy JM (1979) Regulation of biliary cholesterol output in the rat: dissociation from the rate of hepatic cholesterol synthesis, the size of the hepatic cholesteryl ester pool, and the hepatic uptake of chylomicron cholesterol. *J Lipid Res* 20:923–934.

Turley SD, Dietschy JM (1981) The contribution of newly synthesized cholesterol to biliary cholesterol in the rat. *J Biol Chem* 256:2438–2446.

Turley SD, Spady DK, Dietschy JM (1983) Alteration of the degree of biliary cholesterol saturation in the hamster and rat by manipulation of the pools of preformed and newly synthesized cholesterol. *Gastroenterology* 84:253–264.

Turrill FL, McCarron MM, Mikkelson WK (1960) Gallstones and diabetes: an ominous association. *Am J Surg* 102:184–190.

Twiss JR, Carter RF (1964) The relationship of biliary tract disorders to diabetes mellitus. *Am J Med Sci* 224:263–273.

Ulloa N, Garrido J, Nervi F (1987) Ultracentrifugal isolation of vesicular carriers of biliary cholesterol in native human and rat bile. *Hepatology* 7:235–244.

Une M, Inoue A, Kurosawa T, Tohma M, Hoshita T (1994) Identification of (24E)-3$\alpha$,7$\alpha$-dihydroxy-5$\beta$-cholest-24 – enoic acid and (24R,25S)-3$\alpha$,7$\alpha$,24-trihydroxy-5$\beta$-cholestanoic acid as intermediates in the conversion of

$3\alpha,7\alpha$-dihydroxy-$5\beta$-cholestanoic acid to chenodeoxycholic acid in rat liver homogenates. *J Lipid Res* 35:620–624.

Une M, Singhal AK, McSherry CK, May-Donath P, Mosbach EH (1985) Metabolism of $3\alpha,7\alpha$-dihydroxy-$7\beta$-methyl-$5\beta$-cholanoic acid and $3\alpha,7\beta$-dihydroxy-$7\alpha$-methyl-$5\beta$-cholanoic acid in hamsters. *Biochim Biophys Acta* 833:196–202.

Vachell HR, Stevens WM (1906) Case of intrahepatic calculi. *Br Med J* 1:434–436.

Vakil N, Everbach EC (1991) Gas in gallstones: qualitative determinations and possible effects on fragmentation by shock waves. *Gastroenterology* 101:1628–1634.

Valdivieso V, Palma R, Wünkhaus R, Antezana C, Severin C, Contreras A (1978) Effect of aging on biliary lipid composition and bile acid metabolism in normal Chilean women. *Gastroenterology* 74:871–874.

Valdivieso V, Palma R, Nervi F, Covarrubias C, Severin C, Antezana C (1979) Secretion of biliary lipids in young Chilean women with cholesterol gallstones. *Gut* 20:997–1000.

Valdivieso V, Covarrubias C, Siegel F, Cruz F (1993) Pregnancy and cholelithiasis and natural course of gallstones diagnosed in early puerperium. *Hepatology* 17:1–4.

Van Berge Henegouwen GP, Hofmann AF (1978) Nocturnal gallbladder storage and emptying in gallstone patients and healthy subjects. *Gastroenterology* 75:879–885.

Van Berge Henegouwen GP, Van der Werf SDJ, Ruben AT (1987) Fatty acid composition of phospholipids in bile in man: Promoting effect of deoxycholate on arachidonate. *Clin Chim Acta* 165:27–37.

Van de Heijning BJM, Stolk MFJ, van Erpecum KJ, Renooij W, Groen AK, van Berge-Henegouwen GP (1994) Bile salt-induced cholesterol crystal formation from model bile vesicles: a time course study. *J Lipid Res* 35:1002–1011.

Van der Linden W (1961) Some biological traits in female gallstone-disease patients. *Acta Chir Scand* 269(Suppl):1–94.

Van der Linden W (1979) Gallstone formation in animals. In Fisher MM, Goresky CA, Shaffer EA, Strasberg SM (eds): *Gallstones*. New York, Plenum, pp 213–222.

Van der Linden W, Bergman F (1977a) An analysis of data on human hepatic bile. Relationship between main bile components, serum cholesterol and serum triglycerides. *Scand J Clin Lab Invest* 37:741–747.

Van der Linden W, Bergman F (1977b) Formation and dissolution of gallstones in experimental animals. *Int Rev Exp Pathol* 17:173–233.

Van der Linden W, Lindelöf G (1965) The familial occurrence of gallstone disease. *Acta Genet Basel* 15:159–164.

Van der Linden W, Nakayama F (1974) Occurrence of cholesterol crystals in human bile. *Gut* 15:630–635.

Van der Linden W, Nakayama F (1976) Effect of intravenous fat emulsion on hepatic bile. Increased lithogenicity and crystal formation. *Acta Chir Scand* 142:401–406.

Van der Linden W, Simonson N (1973) Familial occurrence of gallstone disease. Incidence in parents of young patients. *Human Hered* 23:123–127.

Van der Linden W, Westlin N (1966) The familial occurrence of gallstone disease. II. Occurrence in husbands and wives. *Acta Genet Basel* 16:377–382.

Van der Linden W, Christensen F, Dam H (1959) Cholecystectomy and gallstone formation in the Golden hamster. *Acta Chir Scand* 118:113–116.

Van der Linden W, Nakayama F, Bergman F (1971) Effect of cholesterol biosynthesis inhibitor AY-9944 on gallstone formation in hamsters. *Acta Chir Scand* 137:355–360.

Van der Linden J, Schwaier A, Weis HJ (1980) Tupaia (tree shrews) – A new animal model for gallstone research. III. Cholesterol metabolism under different diets and CDCA. *Res Exp Med* 178:21–28.

Van der Linden W, Katzenstein B, Nakayama F (1983) The possible carcinogenic effect of cholecystectomy. No post-operative increase in the proportion of secondary bile acids. *Cancer* 52:1265–1268.

Van der Meer R, Termont DS, De Vries HT (1991) Differential effects of calcium ions and calcium phosphate on cytotoxicity of bile acids. *Am J Physiol* 260:G142–G147.

Vandermeeren A, Delhaye M, Cremer M (1993) The management of giant bile duct stones after endoscopic sphincterotomy. *Gastroenterology* 104:A380 (abstract).

Van der Werf SDJ, Huijbregt SAWM, Lamers HLM, Van Berge Henegouwen GP, Van Tongeren JHM (1981) Age dependent differences in human bile acid metabolism and $7\alpha$-dehydroxylation. *Eur J Clin Invest* 11:425–431.

Van der Werf SDJ, Nagengast FM, Van Berg Henegouwen GP, Huijbregts AWM, Van Tongeren JHM (1982) Colonic absorption of secondary bile acids in patients with adenomatous polyps and in matched controls. *Lancet* I:759–761.

Van Erpecum KJ, Van Berge Henegouwen GP, Stoelwinder B, Stolk MFJ, Eggink WF, Govaert WHA (1988) Cholesterol and pigment gallstone disease: comparison of the reliability of three bile tests for differentiation between the two stone types. *Scand J Gastroenterol* 23:948–954.

Van Erpecum KJ, Van Berge Henegouwen GP, Stoelwinder B, Schmidt YMG, Willekens FLH (1990) Bile concentration is a key factor for nucleation of cholesterol crystals and cholesterol saturation index in gallbladder bile of gallstone patients. *Hepatology* 11:1–6.

Van Erpecum KJ, Stolk MF, Van den Broek AM, Renooij W, Van de Heijning BJ, Van Berge Henegouwen GP (1993) Bile concentration promotes nucleation of cholesterol monohydrate crystals by increasing the cholesterol concentration in the vesicles. *Eur J Clin Invest* 23:283–288.

Van Sonnenberg E, Casola G, Zakko SF, Varney RR, Cox J, Wittich GR, Hofmann AF (1988) Gallbladder and bile duct stones: percutaneous therapy with primary MTBE dissolution and mechanical methods. *Radiology* 169:505–509.

Van Sonnenberg E, Zakko SF, Hofmann AF, D'Agostino HB, Jinich H, Hoyt DB, Miyai K, Ramsby G, Moossa AR (1991) Human gallbladder morphology after gallstone dissolution with methyl tert-butyl ether. *Gastroenterology* 100:1718–1723.

Vawter GF, Schwachman H (1979) Cystic fibrosis in adults. *Pathol Annu* 14:357–382.

Veraldi ALM, Groen AK, Oude EI, Elferink RPI, Van der Meer R, Palasciano G, Tytgat GNJ (1991) Cell type-dependent effect of phospholipid and cholesterol on bile salt cytotoxicity. *Gastroenterology* 101:457–464.

Verine HJ, Gevrey JP, Murat JE (1969) *Toxacara canis* as a support for cholelithiasis in the dog. *Vet Rec* 85: 98–99.

Verkade HJ, Wolbers MJ, Havinga R, Uges DRA, Vonk RJ, Kuipers F (1990) The uncoupling of biliary lipid from bile acid secretion by organic anions in the rat. *Gastroenterology* 99:1485–1492.

Vernick LJ, Kuller LH (1981) Cholecystectomy and right-sided colon cancer: an epidemiologic study. *Lancet* 2:381–383.

Verschure JCM (1956) Electro-chromatograms of human bile. *Clin Chim Acta* 1:38–48.

Verschure JCM, Mijnlieff PH (1956) The dominating macromolecular complex of human gallbladder bile. *Clin Chim Acta* l:154–166.

Vezina WC, Paradis RL, Grace DM, Zimmer RA, LaMont DD, Rycroft KM, King ME, Hutton LC, Chey WY (1990) Increased volume and decreased emptying of the gallbladder in large (morbidly obese, tall normal, and muscular normal) people. *Gastroenterology* 98:1000–1007.

Villanova N, Bazzoli F, Taroni F, Frabboni R, Mazzella G, Festi D, Barbara L, Roda E (1989) Gallstone recurrence after successful oral bile acid treatment. A 12-year follow-up study and evaluation of long-term postdissolution treatment. *Gastroenterology* 97:726–731.

Vlahcevic ZR, Bell CC Jr, Buhac I, Farrar JT, Swell L (1970a) Diminished bile acid pool size in patients with gallstones. *Gastroenterology* 59:165–173.

Vlahcevic ZR, Bell CC Jr, Swell L (1970b) Significance of the liver in the production of lithogenic bile in man. *Gastroenterology* 59: 62–69.

Vlahcevic ZR, Bell CC Jr, Gregory DH, Baker G, Juttijudata P, Swell L (1972) Relationship of bile acid pool size to the formation of lithogenic bile in female Indians of the Southwest. *Gastroenterology* 62:73–83.

Vlahcevic ZR, Heuman DM, Hylemon PB (1991) Regulation of bile acid synthesis. *Hepatology* 13:590–600.

Von Dippe P, Drain P, Levy D (1982) Synthesis and transport characteristics of photoaffinity probes for the hepatocyte bile acid transport system. *J Biol Chem* 258:8890–8895.

Von Bergmann K, Becker M, Leiss O (1986) Biliary cholesterol saturation in non-obese women and non-obese men before and after puberty. *Eur J Clin Invest* 16:531–535.

Wagner CI, Trotman BW, Soloway RD (1976) Kinetic analysis of biliary lipid excretion in man and dog. *J Clin Invest* 57:473–477.

Wahlin T (1977) Synthesis of glycoproteins in the Golgi complex of the mouse gallbladder epithelium during fasting, refeeding and gallstone formation. A light microscopic autoradiographic and quantitative electron microscopic study. *Histochemistry* 51:133–140.

Wahlin T, Schiebler TH (1975) Zur Entwicklung des gallenblasenepithels des Meerschweinchens. II. Elektronmikroskopische und enzymhistochemische Untersuchungen. *Histochemistry* 44:253–275.

Wahlin T, Bloom GD, Carlsöö B (1974) Histochemical observations with the light and electron microscope on the mucosubstances of the normal mouse gallbladder epithelial cells. *Histochemistry* 42:119–131.

Wahlin T, Bloom GD, Carlsöö B, Rhodin L (1976) Effects of fasting and refeeding on secretory granules of the mouse gallbladder epithelium. A quantitative electron microscopic study. *Gastroenterology* 70:353–358.

Wahlin T, Thornell E, Jivegård L, Svanvik J (1988) Effects of intraluminal prostaglandin $E_2$ in vivo on secretory behavior and ultrastructural changes in mouse gallbladder epithelium. *Gastroenterology* 95:1632–1635.

Wald A, Van Thiel DH, Hoechstetter L, Gavaler JS, Egler KM, Verm R, Scott L, Lester R (1982) Effect of pregnancy on gastrointestinal transit. *Dig Dis Sci* 27:1015–1018.

Wales EE, Englert E, Peric-Golia L, Straight RC (1982) The spontaneous amorphous black pigment gallstone of the domestic dog. *J Comp Pathol* 92:381–385.

Walker S, Rudolph G, Raedsch R, Stiehl A (1992) Intestinal absorption of ursodeoxycholic acid in patients with extrahepatic biliary obstruction and bile drainage. *Gastroenterology* 102:810–815.

Wang HY, Yao BL (1983) The characteristics of cholelithiasis of 166 cases of Xinjiang region. *Bull Xinjiang Med College* 6:314–326. (In Chinese with an English summary)

Watkinson G (1967) The autopsy incidence of gallstones in England and Scotland. In *Proceedings of 3rd World Congress of Gastroenterology, Tokyo, 1966*, Vol 4. Basel, Karger, pp 157–162.

Wattchaw DA, Hall JC, Whiting MJ, Bradley B, Iannos J, Watts JMK (1983) Prevalence and treatment of gall stones after gastric bypass surgery for morbid obesity. *Br Med J* 286: 763.

Watts JMK, Jablonski P, Toouli J (1978) The effect of added bran to the diet on the saturation of bile in people without gallstones. *Am J Surg* 135:321–324.

Weber AM, Roy CC, Morin CL, LaSalle R (1973) Malabsorption of bile acids in children with cystic fibrosis. *N Engl J Med* 289:1001–1005.

Weens HS (1945) Cholelithiasis in sickle cell anemia. *Ann Intern Med* 22:182–191.

Wei O (1973) Internal organs of a 2100-year-old female corpse. *Lancet* 2:1198.

Weingarten MA, Eilat-Zan'Ani Z, Hart J (1990) Frequency of clinical gallstone disease among Yemenite Jews in Israel. *Isr J Med Sci* 26:200–204.

Weinsier R L, Wilson L J, Lee J (1995) Medically safe rate of weight loss for the treatment of obesity: a guideline based on risk of gallstone formation. *AM J Med* 98:115–117.

Weiss KM, Hanis CL (1984) All "silent" gallstones are not silent. *N Engl J Med* 310:657–658.

Weiss NS, Daling JR, Chow WH (1982) Cholecystectomy and the incidence of cancer of the large bowel. *Cancer* 49:1713–1715.

Wen HY, Liu CZ, Ma L, Lin YI, Cui L (1987) Prevalence of cholelithiasis in adult population in Kunming, Yanan, China. *Collected Abstracts of the Third National Congress of Choletlithsis, Oct 11–13, 1987*, pp 24–25. (In Chinese)

Wenckert A, Robertson B (1966) The natural course of gallstone disease. Eleven-year review of 781 nonoperated cases. *Gastroenterology* 50:376–381.

Werner B, de Heer K, Mitschke H (1977) Cholecystectomy and carcinoma of the colon. An experimental study. *Z Krebsforsch* 88:223–230.

Wheeler HO (1973) Biliary excretion of bile acids, lecithin and cholesterol in hamsters with gallstones. *Gastroenterology* 65:92–103.

Wheeler HO, King KK (1972) Biliary excretion of lecithin and cholesterol in the dog. *J Clin Invest* 51:1337–1350.

Wheeler HO, Ross ED, Bradley SE (1968) Canalicular bile production in dogs. *Am J Physiol* 214:866–874.

Wheeler M, Hills LL, Laby B (1970) Cholelithiasis: a clinical and dietary survey. *Gut* 11:430–437.

Whiting MJ, Watts JM (1984) Supersaturated bile from obese patients without gallstones supports cholesterol crystal growth but not nucleation. *Gastroenterology* 86:243–248.

Whitington PF, Black DD (1980) Cholelithiasis in premature infants treated with parenteral nutrition and furosemide. *J Pediatr* 97:647–649.

Whorewell PJ, Hawkins R, Dewbury K, Wright R (1984) Ultrasound survey of gallstones and other hepatobiliary disorders in patients with Crohn's disease. *Dig Dis Sci* 29:930–933.

Wilbur RS, Bolt RJ (1959) Incidence of gall bladder disease in "normal" men. *Gastroenterology* 36:251–255.

Williams CN, Johnston JL (1980) Prevalence of gallstones and risk factors in Caucasian women in a rural Canadian community. *Can Med Assoc J* 122: 664–668.

Williams CN, Johnston JL, Weldon KLM (1977a) Prevalence of gallstones and gallbladder disease in Canadian Micmac Indian women. *Can Med Assoc J* 117:758–760.

Williams CN, Morse JWI, MacDonald IA, Kotoor R, Riding MD (1977b) Increased lithogenicity of bile on fasting in normal subjects. *Am J Dig Dis* 22:189–194.

Williamson BWA, Percy-Robb IW (1979) The interactions of calcium ions with glycocholate micelles in aqueous solution. *Biochem J* 181:61–66.

Williamson BWA, Percy-Robb IW (1980) Contribution of biliary lipids to calcium binding in bile. *Gastroenterology* 78:696–702.

Wilson MD, Rudel LL (1994) Review of cholesterol absorption with emphasis on dietary and biliary cholesterol. *J Lipid Res* 35:943–955.

Windler EET, Kovanen PT, Chao YS, Brown MS, Havel RJ, Goldstein JL (1980) The estradiol-stimulated lipoprotein receptor of rat liver. A binding site that mediates the uptake of rat lipoproteins containing apoproteins B and E. *J Biol Chem* 255:10464–10471.

Wolpers C (1968) Spontanauflösung von Gallenblasensteinen. *Dtsch Med Wochenschr* 93:2525–2532.

Wolpers C (1974) Morphologie der Gallensteine. *Leber Magen Darm* 4:43–57.

Wolpers C (1987) *Gallenblasensteine. Ihre Morphogenese und Auswahl zur Litholyse.* Basel, Karger.

Wolpers C, Hofmann AF (1993) Solitary versus multiple cholesterol gallbladder stones. Mechanism of formation and growth. *Clin Invest* 71:423–434.

Womack NA, Zeppa R, Irvin GL III (1963) The anatomy of gallstones. *Ann Surg* 157:670–686.

Wood JR, France VM, Sutor DJ (1974) Occurrence of gallstones in foetal sheep. *Lab Anim* 8:155–159.

Wood RJ, Svanvik J (1983) Gall-bladder water and electrolyte transport and its regulation. *Gut* 24:579–593.

Worobetz LJ, Inglis FG, Shaffer EA (1993) The effect of ursodeoxycholic acid therapy on gallstone formation in the morbidly obese during rapid weight loss. *Am J Gastroenterol* 88:1705–1710.

Wosiewitz U, Sabinski F (1993) Chemolysis of residual debris from MTBE–treated cholesterol stones. Gastroentgerology 104:A382 (abstract).

Wosiewitz U, Schroebler S (1978) "Polymer pigments" in human pigment gallstones, *Naturwissenschaften* 65:162–163.

Wosiewitz U, Schenk J, Sabinski F, Schmack B (1983) Investigations on common bile duct stones. *Digestion* 26:43–52.

Wosiewitz U, Güldütuna S, Fischer H, Leuschner U (1989) Pigment gallstone dissolution in vitro. Solubilization of brown bilirubinate and black polybilirubinate stone material by buffered solvents containing ethylenediaminetetraacetic acid, bile salts and reducing thiols. *Scand J Gastroenterol* 24:373–380.

Xia LF (1987) Prevalence of gallstones in Guiyang, Guizhou, China. *Collected Abstracts of the Third National Congress of Cholelithiasis, Nanjing, China Oct, 11–13, 1987*, pp 19–20. (In Chinese)

Xian YY, Beiwen J, Feng ZY, Xiu JL (1992) Bile secretory immunoglobulin A in biliary infection and cholelithiasis. *Gastroenterology* 102:1000–1008.

Xu QW, Shaffer EA (1993) Cisapride improves gallbladder contractility and bile lipid composition in an animal model of gallstone disease. *Gastroenterology* 105:1184–1191.

Xu GR, Salen G, Batta AK, Shefer S, Nguyen LB, Niemann W, Chen TS, Arora-Mirchandani R, Ness GC, Tint GS (1992) Glycocholic acid and glycodeoxycholic acid but not glycoursodeoxycholic acid inhibit bile acid synthesis in the rabbit. *Gastroenterology* 102:1717–1723.

Xu GR, Salen G, Shefer S, Batta AK, Ness GC, Nguyen LB, Zhao ZH, Chen TS, Niemann W, Tint GS (1993) Different feedback regulation of hepatic cholesterol and bile acid synthesis by glycodeoxycholic acid in rabbits. *Gastroenterology* 105:1192–1199.

Yalow RS, Berson SA (1960) Immunoassay of endogenous plasma insulin in man. *J Clin Invest* 39:1157–1175.

Yamakawa T, Komaki F, Shikata J (1978) Experience with postoperative choledochoscopy via the T-tube sinus tract. *World J Surg* 2:379–385.

Yamasaki T, Chijiiwa K, Endo M (1993) Isolation of mucin from human hepatic bile and its induced effects on precipitation of cholesterol and calcium carbonate in vitro. *Dig Dis Sci* 38:909–915.

Yamase H, McNamara JJ (1972) Geographic differences in the incidence of gallbladder disease. Influence of environment and ethnic background. *Am J Surg* 123:667–670.

Yamashita N, Yanagisawa J, Nakayama F (1988) Composition of intrahepatic calculi. Etiological significance. *Dig Dis Sci* 33:449–453.

Yamashita H, Kuroki S, Nakayama F (1990) Assay of cholesterol $7\alpha$-hyroxylase utilizing silica cartridge column and $5\alpha$-cholestane-$3\beta$,$7\beta$-diol as internal standard. *J Chromatogr* 496:255–269.

Yamazaki K, Powers S P, LaRusso N F (1988) Biliary proteins: assessment of quantitative techniques and comparison in gallstone and nongallstone subjects. *J Lipid Res* 29:1055–1063.

Yang JX, Gao L (1987) Prevalence of gallbladder stone cases in Beijing. *Collected Abstracts of the Third National Congress of Cholelithiasis, Nanjing, China, Oct. 11–13, 1987*, pp 25. (In Chinese)

Yang H, Petersen GM, Roth MP, Schoenfield LJ, Marks JW (1992) Risk factors for gallstone formation during rapid wight loss. *Dig Dis Sci* 37:912–918.

Yang B, Taylor RC, Morris MD, Wang XZ, Wu JG, Yu BZ, Xu GX, Soloway RD (1993) Normal coordinate analysis of bilirubin vibrational spectra: Effects of intramolecular hydrogen bonding. *Spectrochim Acta* 49A:1735–1749.

Yellin TO, Klaiber MS, Webb E (1973) Lithogenic effects of cholic acid and chenodeoxycholic acid in the cholesterol fed mouse. *Biochim Biophys Acta* 320:478–485.

Yio XY, Jin B, Yin FZ, Li XJ (1992) Biliary secretory immunoglobulin A in biliary infection and cholelithiasis. *Gastroenterology* 102:1000–1008.

Yoshida T, Honda A, Tanaka N, Matsuzaki Y, He B, Osuga T, Kobayashi N, Ozawa K, Miyazaki H (1993) Simultaneous determination of mevalonate and $7\alpha$-hydroxycholesterol in human plasma by gas chromatography-mass spectrometry as indices of cholesterol and bile acid synthesis. *J Chromatogr* 613:185–193.

Young DL, Manson KC (1972) Effect of bile salts on hepatic phosphatidylcholine synthesis and transport into rat bile. *J Lipid Res* 13:244–252.

Yu P, de Petris G, Biancani P, Amaral J, Behar J (1993) Abnormal calcium channel function in smooth muscle from human gallbladder with cholesterol stones. *Gastroenterology* 104:A606 (abstract).

Zahor Z, Sternby NH, Kagan A, Uemura K, Vanecek R, Vichert AM (1974) Frequency of cholelithiasis in Prague and Malmö. An autopsy study. *Scand J Gastroenterol* 9:3–7.

Zaki OA, Kamel R (1967) Incidence of cholelithiasis in Egyptians and its relationship with cholesterol. *Br J Surg* 54:713–717.

Zakko SF, Ramsby GR, van Sonnenberg E, Hofmann AF (1989) Percutaneous contact dissolution of gallbladder stones using a microprocessor assisted solvent transfer system and methyl tert-butyl ether (MTBE): experience in 16 patients. *Gastroenterology* 96:A676 (abstract)

Zhu XG, Greeley GH, Newman J, Wiener I, Fagan CJ, Thompson JC (1985) Correlation of in vitro measurements of contractility of the gallbladder with in vivo ultrasonographic findings in patients with gallstones. *Surg Gynecol Obstet* 161:470–472.

Zucker KA, Bailey RW, Gadacz TR, Imbembo AL (1991) Laparoscopic guided cholecystectomy. *Am J Surg* 161:36–44.

# Index